The Natural History of Rabies

VOLUME I

Painting of a rabid dog biting a man. Arabic (Mesopotamian), A.D. 1224; Baghdad school, by Abdallah ibn al-Fadl. (Courtesy of the Smithsonian Institution, Freer Gallery of Art, Washington, D. C.)

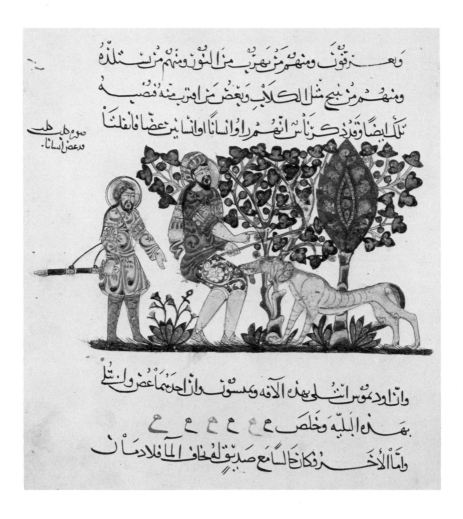

And they make music, and some of them run away from the light while others enjoy it. Others howl like dogs and bite whomever approaches them, who in turn get afflicted also. Some people mentioned that they saw one or two men bitten and loose, and that Odimus and Hemson were affected by the disease and that one of them succumbed to the disease after being bitten and then expired; the other, however, was staying with a friend and manifested fear of water and ran. (Translation, courtesy of Mr. A. E. Najjar.)

The Natural History of Rabies

VOLUME I

Edited by GEORGE M. BAER

Viral Zoonoses Branch
Center for Disease Control
Lawrenceville Facility
Public Health Service
United States Department of
   Health, Education, and
   Welfare
Lawrenceville, Georgia

ACADEMIC PRESS   New York   San Francisco   London   1975
A Subsidiary of Harcourt Brace Jovanovich, Publishers

ACADEMIC PRESS, INC.
111 Fifth Avenue, New York, New York 10003

United Kingdom Edition published by
ACADEMIC PRESS, INC. (LONDON) LTD.
24/28 Oval Road, London NW1

Library of Congress Cataloging in Publication Data

Baer, George M
    The natural history of rabies.

    Includes bibliographies and index.
    1.   Rabies.   I.   Title.   [DNLM: 1.   Rabies—History.
2.   Rabies virus.   WG550 B141n]
RC148.B33   616.9'53   74-10215
ISBN 0–12–072401–4 (v. 1)

PRINTED IN THE UNITED STATES OF AMERICA

Contents

Chapter 1 **History of Rabies**
           James H. Steele

PART I THE VIRUS

Chapter 2 **Morphology and Morphogenesis**
           Frederick A. Murphy

Chapter 3 **Antigenic Composition of Rabies Virus**
           H. G. Aaslestad

Chapter 4   Chemical Composition and Structure of Rabies Virus

Frantisek Sokol

Chapter 5   Hemagglutinin of Rabies Virus

Pekka Halonen

Chapter 6   Passive Hemagglutination Test

Patricia M. Gough and Richard E. Dierks

Chapter 7   Concentration and Purification

Lothar G. Schneider

Chapter 8   Rabies Virus Antigenic Relationships
R. Shope

PART II PATHOGENESIS AND PATHOLOGY

Chapter 9   Growth of Rabies Virus in Cell Culture
T. J. Wiktor and H F. Clark

Chapter 10   Pathogenesis to the Central Nervous System
George M. Baer

Chapter 11 **Spread of Virus within the Central Nervous System**

Lothar G. Schneider

Chapter 12 **Electron Microscopy of Central Nervous System Infection**

Seiichi Matsumoto

Chapter 13 **The Pathology of Rabies in the Central Nervous System**

Daniel P. Perl

Chapter 14 **Spread of Virus from the Central Nervous System**

Lothar G. Schneider

Chapter 15   Electron Microscopy of Extraneural
             Rabies Infection

             Richard E. Dierks

Chapter 16   Lipotropism in Rabies Virus Infection

             S. Edward Sulkin and Rae Allen

Chapter 17   Latency and Abortive Rabies

             J. Frederick Bell

Chapter 18   Interferon and Rabies Virus Infection

             S. Edward Sulkin and Rae Allen

PART III DIAGNOSIS

Chapter 19   **Animal Inoculation and the Negri Body**
              P. Atanasiu

Chapter 20   **The Fluorescent Antibody Test in Rabies**
              Robert E. Kissling

Chapter 21   **The Serum Neutralization, Indirect
              Fluorescent Antibody, and Rapid
              Fluorescent Focus Inhibition Tests**
              J. B. Thomas

List of Contributors

Numbers in parentheses indicate the pages on which the authors' contributions begin.

H. G. AASLESTAD* (63), *The Wistar Institute of Anatomy and Biology, Philadelphia, Pennsylvania*

RAE ALLEN (319,355), *Department of Microbiology, The University of Texas, Southwestern Medical School at Dallas, Dallas, Texas*

P. ATANASIU (373), *Rabies and Rhabdovirus Research Department, Pasteur Institute, Paris, France*

GEORGE M. BAER (181), *Viral Zoonoses Branch, Center for Disease Control, Lawrenceville Facility, Public Health Service, United States Department of Health, Education, and Welfare, Lawrenceville, Georgia*

J. FREDERICK BELL (331), *Rocky Mountain Laboratory, National Institute of Allergy and Infectious Diseases, National Institutes of Health, Public Health Service, United States Department of Health, Education, and Welfare, Hamilton, Montana*

H F. CLARK (155), *The Wistar Institute of Anatomy and Biology, Philadelphia, Pennsylvania*

RICHARD E. DIERKS† (115,303), *Veterinary Medical Research Institute, College of Veterinary Medicine, Iowa State University, Ames, Iowa*

PATRICIA M. GOUGH (115), *Veterinary Medical Research Institute, College of Veterinary Medicine, Iowa State University, Ames, Iowa*

PEKKA HALONEN (103), *Department of Virology, University of Turku, Turku, Finland*

* Present address: N.C.I. Frederick Cancer Research Center, Frederick, Maryland.
† Present address: Veterinary Science Department, Montana State University, Bozeman, Montana.

ROBERT E. KISSLING (401), *Virology Division, Center for Disease Control, Public Health Service, U. S. Department of Health, Education, and Welfare, Atlanta, Georgia*

SEIICHI MATSUMOTO (217), *Virology Division, Institute for Virus Research, Kyoto University, Kyoto, Japan*

FREDERICK A. MURPHY (33), *Virology Division, Center for Disease Control, Public Health Service, U. S. Department of Health, Education, and Welfare, Atlanta, Georgia*

DANIEL P. PERL (235), *Department of Medical Sciences, Brown University, and The Miriam Hospital, Providence, Rhode Island*

LOTHAR G. SCHNEIDER (125,199,273), *Department of Comparative Rhabdovirus Research, Federal Research Institute for Animal Virus Diseases, Tübingen, West Germany*

R. SHOPE (141), *Yale Arbovirus Research Unit, Department of Epidemiology and Public Health, Yale University School of Medicine, New Haven, Connecticut*

FRANTISEK SOKOL* (79), *The Wistar Institute of Anatomy and Biology, Philadelphia, Pennsylvania*

JAMES H. STEELE (1), *Institute of Environmental Health, School of Public Health, University of Texas, Houston, Texas*

S. EDWARD SULKIN* (319,355), *Department of Microbiology, The University of Texas Southwestern Medical School at Dallas, Dallas, Texas*

J. B. THOMAS† (417), *Microbiological Industries, Inc., Highland Home, Alabama*

T. J. WIKTOR (155), *The Wistar Institute of Anatomy and Biology, Philadelphia, Pennsylvania*

---

* Deceased.
† Present address: Flow Laboratories, Rockville, Maryland.

Preface

Rabies is a unique virus in that it manages to exit in the saliva when its host is stimulated to bite — a mean accomplishment. Most people are not aware that the dog is still by far the worst offending species for man and that rabid vampire bats cause hundreds of thousands of cattle deaths in the Americas annually. With few exceptions the disease is no less a worldwide problem than it was centuries ago.

This two-volume treatise should serve to underline those aspects of the virus for which control methods are known (and often not applied) and those requiring further investigation (many, indeed, in order to bring us out of the virological dark ages). This volume deals with the more fundamental aspects of the virus. Chapters in Part I emphasize virus characteristics: morphology, chemistry, physical makeup, and relationships to related viruses. Part II deals with virus growth. The chapters on *in vivo* pathogenesis begin with the entrance of the virus, then go on to its spread in the central nervous system and its subsequent exit. Also included is a chapter on latency, still a subject of much disparate opinion. Chapters in Part III cover current diagnostic methods, including those used for determination of virus presence and those used for antibody titration.

Each chapter emphasizes a special area of the disease, and there is a danger that such areas assume unwarranted importance compared to the whole. The thundering words Ortega y Gasset wrote in 1929 come to mind:

> The 19th century begins its destinies under the direction of those that still live encyclopedically, although their training is already of a specialized character. But when, in 1890, a third generation takes the intellectual command of Europe, we find a type of scientist unique in history. He is a man who, of all that a discreet person should know, knows only a certain science, and even of that science really only knows that small portion in which he is an active investigator. He actually proclaims it a virtue not to know anything outside the narrow field in which he specializes, and accuses those having curiosity for general knowledge of "dilettantism."
>
> But this creates an extraordinarily strange class of men. The investigator who discovers something new in nature necessarily has a sense of dominion and

self-confidence. With apparent justification he thinks of himself as "a man who knows." And, in reality, there is within him a piece of something that, together with other absent pieces, really constitutes knowledge. The specialist "knows" his minimum corner of the universe very well, but ignores the very roots of all the rest.

I have said that he is thus a figure without counterpart in history. Because before now men could be divided, simply, into wise or ignorant, into more or less wise and more or less ignorant. But the specialist cannot be placed under either of these two categories. He is not wise, because he ignores all except his specialty; but neither is he ignorant, because he is a "man of science," and knows very well his tiny piece of the universe. We would have to call him a wise ignoramus, an extremely serious situation, since he is thus an individual who will behave, in all those fields which he ignores, not as ignorant, but with all the petulance of one who is wise in his special area.

But specialization, which has made possible the progress of experimental science for a century, is approaching an era in which it cannot progress alone, unless it results in the next generation's building new and stronger bonds. But if the specialist is not aware of the internal physiology of the science he cultivates, he especially ignores the historic conditions for his existence, that is, how society—and mens' hearts—must be organized for there even to continue to be researchers.

> Reproduced with permission from _La Rebellion de las Masses_, by Ortega y Gasset (1929), Revista de Occidente, Madrid. (Translated by the editor.)

This book was conceived by Dr. Goeffrey Bourne, distinguished scientist and director of the Yerkes Regional Primate Center, Emory University, Atlanta, Georgia, and I thank him for this wonderful opportunity and also for his continued help. Many people have assisted me in preparing this treatise and revising it for final publication, too many to acknowledge individually. Most special thanks for its publication are due Mrs. Barbara B. Andrew, my tireless secretary, who worked after hours on many evenings and weekends, typing draft after draft, to put it in final form.

GEORGE M. BAER

Contents of Volume II

The Natural History of Rabies

VOLUME I

CHAPTER 1

History of Rabies

James H. Steele

Rabies has a long and interesting history that is lost in antiquity. Plutarch asserts that according to Athenodorus it was first observed in mankind in the days of the Asclepiadae, the descendants of the god of medicine, Asculapius. Acteon, the famous hunter of myth who was torn to pieces by his hounds when he surprised Diana and her attendants at the bath, was thought to have been destroyed by rabid dogs. In the Iliad, Homer is thought to refer to rabies when he mentions that Sirius, the dog star of the Orion, exerts a malignant influence upon the health of mankind. The dog star, Sirius, was associated with mad dogs all through the eastern Mediterranean and Egypt, and later Rome. Homer further uses the term "raging dog" in the epithets that are thrown at Hector by Teucrus. The Greeks had a special god in their mythology to counteract the effect of rabies, his name being Aristaeus, son of Apollo. Artemis is represented as the healer of rabies.

The Greeks called rabies Lyssa or Lytta which meant madness. The disease in man was described as hydrophobia in which the sick person is tormented at the same time with thirst and the fear of water. The Latin word "rabies" comes from an old Sanskrit word *rabhas* which translated means "to do violence." The German word *tollwut* originates with the Indogermanic *Dhvar*, to damage, and *wut* from middle German *wuot* which is rage. The French word for rage is derived from the noun *robere*, to be mad.

Democritus is thought to have made the first recorded description of canine rabies some 500 years B.C. *Aristoteles*, in the fourth century B.C., wrote in the *Natural History of Animals*, Book 8, Chapter 22, "that dogs suffer from the madness. This causes them to become very irritable and all animals they bite become diseased." Fleming states that Aristotle believed that mankind was exempt from its attacks.

1

This is indeed strange when hydrophobia was already known as a disease of men. Hippocrates is supposed to refer to rabies when he says that persons in a frenzy drink very little, are disturbed and frightened, tremble at the least noise, or are seized with convulsions. He is said to have recommended boxwood (*Buxus*) as a preventive. Plutarch also writes about the dangers of rabid dog bites, and that the illness can be spread by the bite of a rabid dog. Others who mention rabies in ancient times include Zenophon, in the *Anabasis*, Epimarchus, Virgil, Horace, and Ovid. Lukian, a Roman writer, was of the belief that not only was the disease spread by biting dogs but that persons who became rabid could spread the disease by biting other persons, and could affect a whole group of people (Smithcors, 1958a).*

The infectivity of the saliva of rabid dogs is described by Cardanus, a Roman writer. The Roman writers described the infectious material as a poison for which the Latin was "virus." Another cause of rabies which is first mentioned by Pliny and Ovid is the so-called dog tongue worm. To prevent rabies, in ancient medical times, the attachment of the tongue (the frenum linguae, a mucous membrane) was cut and a fold removed in which the worm was thought to be. This idea was to persist until the nineteenth century when Pasteur demonstrated the cause of rabies beyond doubt.

Celsus, although a physician, appears to have made rabies his particular study in the first century. He was emphatic that the bites of all animals that contained virus were dangerous to man and beast. Indeed, it was fully recognized by Celsus and his contemporaries that the saliva alone contained the poisonous agent. In his description of wounds he says, "I have spoken concerning those wounds which are mostly inflicted by weapons, so it follows that I may speak concerning those which are made by the bite, sometimes of a man, sometimes of an ape, often of a dog, and sometimes of wild animals or of serpents. But every bite has mostly some venom" (*autem omnis morsus habet fere quoddam virus*). Of the malady itself he writes "The Greeks call it *hydrophian*, a most wretched disease, in which the sick person is tormented at the same time with thirst and the fear of water, and in which there is but little hope" (Smithcors, 1958a).

He recommends the practice of resorting to caustics, burning, cup-

---

* A near such episode occurred in Southern California in the 1950's when a patient who was suffering from rabies escaped from a hospital in a restraining gown. In bringing him under control, he attempted to bite nurses, doctors, and policemen. Fortunately no one was bitten severely but many persons took antirabies vaccine because they were uncertain of their exposure.

ping, and also sucking the wounds of those bitten by rabid dogs. He points out that there is no danger in sucking wounds except if there should be an abrasion or sore on the lips or in the mouth. If the wound is serious the cupping instrument is to be applied; if slight, a plaster can be used. Afterward, if the wound does not involve a nerve or muscle, the wound is to be cauterized. If it cannot be burnt, bloodletting should be attempted. Then the wound should be treated as a burn. But if it cannot be burnt then use those medicines which violently corrode, after which the ulcer will be healed in the usual way.

These sagacious precautions not only show the disease was well understood but that it was more or less prevalent and taxed the medical skills of the times. Hot and cold baths were also other measures recommended by Celsus. He states that when the disease appears, "The only remedy is to throw the patient unexpectedly into a pond, and if he has not a knowledge of swimming to allow him to sink, in order that he may drink, and to raise and again depress him, so that though unwillingly, he may be satisfied with water; for thus at the same time both the thirst and dread of water is removed."* Celsus also mentions the danger of cold water lest they destroy the enfeebled body. In those cases, the patient should be put into hot oil. In some cases, he says hot baths should be given immediately after the bite of a rabid dog allowing the patient to sweat while he still has the strength. In doing this the wound is also opened and the virus distils out. Then large quantities of pure wine should be taken which is antagonistic to all poisons. When this has been done for 3 days the person should be free from danger. Celsus also recommends salt as an application to wounds caused by the bites of dogs.

Virgil, in his *Georgics*, classes rabies among the diseases caused by a pestilential state of the air. Pliny in his hearsay story of the dog tongue worm states further, if the worm is removed and carried three times around a fire and is given to an exposed person, this will prevent him or her becoming mad. Many other tales of the prevention and treatment of disease are found in Fleming. These include eating a cock's brain or a cock's comb pounded and applied to the wound, and using goose grease and honey as a poultice. The flesh of a mad dog is sometimes salted and taken with food as a remedy. In addition, young puppies of the same sex as the dog that inflicted the wound are drowned, and the person bitten eats their liver raw. The

---

* This formidable treatment was continued until the nineteenth century according to Fleming who cites a cooper of Ghent being cured by submersion in the sea. He was dropped in the ocean from a ship and allowed to sink with the aid of irons. After a couple of submersions he was brought to the deck and revived, and lived.

urine of mad dogs was also considered poisonous by the ancients. If trod upon it was considered injurious, more so if a person had an ulcerous sore. In these cases, horse dung sprinkled with vinegar and warmed should be applied. Other treatments stretch the imagination. They include applying the ashes of a dog's head to the wound, they were also used in a potion and some even recommended eating the dog's head. Others were the placing of a maggot, taken from the carcass of a dead dog, on the wound. The hair or ashes of the hair of the tail of the dog that inflicted the wound were also inserted into the wound.*

Another story of antiquity which has lived down to this day in some parts of the world, and is related by Columella, is that it was believed among shepherds that if, on the fortieth day after the birth of a pup, the last bone of the tail is bitten off, the sinew will follow with it. After this the tail will not grow, and this will prevent the dog from getting rabies.

Writers of the early Christian era had much to say about rabies, describing it both in dogs and man. This is true of all of the Roman empire but especially Greece and Crete where the disease was widespread. Sicily must have had much disease from the frequent references. The administration of fluids is discussed by many writers. Some recommend snow, others the use of a straw in a dark room and, if no oral methods succeed, the use of enemas. Treatment of lower animals is described in the third century by Vegetius Renatus, one of the early writers on veterinary medicine. He recommended as an antidote for cattle that have been bitten by a mad dog, to give the cattle the boiled liver of the dog to eat, or to make it into balls and force it down as medicine. In the sixth century there are further accounts of the disease. Aetius, a physician of Mesopotamia, has left an accurate description of the dog disease. The symptoms were manifested by the dogs becoming mute, then delirious and incapable of recognizing their masters and surroundings. They refuse food, are thirsty but do not drink, and usually pant. They breathe with difficulty, keep the mouth open with the tongue hanging out, and discharge abundance of frothy saliva. Their ears and tail hang down, they move slowly and are dull and sleepy. When they run it is faster than usual, and in an irregular and uncommon manner.

A century later Paulus Aegiurata, a Greek physician, offers a good account of hydrophobia. He follows previous authors in enumerating the symptoms and distinguishes between the disease due to the bite

---

* This form of therapy brings to mind the recommendation of baccanals of centuries past and present to seek relief by resorting to the potion which hung them over.

of dogs and that remediable, simple nervous hydrophobia arising from other causes. The inoculated hydrophobia was always fatal.

Native Syrian doctors believed at the beginning of the ninth century that the disease was incurable. They attempted to give water in a globule of honey which was to be put in the mouth.

Rhazes, a celebrated Arab physician, mentions hydrophobia and says that a certain man barked by night like a dog and died.* He also described a patient who, when he beheld water, was seized with trembling and rigors, but when the water was removed the symptoms ceased.

The Arab physician, Avicenna, of the eleventh century speaks of rabies. He directs that the wound be kept open for 40 days and that ordinary blisters be placed on it. He alludes that hydrophobous persons bark like a dog and that they have a desire to bite people; that patients who attempted to drink suffocated, and the illness terminated in apoplexy. Altogether his observations mark a step forward in understanding the disease. He describes a dull redness, or erythema, which had been designated rabic roseola. There have been other cutaneous symptoms in man which received the names of rabic pleiads and rabic bubo.

The earliest mention of the disease in Great Britain is in the laws of Howel the Good, of Wales, which were revived in 1026. In them, an outbreak is alluded to as a most noteworthy event and that during that year there was a madness among the dogs.

From this period the literature of rabies gradually expands and with the progress of medicine the remarks become more valuable and comprehensive, though, so far as the successful prevention or attempts at curing the malady are concerned, little progress appears to have been made.

The Sorbonne condemned all superstitious practices for the treatment of rabies in a declaration June 10, 1671, and as early as the fifteenth century the celebrated theologian, Gerson, had pronounced against them. There was a great faith in the miracles of St. Hubert which was practiced as late as the nineteenth century, even though it had been pointed out that many who went to the shrine near Liége, Belgium, died of madness. In a critical history of superstitious customs published in 1709 by Father LeBrun, he states those that are cured have either not been bitten by mad dogs or have had other ailments distinct from hydrophobia; or, it has been the strength of their

---

* Habel (personal communication) describes such a patient near Washington, D. C. in the 1940's who made barking sounds and died of rabies. See also the frontispiece of this volume.

constitutions or the physical remedies which have cured them and not the miracle denied by the most skilled theologians and medical people. He treats the practice of the miracle as eminently superstitious and refutes the system.

The clergy of St. Hubert of course replied to the attack, but by arguments which failed to meet the objections raised, and the question appears since to have rested where all such questions remain — the world of common sense denies the miracle, the superstitious and priest-led affirm it.

In many Rhine villages there were what are called the Keys of St. Hubert which consisted of an iron, heated red hot and applied to the animals bitten by mad dogs. It never appears to have been in the form of a key. In St. Hubert itself the amulet was an iron ring inserted in the wall of one of the houses in the principal street. It no longer exists, but in the nineteenth century the belief in the potency of St. Hubert among the peasantry was as strong as ever. In other towns such as Liége there was also an iron ring, while in Utrecht there was an iron cross. Figure 1 shows a photograph of a statue of St. Hubert from the chapel of Our-Lady-on-High (Notre Dame du Haut), Moncontour, Brittany, France. It is one of seven statues of healing saints (St. Guerissant) in that chapel. Note the figure of the dog at the feet of the saint and the cautery ring held in the right hand.

Up until the middle ages epizootics were rare. Most cases were singular bites of rabid dogs, and occasionally of wolves, badgers, foxes, and even bears. Fleming tells of the invasion of Lyon by a rabid bear about the year 900 which bit some 20 people who attempted to kill the bear. Six people developed madness and were smothered to death in the next 27 days.

The first large outbreak is that described in Franconia in 1271 when rabid wolves invaded towns and villages attacking herds and flocks, and that no fewer than 30 persons died following bites inflicted on them. In 1500, Spain was said to be ravaged by canine rabies. By 1586 there were epizootics of rabies among dogs in Flanders, Austria, Hungary, and Turkey. In 1604, canine rabies was widespread in Paris and caused great alarm. In the 1700's rabies appeared in many parts of Europe. From 1719 until 1721 rabies was uncommonly frequent, especially in France and Silesia. It continued to be a problem in central Europe where it erupted among the wolves and foxes. In England the disease appeared in 1734–1735 where many mad dogs were seen in the late summer.

Fleming, according to Hughes, states that in 1741 many dogs went

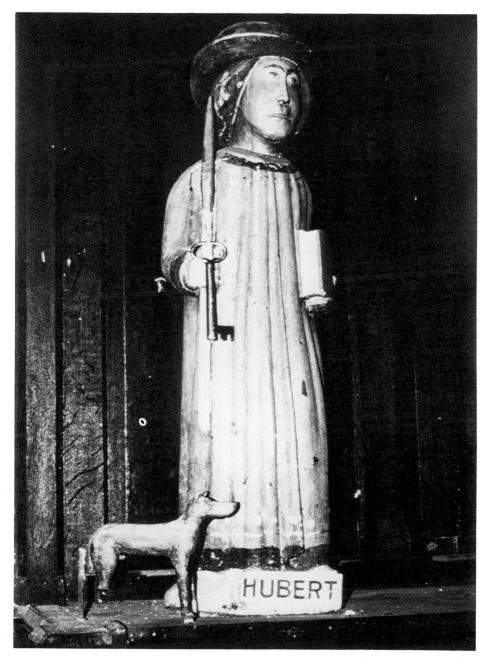

Fig. 1. Statue of St. Hubert, Chapelle Notre Dame du Haut, Moncontour, Brittany, France. (Courtesy of Dr. M. Hattwick.)

mad in Barbados where even cattle were affected. A correspondent writing from Charles Town, South America, under the date of November 10, 1750, says that since the first of the year a kind of madness has appeared in the dogs, first in the country and later in the city. Previously, no mad dogs had been reported in the province. He reports no persons bitten but says that the disease spread rapidly among the dogs. If the dogs were not killed they died in 2 or 3 days. He also states that some hogs were seized in the same way.

In 1752 rabies appeared about St. James in London and orders were issued to shoot all dogs on sight. Such orders were also issued in country towns. The years 1759–1760 saw a serious outbreak of disease in and around London. The city officials issued orders for all dogs to be confined for a month and ordered the destruction of all dogs on the streets with a reward of two shillings for each dog killed. Great cruelty was the result of this bribe to slay unfortunate dogs, and the most barbarous scenes were enacted by the brutal rabble which received a premium for their savage behavior. The London outbreak lasted until 1762.

In 1763 rabies appeared in France, Italy, and Spain. Dogs were slaughtered by the hundreds by the authorities. In Madrid 900 dogs were killed in 1 day. In 1768 rabies was already alarmingly frequent in Boston and other towns in North America. The archives of the State of Virginia contain references to rabies in dogs as early as 1753 and those of North Carolina as of 1762. The 1768 outbreak is considered the first major epizootic in North America. The epizootic continued until 1771 when foxes and dogs carried the disease to swine and domestic animals. The malady was so unusual that it was reported as a new disease.

By 1774 the disease was general in England and people were discouraged from keeping dogs. Paupers were not allowed to keep dogs. Up to five shillings were paid for every mad dog killed.

From 1776 to 1778 the French West Indies was visited for the first time by rabies and in epizootic form. At Guadaloupe the dogs were attacked with dumb madness. Subsequently a furious disease followed. Many cattle were bitten and died. Likewise many human beings were bitten and died. Many dogs died of dumb rabies but others became mad and bit everything that came in their way.

In 1779 rabies was very common in Philadelphia and Maryland. It first appeared in Jamaica and Hispaniola (Haiti and Dominican Republic) in 1783 and continued until 1784. Many persons were bitten and died. Domestic animals including horses, swine, and goats perished from the disease. The disease was so extensive in Kingston that all dogs were ordered killed. Likewise thousands of dogs were killed in Port au Prince.

Canine madness was raging all over colonial states of North America in 1785 and continued until 1789. That year a man died in New York of hydrophobia after skinning a cow that died of rabies. The disease appeared in Rhode Island as an epizootic among dogs and domestic animals in 1797. The disease reappeared in the eastern United States in 1810 and in Ohio it assumed an epizootic character affecting dogs, foxes, and wolves.

In the nineteenth century rabies appears to have become more widespread in Europe, especially France, Germany, and England. An extensive fox outbreak occurred in the Jura Alps in eastern France beginning in 1803 (Smithcors, 1958b). This was reported as the largest outbreak that had ever been seen. Hundreds of dead foxes were seen in the districts at the foot of the Jura Alps. Many people, dogs, pigs, and other animals were bitten. The epizootic continued unabated until 1835, and in the interval spread all over Switzerland. In 1804 the disease appeared in the west German states. In 1819 the disease spread into the upper Danube and Bavaria, and by 1825 had entered the Black Forest. In 1821–1822 it was widespread in the forests of Thuringia. In the Voralberg, upper Austria, 17 cows and goats died from fox-inflicted rabies in the summer of 1821. In 1824 it was common among the foxes of Upper Hesse. It reached Lower Hesse and Hanover the following year. As late as 1836 a man and a girl were bitten by a rabid fox in the district of Rottenburg. The girl died of rabies. In 1837 mad foxes were killed at Ulm. The fox rabies did not spread to north Germany such as it has in modern times. In some places all the foxes died and there was panic among the villagers.

At Crema, Italy, in 1804 a mad wolf descended from the mountains and bit 13 persons of whom nine died of hydrophobia. In 1806 rabies was very common in England and abounded in the vicinity of London. It continued as an epizootic for 2 years becoming less prevalent but never disappearing. In the winter of 1807 it was a serious problem in Dover where many human cases recurred. Until 1823 it was more or less prevalent in London and suburbs every year.

In 1803 rabies appeared for the first time in Peru, spreading as an epizootic from north to south. Forty-two persons are said to have died in Ica, 12–90 days after being bitten. These patients were violently ill and threatened to attack the attendants looking after them. None survived more than 5 days after the onset of their frenzy.

The slaughter of dogs in Lima saved the city from the epizootic—this practice continued for a number of years. The disease remained active for many years reaching Arequipa in 1807. All kinds of animals were affected including horses, donkeys, cattle, swine, goats, and even fowl as well as dogs and cats. By 1808 the epizootic subsided but the disease remained enzootic.

Fleming (1872) states that rabies was introduced into La Plata, Argentina, in 1806 by sporting dogs belonging to English officers. The disease is enzootic in that area to this day.

Rabies was common in the Ukraine in 1813. Fourteen persons are stated to have had the disease. As with all diseases, rabies follows the wars around. No doubt the disruption by the Napoleonic war contributed to its spread in Europe. In 1815 rabies was much more frequent than usual in Austria and particularly Vienna. Previously there had been only four or five cases of sporadic rabies among the dogs in Vienna and its suburbs between 1808 and 1814. The disease assumed epizootic proportions in October 1814 with five cases, increasing to fifteen by December. In 1815 there were 46 dog cases in Vienna. Likewise there was an epizootic in Copenhagen in 1815.

In 1819 the Duke of Richmond, then Governor General of Canada was bitten by a captive fox near Ottawa and died shortly thereafter of hydrophobia. In 1822 rabies was common in Holland and in 1824 was epizootic in Sweden, extending to foxes, wolves, dogs, cats, and reindeer. It was likewise general in Norway and Russia as well as England. From 1823 to 1828 there were more cases than usual in Berlin. In 1828 the English Registrar-General Report lists 28 persons dying from hydrophobia.

During the 1830's the disease was frequent in Saxony and again in Vienna and England. In 1831–1832 Posen was affected. Pomerania also suffered from the disease. In 1834 the Canton of Thurgau ordered the destruction of all foxes as rabies continued among these animals. In Zurich animals were attacked and in Lausanne sheep were attacked.

Rabies invaded Chile in 1835 where it became prevalent, and men were bitten and died of the disease.

Vienna was invaded again by an epizootic in 1838 which was to last until 1843. In 1838 there were 17 cases; in 1839, 63 cases; in 1840 only 42, but in 1841 no fewer than 141 cases were reported—an unprecedented number which caused much alarm. The following year, 1842, there were 42 cases and in 1843 only two dog cases.

The 1840's saw the disease still rampant in Germany. In Wurtemburg there was an epizootic from September 1839 to the end of 1842 which was believed to have begun with foxes. From the first of January 1840 until the end of February 1842 rabies was observed in 251 dogs.

For 1839–1840 the Veterinary School of Lyons reported few cases of rabies — but in the next report 1840–1841 rabies is seen in great numbers. Out of 64 suspect cases 33 developed symptoms and died. Professor Rey states that they were able to transmit the disease through several animals by the inoculation of saliva. In 1804 Zinke had first demonstrated that rabies could be transmitted by saliva. His experiments were crude however and not entirely convincing; hence, repetition added to the authenticity of his experiments.

Zinke's experiment was quite simple. He took saliva from a mad dog as soon as it had been killed and, by means of a little paint brush, painted the saliva into incisions he had made on the foreleg of a 1-year-old dachshund. He painted as much saliva on the wounds as the paint brush would hold. The dog according to his report remained lively and ate and drank until the seventh day. On the eighth day the dog ignored his food, did not drink, was sad and crawled into the corner of his cage. By the tenth day the dog had overt rabies. Zinke wrote quite extensively on rabies as to its source, pathogenesis, and treatment. One author he quotes is Hayworth who advised extensive irrigation of the wound with warm water for several hours, whereas other authorities urged the use of the hot iron or blistering agents. Some even advocated quicksilver and other metals. He closes his booklet with the admonition that one should take care not to be contaminated with saliva, and not to touch anything with bare hands that had been in the mouth of the patient. Everything in contact with the patient should be burned or buried deep in the ground. The book is a curious mixture of ancient superstition and sound modern ideas, especially the extensive irrigation of the wound.

Another experimenter, Hugo Alt Graf zu Salm-Reifferschied (1813), was able to transmit rabies among dogs by saliva from a rabid animal which was inoculated. He also claimed that food smeared with contaminated saliva caused rabies. He was convinced that the saliva contained the infectious agent.

Krugelstein reported in 1826 in an extensive book, 640 pages, on every phase of rabies. He likewise thought that the causal agent was in the saliva but he believed that the agent appeared *de novo* under various conditions. Neither he nor Zinke had any idea of a living agent. On the other hand he says that rabies is without doubt a disease of the nervous system. Further he states that if any nerve ending is infected by the saliva poison, it sickens locally and sends the poison along the sympathetic nerves until it reaches the coeliac plexus where the poison affects the entire nervous system. From there it spreads by the way of the spinal cord and the disease reaches its acme. This is an interesting thought for the period in which it was written. He sought diligently for changes in the nerve system, but with his crude methods could only find congestion. As to treatment, he lists 60 medicaments in addition to bloodletting, drinking blood, galvanism, magnetism, and applying pressure on the carotids. We can be thankful that suffocation was no longer listed.

The Swedish epizootic of 1824 led to an interesting paper by Ekstrom (1830). In his paper he recommends that treatment should consist of making deep incisions of the wounds and surrounding parts. These were then to be washed diligently for several minutes either with water or diluted muriatic acid, or solution of muriate of lime. After the wound was clean and dried, a hot iron or strong muriatic acid was to be applied. This is the first instance of the use of acid. Later, in 1899, Follen Cabot reported on the use of nitric acid following its experimental use in guinea pigs. Webster in 1942 asked what nitric acid did to rabies virus when applied to a dog bite wound. Today we recognize soap and water as the best method of dealing with a wound from a rabid animal.

Bouchardat was another reporter of the nineteenth century that put to rest many therapeutic claims in his extensive reports of 1852 and 1854. He was also among the first to think about inoculations against rabies and had an early influence on Pasteur. He attempted many experiments at the Lyon Veterinary Faculty.

During 1841–1842 rabies was epizootic in Lyon. The Veterinary School reported that they had never seen so many rabid animals. Out of 104 dogs that died in the hospital from various causes, 62 perished from rabies. Eight persons died following bites of rabid dogs. The Lyon's Veterinary School had records of rabies going back to 1800 — during that 30-year period 779 dogs had died of rabies in the hospital. In 1843 only 14 cases were seen at the School (Billings).

An unusual outbreak of cattle rabies occurred in the district of Heyden, Reinland, in 1843–1844. The affected animals were vicious and attacked each other with their horns. They kept up a continuous bellowing and foamed at the mouth. The hind parts were weak and the weakness increased so rapidly that on the third day the animals were on the ground and could not rise. The muscles of the face, shoulders and thighs were contracted at intervals by spasms. There was no unusual thirst and the ability of swallowing remained unimpaired. Any fluids poured into the mouth were sucked down, although some animals had choking motions and a twitching of the muscles of the face. The disease was usually fatal about the fourth day. The officials in charge believed the disease to be spontaneous rabies, as they could not discover any evidence of dog bites among the cattle.

In 1847 rabies appeared at Roscommon, Ireland where many dogs were affected. The disease also appeared in Malta that year, supposedly for the first time.

Canine rabies raged as an epizootic in Northern Germany in the 1850's. At Hamburg, 267 cases were seen among dogs in 1851 after an absence of 23 years. Active measures included the restraint of all dogs and the killing of all stray dogs. The total number killed exceeded 1400; in addition, some 300 or 400 were killed by their owners. The epizootic continued until 1856. By that time nearly 600 rabid dogs were reported in Hamburg.

A rabid wolf caused much damage in France in 1851 in the vicinity of Hue-Au-Gal where during a single day 46 persons and 82 head of cattle were bitten. The consequences were that many persons died; all of the cattle were purposely destroyed.

Another wolf episode occurred in the Turkish territories in the town of Adalia where the people were defenseless because of the governor's seizure of all weapons. The wolf bit several people in the town and then fled to a garden where several hundred individuals were camping during the silkworm harvest. There, 128 persons were severely wounded. From the garden the wolf attacked a flock of sheep, killing 85 of them. It was not until the following day that the wolf was killed with weapons returned to the people. How many people died is not stated in Fleming's *Rabies and Hydrophobia* although he states that several of those bitten died raving mad.

In England in 1856 rabies was prevalent among dogs and a herd of deer. The disease appeared among the deer after a mad dog had been in the community. Nearly 100 deer died of the disease. The symptoms included foaming at the mouth, biting one another, tearing off the hair and flesh, and when confined, biting at whatever they came in contact with. Several dogs also died at the same place, exhibiting symptoms of rabies. The disease was not suspected of being rabies until a child was bitten and an investigation was made by the local board of health. Their conclusion was that the disease was rabies and people should take precautions.

Another outbreak was reported in Berkshire, England, where a flock of sheep was attacked by a mad dog. About 20 sheep were wounded and four killed. Of the 20 sheep nearly all died after several weeks, during which many lambed. The lambs were not affected. The diseased ewes trotted backward and forward, and repeatedly bit at the fence, foamed at the mouth, and tore mouthfuls of wool out of one another.

Rabies appeared in Hong Kong for the first time in 1857. An English bloodhound suddenly became rabid and bit several people; one man died of hydrophobia. This appears to be the only case reported for many years. Rabies was reported in China in 1860 when a man died of hydrophobia near Canton. In 1861 Fleming reports that the disease was present at Tientsin near Peking and that the natives died of hydrophobia caused by the bites of rabid dogs. The disease appeared in Shanghai in 1867 in English dogs. Several persons were bitten. Two Europeans bitten by their own dogs died of hydrophobia. Rabies became very common among dogs of European residents, and of several people who were bitten, all were treated and survived. In the winter of 1869 a Scotch Terrier became rabid at Chinkiang and bit a buffalo which subsequently died.

Hydrophobia appears to be well known to Chinese physicians and there was a formidable list of cures. Among these was one said to be infallible, composed of musk and cinnabar. These were combined and suspended in rice spirits. Calm sleep and copious perspiration were supposed to follow, otherwise a second dose of the material is given, and a sure cure was to follow.

In 1858 the disease was so extensive in Algeria that the Governor General issued a circular relative to preventive measures.

By 1860 (Smithcors, 1958b) rabies had spread all across America and was attributed to the large number of idle dogs everywhere which were free to prowl around. There is no mention of skunks and foxes during this period (Billings, 1884).

In the 1860's rabies was epizootic in many parts of Europe. Vienna appeared to be the center of the epizootic. Both furious and dumb rabies were seen at the Imperial Veterinary Institute. A boy bitten by a dog diagnosed as rabid died 4 weeks after the exposure. Three other persons bitten by the same dog had their wounds cauterized and escaped the disease. The boy's wounds were not cauterized because they were so extensive.

The disease reappeared in Saxony after 10 years. The city of Dresden had not seen a case from 1853 to 1863. In 1863 it began to spread gradually and soon the whole country was affected; 10 cases were reported. In the following year there were 33 cases; in 1865, 227; in 1866, 287.

About 1862, Sir Samuel Baker, exploring the Nile tributaries of

Abyssinia (Ethiopia), reports that rabies was epizootic in that country. To prevent the disease, a grass hut was filled with straw and fired, after which each dog was brought by its owner and thrown into the flames. The dogs were able to escape although they would be badly frightened and scorched.

In 1864, there were 12 hydrophobia deaths in England. There was an extensive outbreak in Lancashire. In Liverpool, a thousand dogs were destroyed. There were seven human deaths in Ireland but none in Scotland.

In the middle of 1865, rabies was epizootic in and around London. Many persons were bitten and three deaths occurred from hydrophobia. The total human deaths in 1865 was 19 for England. In 1866, rabies was widespread in England, especially in Lancashire. The Registar-General reported fewer than 36 deaths, of which 11 were in London, 13 in Lancashire, three in Northumberland, and others scattered. In 1867 the Metropolitan Streets Act was passed which enabled the police to seize all vagrant dogs. In June 1868, the Act was put in force and rabies was greatly decreased in and around London.

Rabies appeared in Belgium in 1868 where the disease had been rare. It commenced in January and reports were received from several provinces. Up to May, 32 dogs, a horse, and a cat were diagnosed as being rabid at the Cureghem Veterinary School near Brussels. Two human cases were seen.

In 1869, rabies was noted in Paris and the transmission of disease from a cat to a human being was reported. A few years earlier, 1865, Trousseau had published his masterful clinical description of rabies. He was of the opinion that a specific virus was the cause of the disease which was transmitted only by the bite of a rabid animal. With the methods available he found no special anatomic lesions. As to treatment, he advised cauterization with a hot iron. He raised the question of the value of curare to relax the patient. He also gives the old Chinese formula, which was supposed to be infallible, of musk and cinnabar.

Early in 1869, a rabies epizootic began to spread from Lancashire to Yorkshire and to the borders of Scotland. Two human deaths occurred in March, 1869, where six rabid animals were destroyed in Preston. In September, several cases occurred at Yorkshire and a boy aged 3 years died of hydrophobia. At Newburgh in the same month, a mad dog bit a man and several animals; the man died. Animals and human beings continued to be bitten during this epizootic with the loss of life. Dogs, cats, pigs, sheep, cows, and horses died of the disease. In 1870, many men and children died of hydrophobia in

England and one case occurred in Dundee, Scotland. Officials recommended that all animals exposed to a rabid animal be destroyed. Hundreds of dogs were killed during the 1870's when rabies was so rampant in England. The alternative was to confine an exposed dog for 10 months.

Rabies was also a serious problem on the continent during periods of epizootics in France, Germany, and Austria. In 1871, rabies reappeared in Barbados, West Indies. The custodian of the library was severely bitten while separating two dogs which were fighting. Afterward he died of rabies. In addition, three children died of the disease in one family. In another family two children died of rabies. Gibraltar had an outbreak of rabies in 1870. Of 13 people bitten, 11 died. Algeria had many cases of rabies in man and animals in the 1860's and 1870's. The French were of the opinion that the disease was indigenous before their occupation.

Russia had an increase of rabies in the 1860's and 1870's. In 1863 only eight, with seven suspected, dogs were rabid but three people died in St. Petersburg. From that year up to 1874 there was a varying increase. In 1874, 49 persons were bitten by rabid dogs and eight people died. Altogether in 12 years, 2724 people were bitten; of 1895 dogs, 1066 were healthy, 198 rabid, 103 suspected, and 528 dogs were affected with various other diseases. In St. Petersburg during that period, 47 people died from rabies. The rabies problem was extensive in Russia.

The Registrar-General reported 74 deaths in 1874 in Great Britain, and 47 in 1875 in England. The *Lancet* remarks "It is an undoubted fact that hydrophobia has been increasingly fatal in England in recent years. The annual death rate from this disease to a million living, which according to the Registrar-General's report, did not exceed 0.3 in the five years 1860-65 rose successively to 0.9 and 1.8 in the two succeeding five years and further increased to 2 per million in 1875. In London, six deaths from hydrophobia were reported in both 1875 and 1876, and in the first 29 weeks of 1877, ending July 21, nine cases have already been recorded." The British rabies problem was serious.

Hill reports that in 1886 rabies was made a notifiable disease under the Contagious Diseases (animals) Act and in 1887 the Rabies Order gave local authorities power to muzzle, control, seize and detain, and dispose of stray dogs. The local authorities were lax in enforcing this legislation and in 1890 the Rabies Order (muzzling of dogs) brought the disease under central control. The muzzling orders reduced the number of cases of rabies in dogs from 129 in 1890 to 38 in 1892. There was considerable opposition from the public to the muzzling orders and they were withdrawn and control was handed back to the local authorities. The situation became acute again and in 1895 there were 727 cases of rabies recorded, and in 1896, 463 cases were reported. A new Rabies Order and the control of the Importation of Dogs Order came into operation in 1897. These measures succeeded in eradicating the disease in 1902. Fortunately, Great Britain did not have a sylvatic reservoir of disease, but regardless, the eradication of the disease by dog control was a great achievement. The country remained free until 1918 when rabies reappeared at Plymouth in a dog illegally brought back from the continent. The epizootic spread to Devon and Dorset where 129 cases were reported. Another 190 cases occurred in other parts of the country. Whether all these were attributable to the case at Plymouth or could be attributed to other dogs brought home by returning soldiers could not be ascertained. The disease was eradicated by 1922. Since 1922 nearly 100,000 dogs and cats have been imported and have undergone quarantine; 27 cases have been confirmed in quarantine; 25 dogs, one cat, and one leopard cub. Nearly all were observed within 1 month of landing, but two cases occurred between 6 and 7 months, and one at almost 8 months. Fortunately none of these latter animals had been released after 6 months quarantine. In addition, a case of rabies occurred in a rhesus monkey imported for medical research in November 1965. In 1969 a case occurred in a dog imported from West Germany, which had been in quarantine for 6 months. It died 2 weeks after being released, before it died, it bit a cat and its owner. A further case was confirmed at Newmarket, almost 9 months after landing and 3 months after release from quarantine (Hill). These cases will be discussed in detail under quarantine control measures.

Smithcors (1958c) reports, following the Civil War, rabies was widespread in most of the United States. Mad dogs were reported in many urban areas as well as rural areas. Sylvatic rabies had been recognized in the eastern states in the eighteenth century. In the nineteenth century the disease was seen in foxes throughout the eastern part of the country. With the movement west of the population, rabies appears to have gone with the pioneers. Skunk rabies was reported by the mountain men on the Great Plains in the 1830's. It was first reported in California in the 1850's. The United States Army reported serious skunk rabies was so common that the early settlers on the Great Plains referred to skunks as hydrophobia cats, or phobey cats. At the turn of the twentieth century rabies was a dreaded disease throughout the United States. Control measures were not effective as the public would not accept dog control and muzzling. It was not until dog vaccination could be successfully performed by a single inoculation that the fear of dog rabies was to be alleviated. The sylvatic problem remains with no solution visible. There are thousands of rabid skunks and foxes reported each year and there are probably thousands more than go unreported.

Madstones (or moonstones) have long been used as a means of warding off rabies. The original amulets — apparently "hair balls" from the stomach of white deer (or their gallstones), gallstones of white cows, or any smooth white stones — were used by the frontiersmen and early settlers. The origin of the special effects of amulets is lost in antiquity. Gallstones in sheep and cattle are rare and therefore were thought to have special attributes among which was preventing rabies if one were attacked by a rabid animal. Some people boiled the stone in milk to "prepare" it for a particular application. If the milk turned to a color other than white, the boiling was continued to free it of impurities from previous applications, but if the milk stayed white the stone was ready for use (T. E. Sellers, Sr., personal communication). The longer the stone "stuck" on the wound the better. In some cases where rabies appeared in humans, the madstone was used to treat the person by placing it in his possession or on the wound.

Fleming uses the example of rabies in Algeria and Peru in support of the theory of the spontaneous origin of rabies in many cases of the world. Fleming was a strong proponent of spontaneous disease, citing glanders, farcy, and strangles in the horse, anthrax in cattle, typhus in pigs, and distemper in dogs as examples of the spontaneous appearance of disease. He does accept the inoculation of a virus by a bite as the cause of disease but the origin of the virus is when he falls back on spontaneous generation — not unlike our concepts of certain chronic diseases.

Galtier in his studies on rabies reported in 1879 that he was able to transmit rabies to rabbits and from rabbit to rabbit. He does not state the method of transmission. The symptoms were paralysis and convulsions. The average incubation period was 18 days. This appears to be the first report on the transmission to rabbits, unfortunately without much needed detail. The work of Pasteur was on the other hand definitive. A little later, Maurice Raynaud reported that he took saliva from a rabid patient and injected it subcutaneously into a rabbit's ear. Four days later the rabbit was stricken with a sort of paralysis and died during the night. Fragments of submaxillary salivary gland inoculated into other rabbits subcutaneously are said to have reproduced the disease, as they died on the fifth and sixth day. An autopsy showed only congestion of the lungs. These observations are not convincing but are mentioned as leading up to Pasteur's great work.

Pasteur published his first report on rabies during 1881, a period when many scientists were attempting to transmit rabies from man to animals, and animals to animals. Pasteur's first experiments with saliva from a child dead of rabies produced a pneumococcus septicemia in the rabbit. This was recognized by Pasteur while other investigations thought they had produced rabies even though the rabbits died in 48 hours. Pasteur with his extraordinary acumen and experimental ability resolved the question in his report. Both the symptoms and histologic changes led him to the conclusion that "the central nervous system and especially the bulb which joins the spinal cord to the brain are particularly concerned and active in the development of the disease." He then reported success in producing rabies by the injection of central nervous system material and spinal fluid. The seat of the virus is not then solely in the saliva. Pasteur was bothered by the experimental difficulties of the long incubation period. He soon found that by injecting brain material from rabid animals directly into the brains of dogs the incubation period was shortened to 1 or 2 weeks, or at the most 3 weeks. This was an important advance in experimental rabies studies.

Pasteur reported further on his fundamental studies. He pointed out that saliva was not a satisfactory source of virus for experimental work since its effects were uncertain and the incubation period might be very long. He again referred to the certainty and rapidity with which rabies could be produced by direct intracerebral injections of central nervous system material from rabid animals. He pointed out that virus was not only found in the lower centers of the brain but in the spinal cord as well. He differentiated dumb rabies characterized by paralysis and furious rabies in which the animal attacked everything. He found that inoculation into the bloodstream first affected the spinal cord and was likely to produce the dumb type rather than the furious. He also found that an animal which recovered after early symptoms of rabies was immune to later inoculations, and that some dogs seemed to have a natural resistance. Finally he produced rabies by the intracerebral injection of all parts of the brain of a cow dead of rabies.

In 1884, a year of much rabies in France, Pasteur made a more definitive report. Intravenous injections as previously reported usually produced a paralytic type of rabies, and dogs sacrificed at the first symptom of paralysis revealed the spinal cord containing virus when there was no evidence as yet of any virus in the bulb. Pasteur also demonstrated virus in pneumogastric and sciatic nerves, and in the salivary glands with the conclusion that the entire nervous system is susceptible. Virus preserved its virulence in spinal cords kept at 0°–12°C. Pasteur was unable to cultivate any bacteria from the nervous system, but he stated that "one is tempted to believe that a microbe of infinite smallness, having the form neither of a bacillus nor a micrococcus is the cause." How right he was when the electron microscope has revealed the virus as being bullet shaped. He reported observations to show that the clinical type of rabies produced depended somewhat upon the dose of infective material, and he believed that injections of small amounts of virus did not produce immunity. He discussed the hypothesis of the passage of virus from the periphery to the central nervous system via the nerves as against the distribution of virus by the bloodstream and, whether or not the former was correct, he regarded the latter as proved. Finally and most important, he discussed the theoretical basis of immunizing injections and made a general statement that he had already achieved some success.

Later in the year, Pasteur, in collaboration with Chamberland and Roux, made another report to the Academy of Science dealing primarily with the problem of attenuation of virus. If one passed rabies virus from dog to monkey and then from monkey to monkey, the virulence of the virus fell off at each passage. If the virus was then returned to dog, rabbit, or guinea pig it remained attenuated. It did not immediately resume the virulence of street virus in the dog. Even intracerebral inoculation might not produce the disease, although it established nonetheless a state refractory to rabies. But if the virus was passed back to the dog, it was much more virulent than street virus and, if inoculated into the bloodstream, it always caused fatal rabies. By using a series of injections of attenuated virus, he made dogs immune or at least refractory. He alluded in a general way to some favorable observations on immunization of man, taking advantage of the long incubation period.

Although Pasteur had alluded to his method of prophylaxis of rabies in earlier papers, he gave his first detailed report in 1885 to the Academy of Science. The first step was the intracerebral inoculation of street virus into a rabbit and the passage through successive rabbits. The incubation period gradually became shorter until it reached a fixed time of 7 days. The cords of these rabbits contained virus throughout their length, which gradually diminished in virulence as the cords were suspended in dry air.* The actual immunization was carried out by injecting into a dog subcutaneously a syringe of broth to which was added a tiny bit of rabbit cord, beginning with one dried long enough to be avirulent and successively using more virulent material until finally a virulent cord is reached. The dog was by this time refractory to rabies, as demonstrated in 50 dogs. At about this time there arrived from Alsace a boy of 9 years, Joseph Meister, who had been bitten 14 times by a rabid dog. The boy was examined by Doctors Vulpian and Grancher who thought the child had received a fatal inoculation of rabies virus. Pasteur goes on to say "The death of this child seemed inevitable, and I decided, not without lively and cruel doubts, as one can believe, to try in Joseph Meister, the method which has been successful in dogs. Consequently on July 6 at 8 o'clock in the evening, 60 hours after the bites, in the presence of Doctors Vulpian and Grancher, we inoculated under a skin fold in the right hypochondrium of the little Meister a half syringe of the cord of a rabid rabbit preserved in a flask of dry air for 15 days." Thirteen successive inoculations were made with cords of increasing virulence. The little boy never developed rabies.

Pasteur with the penetrating curiosity which was so characteristic of him was not satisfied with practical results but wished to understand the mechanism of his method. He concluded that the dried cords contained fewer and fewer live virus particles which were not however attenuated in individual virulence. Thus the method consisted in essence of injecting larger and larger quantities of virus each day.

An interesting discussion followed the paper at the Academy of Science. Vulpian said "Rabies, that terrible malady against which all therapeutic attempts have so far failed, has finally found its remedy." Others expressed themselves with equal enthusiasm, and Pasteur closed the meeting with gracious acknowledgment of what had been said.

A year later in 1886 Pasteur reported the results of treatment in 350 cases. Only one person developed rabies, a child bitten on October 3 that was not brought for treatment until November 9. According to contemporary statistics one-half of those bitten should have developed disease. In no case did the injections produce local inflammation, abscess, and other untoward effects. Pasteur concluded

* Earlier, Pasteur had observed that the organisms of fowl cholera *Pasteurella multocida* were modified or attenuated when they remained at room temperature for some days and could be used to immunize fowl.

"The prophylaxis of rabies is established. It is time to create a center for vaccination against rabies." A commission was appointed by the Academy of Science to implement Pasteur's proposal. The commission proposed that an establishment, to be called the Pasteur Institute (Institut Pasteur), be founded for the treatment of both the French people and foreigners. Within a decade there were Pasteur Institutes throughout the world. These institutes were to become the center of scientific investigation in many countries.

Pasteur made further progress reports. By late 1886 over 700 persons had now been treated including 38 Russians bitten by rabid wolves. Three of this group died, and Pasteur points out the great virulence of wolf bite compared with that of the dog. In another report Pasteur recognizes that the treatment was not always successful, especially in face bites. He noted that most of the fatal cases were in children bitten about the face. He was not sure that the treatment was adequate for this type of case. He decided to modify the procedure to make it more rapid and more effective by giving more injections daily and continuing the treatment longer. The standard treatment at this time was 10 daily injections beginning with material dried for 14 days and concluding with the 5-day cord.

Detailed reports that appeared each year from Pasteur Institute cited some failures. In 1898, for example, Pottevin reported 20,166 persons treated with 96 deaths or a mortality of 0.46%. Recent figures from India state that about 0.5% of the treated cases die.

Roux, in a later report, 1887, found that glycerin was an excellent preservative for rabies virus. He found that fresh material from the brain would yield virus after 4 weeks. This was an important observation in a period when frequently the specimens from rabid animals were putrid. Chalmette, following his suggestion in Indochina, kept a supply of desiccated cord preserved in glycerin on hand at the Saigon Pasteur Institute at all times so as to be prepared to give antirabies treatment. Various other methods of attenuating virus including phenol, formalin, and ether were to be used in the next century.

About this time there was considerable discussion as to the route whereby rabies virus reaches the nervous system: (1) by the bloodstream and (2) by the nerves. Pasteur had shown that inoculation by bloodstream and intracerebral inoculation were effective. DiVestea and Zagari (1889) brought forward clinical and experimental evidence that rabies virus was spread from the bite to the central nervous system by passage along the nerves. They had shown, for example, that inoculation of fixed virus into the sciatic nerve of a rabbit and a dog caused death with the same symptoms as those of intracerebral inoculation. Furthermore, death could be prevented by cutting and cauterization of the nerve after injection. Finally the type of clinical phenomenon produced seemed to depend on the location of the inoculation nerve and where it entered the central nervous system. Roux agreed with these observations but had certain reservations. For example, he stated "One sees then that inoculation into the nerves does not always produce rabies with the certainty of trepanation." Meanwhile Nocard and Roux showed that large intravenous injections of rabid spinal cord could be given with impunity to sheep and goats, although immunity was conferred. Helman, another worker at the Pasteur Institute, concluded that rabies virus produced infection on inoculation only if introduced directly into the nerve cells, if introduced into subcutaneous tissue it could give immunity. All this shows how exceedingly complex and confused the subject was. Webster found in 1937 that virus injected under the skin of Swiss mice is first detected 5 or 6 days later in the central nervous system at the site in direct connection with the inoculated areas. This finding, like others, is consistent with the view that the virus does travel by way of the nerves.

Negri, who discovered the bodies which bear his name, in 1903 thought he had uncovered a microorganism which should be included among the protozoa (1903a). This would be natural as Negri was working in the laboratory of Golgi in Pavia where studies of malaria were being intensively pursued. These alleged parasites that Negri observed were seen especially in the dog. Negri observed them also in one human case. The site of predilection was in the horn of Ammon. In this region, especially in the larger nerve cells, the bodies are present in large numbers. They exhibit the form of small, sharply outlined structures. They were also found in the spinal ganglia and in the spinal cord of dogs in which rabies occurred naturally or experimentally, and in rabbits experimentally inoculated. The bodies are of various size, from 1 μm up to 10 or 15 μm or even as large as 27 μm by 5 μm. They were stained best with eosin methylene blue. Four to six parasites may be found in one cell. Negri thought he saw evidence of the multiplication of these bodies. In another paper Negri (1903b) used the presence of Negri bodies as a practical diagnostic test for rabid animals and laid the ground for the long-used test.

The study of events leading to the discovery of the causal agent of rabies is exciting. Pasteur himself had speculated that the agent was a tiny one, unlike ordinary bacteria. Babes reviewed various claims of a bacterial agent in 1887, and himself isolated several organisms from the nervous system of rabid animals, with cultures of which he claimed to reproduce rabies; but, interestingly enough, he thought that the causal agent was a minute body perhaps carried in the bacteria. Babes later confirmed, in 1906, the Negri bodies in rabies but concluded that they represent a reaction to infection and were not parasites although they might contain them. The causal agent, Babes concluded, must be more widespread in the nervous system as the fluorescent antibody test has revealed. In 1909 Negri redescribed his bodies still insisting they were parasites and pointing out the Calkins had named them *Neurocytes hydrophobial*. Calkins, it should be recalled, worked on the Guarnieri bodies of smallpox and concluded that they too were living parasites. Meanwhile Remlinger, in 1903, claimed to have produced rabies in rabbits with Berkefeld V filtrates of central nervous system material from rabid dogs and rabbits. Finally J. Koch and P. Rissling described small coccus-like bodies in the gray matter of the central nervous systems of rabid dogs which they thought might be of etiological significance. Like Babes, they did not accept the Negri bodies as parasites. Later confirmation of the filtrability of rabies virus of course rules out the bodies of Negri and of Koch as causal agents, whatever diagnostic value they may have. The nodules described by Babes, which seem to be leukocytic accumulations in relation to blood vessels, are now thought to be common to neurotropic virus infections. Indeed the Negri body is perhaps the only specific anatomic change. The last contribution in this field is by T. F. Sellers who developed a useful and widely used method of demonstrating Negri bodies by impression preparations of brain tissue specially stained (1927).

Remlinger was the first to give a comprehensive review of the paralyses occurring with antirabies therapy. He gave abstracts of 26 cases between 1888 and 1905. He attempted to analyze the whole problem and discussed various explanations, including the introduction of nonviral toxic substances. He leaned toward a "rabic toxin" as the explanation. Years later in 1935 he discusses paralytic accidents as a Landry-like ascending paralysis. It was assumed that the accidents were true rabies of a type different from the laboratory-proven rabies. Remlinger in this paper discusses the question of whether these accidents of therapy are actually rabies, especially the mild nonfatal ones. No final answer was reached although he concluded that with exception of certain paralyses following dead vaccine, the accidents of antirabic therapy are largely due to fixed virus, a view not accepted today.

Stuart and Krikorian concluded in 1928 that in the basic nerve substance of all antirabies vaccines there seems to exist some deleterious component which is capable of producing neuroparalytic disorders. They actually showed that paralytic accidents can be produced experimentally by the repeated inoculation of nerve substance normal or rabid, homologous or heterologous. Later T. M. Rivers *et al.* showed that repeated intramuscular injections of brain extracts and emulsions into monkeys might be followed by an inflammatory reaction, with demyelinization. Similar findings were described by a series of other investigators. In 1949 Bell *et al.* described a rabies vaccine freed of the factors causing allergic encephalitis. They were successful in removing the factors. Today many experimental vaccines are being prepared without extraneous materials that cause allergic reactions. These will be discussed in other chapters.

Fermi, in a review of a large number of experiments (1907), pointed out that it was difficult to demonstrate rabies virus in the saliva. Bartarelli showed that virus reached the salivary gland in rabid dogs by peripheral travel along nerves. His demonstration consisted in severing first the nervous and then the vascular connections of the paratid gland after which the animal was inoculated with rabies virus. The glands from animals in which the nervous, but not the vascular, connections were left intact produced rabies in other animals. Meanwhile Roux and Nocard showed that rabies virus could be found in the saliva of rabid dogs 2 or 3 days before the least clinical symptom. J. Nicholas found saliva virulent as long as 6 days before the animal showed any recognizable clinical signs of rabies.

Fermi, in another report in 1908, points out various defects in Pasteur's vaccination regime. He introduced a new method in which the vaccine was treated with carbolic acid. One hundred percent of the test animals were saved whereas 100% of untreated controls died. He mentions as advantageous the uniformity of the vaccine and simplicity of preparation instead of the complicated and useless Pasteur method of attenuation. This vaccine can be preserved and sent anywhere so as always to be available. Later Sir David Semple in a masterful article on the practical aspects of rabies in 1919 described a method for preparing a dead carbolized vaccine and reported the cases of 2009 Europeans in India who were treated, with only 0.19% failure. If immunization is complete before the virus traveling along peripheral nerves reaches the central nervous system the patient survives, otherwise he or she dies. Hence, slight bites at the periphery with a long incubation period are more favorable for immunization than severe bites on the face with a brief incubation.

L. T. Webster in a 1939 critical review gives an elaborate review of all the reported laboratory experiences in rabies vaccination. He concludes, "All workers save Fermi have failed to demonstrate a significant protective effect of vaccination following experimental exposure to rabies virus by any route." On the other hand, vaccine, virulent or nonvirulent, given before exposure has been found effective under limited conditions. These rather gloomy conclusions do not seem in harmony with reports of human vaccination. There have been spectacular advances in the prevention of experimental rabies since 1940 which are discussed in other chapters.

A big advance in the diagnosis of rabies was the mouse inoculation test by Webster and Dawson in 1935. They found that mice were quite susceptible to neurotropic viruses. Using such animals they found that rabies was readily produced by intracerebral inoculation of fresh dog brain containing Negri bodies. Rabies could occur within 7 days but in some cases prolonged incubations up to 28 days were reported by later investigators. Leach confirmed the practical value of Webster's mouse test and indeed found it positive in 12% of brains reported negative for Negri bodies, whereas only three specimens among 338 reported gave a negative mouse test.

The mouse test showed that only 85–95% of rabies-positive cases were found by Negri body examination alone. The mouse test was to become the standard test for all Negri body negative tests, and is used to this day except where the fluorescent antibody test has replaced it. They also developed a mouse protection test for the quantitative measurement of antibodies against rabies. The final outcome to these investigations was a mouse test for measuring the immunizing potency of antirabic vaccines in 1939. Webster using the mouse test was able to appraise the potency of vaccines showing that virulent virus injected intraperitoneally as a vaccine immunized mice within 10 days for a period of at least 9 months. Demonstrable neutralizing antibodies accompanied this immunity. Virus given subcutaneously failed to immunize as effectively. He found that commercial vaccines with virulent virus gave results similar to those obtained with laboratory virus, but commercial vaccines inactivated with phenol generally failed to immunize mice. The great variation in the potency of vaccines led to the development of the Habel test which provided a standard for all vaccines in 1948. Similar results were obtained with commercial phenolized vaccines in dogs. This situation was likewise corrected by the Habel test.

An unusual event of the twentieth century was the discovery of bat rabies in Brazil and later Venezuela and Trinidad. The Trinidad outbreak is so unusual that it deserves a place in history. A carrier state is so common with viral infections that one naturally asks whether there are asymptomatic carriers of rabies virus. The vampire bat of Trinidad and other countries has been shown in the past to be such a carrier. The earlier phases of this interesting study was told by E. W. Hurst and J. L. Pawan in 1931 following an outbreak of rabies in Trinidad without history of bites and with symptoms of acute ascending myelitis. In 1936 Pawan first showed that human beings bitten by vampire bats developed sensory symptoms at the bitten site followed by paralysis and death. The unusual epidemic involving almost 100 persons has never reoccurred in Trinidad but lesser cases have in other countries. The bats biting the people were shown to be rabies infected, and died—but strangely some survived, and Pawan reported that some might become carriers capable of spreading infection by their bites for prolonged periods. Bat rabies will be discussed in detail in other chapters.

Webster and Clow were the first to propagate rabies virus in tissue culture as far back as 1936. The medium consisted of Tyrode solution containing normal monkey serum plus a suspension of minced mouse embryo brain. The inoculum consisted of brain from a mouse prostrate on the seventh or eighth day following an intracerebral injection of rabies virus. Material passed through such culture medium as often as 88 times, and the supernatant was still found to be virulent.

Galloway and Elford (1936) were the first to report on the size of the rabies virus, finding it about 100—150 mm. Thus it falls among the larger viruses. Later the shape of the virus was found to be like a bullet.

The growing of rabies virus in the developing chick embryos was a major breakthrough in 1940. Two groups of workers, Bernkopf and Kligler (1940) and Dawson (1939), succeeded at about the same time in growing rabies virus in the chick embryo. Kligler and Bernkopf inoculated the chorio-allantois, Dawson the brain of the embryo. Bernkopf and Kligler in a later appearance describe their work in more detail and point out that the chick embryo virus after many passages showed greatly reduced virulence for rabbits. Dawson also found the virulence greatly reduced for the rabbit. Later H. Koprowski and H. R. Cox (1948) adapted these methods for the production of a chick embryo origin vaccine which was to give a solid basis to the control of canine rabies, and reduce the disease to near zero in human beings. The discussion of urban rabies control will bring out the great advances made with the CEO vaccine in the 1950's and 1960's.

Koprowski, in a 1949 review of control measures, points out that dog rabies control by vaccination was pertinent to rabies control in man. Umeno and Doi were the first to attempt rabies control in 1920 with a single dose Semple type vaccine in dogs. Their success led to similar efforts in the United States that varied widely in their effects, which were not understood until Webster's experiments with commercial phenolized vaccine. Koprowski and Black were successful in the production of a single inoculation for the immunization of dogs with chick embryo vaccine. Tierkel *et al.* first put this to effective control in Memphis in the 1950's. Since then the record speaks for itself.

References

Alt-Graf zu Salm-Reifferschied, H. (1813). *Allg. Anz.* 1, 2.

Babes, V. (1887). *Arch. Path. Anat.* 111, 562.

Babes, V. (1906). *Presse Med.* 14, 669.

Bartarelli, E. (1904). *Zentralbl. Bakt.* 37, 213.

Bell, J. F., Wright, J. T., and Habel, K. (1949). *Proc. Soc. Exp. Biol. Med.* 70, 457.

Bernkopf, H., and Kligler, I. J. (1940). *Proc. Soc. Exp. Biol. Med.* 45, 332.

Billings, F. S. (1884). "The Relation of Animal Diseases to the Public Health The Dog: Rabies of the Dog, Phenomena of Canine Rabies, Prevention," pp. 139–153. Appleton, New York.

Bouchardat, A. (1852). *Bull. Acad. Med., Paris* 18, 6.

Bouchardat, A. (1853). *Bull. Acad. Med., Paris* 20, 714.

Cabot, F. (1899). *M. News,* 74, 321.

Chalmette, A. (1891). *Ann. Inst. Pasteur, Paris* 8, 633.

Dawson, J. R. (1939). *Science* 89, 300.

DiVestea, A., and Zagari, G. (1889). *Ann. Inst. Pasteur, Paris* 3, 237.

Ekstrom, D. D. (1830). *London M. Gas.* 6, 689.

Fermi, C. (1907). *Zentralbl. Bakt.* 44, 26.

Fermi, C. (1908). *Infectionskr.* 58, 232.

Fleming, G. (1871). "Animal Plagues." Chapman & Hall, London.

Fleming, G. (1872). "Rabies and Hydrophobia," pp. 7–68 and 85–92. Chapman & Hall, London.

Fleming, G. (1882). "Animal Plagues," Vol. II. Bailliére, London.

Galloway, J. A., and Elford, W. J. (1936). *J. Hyg.* 36, 532.

Galtier, V. (1879). *C. Acad. Sci.* 89, 444.

Helman, C. (1889). *Ann. Inst. Pasteur* 3, 15.

Hill, F. J. (1971). *Proc. Roy. Soc. Med.* 64, 231–233.

Hurst, E. W., and Pawan, J. L. (1931). *Lancet* 221, 622.

Kligler, I. J., and Bernkopf, H. (1939). *Nature* 143, 899.

Koch, J., and Rissling, P. (1910). *Infectionskr.* 65, 85.

Koprowski, H., and Cox, H. R. (1948). *J. Immunol.* **60**, 533.
Koprowski, H. (1949). *Can. J. Pub. Health* **40**, 60.
Koprowski, H., and Black, J. (1950). *J. Immunol.* **64**, 185–196.
Krugelstein, F. (1826). "Die Geschichte der Hundswuth und der Wasserscheu und deren Behandlung." Gotha.
Negri, A. (1903a). *Zeit. Hyg. Infectionskr.* **43**, 507.
Negri, A. (1903b). *Boll. Soc. Med. Chir. Pavia.* **3**, 88.
Negri, A. (1909). *Zeit. Hyg. Infectionskr.* **63**, 421.
Nocard, M., and Roux, E. (1888). *Ann. Inst. Pasteur, Paris* **2**, 341.
Pasteur, L. (1881). *C. R. Acad. Sci.* **92**, 1259.
Pasteur, L. (1882). *C. R. Acad. Sci.* **95**, 1187.
Pasteur, L. (1884). *C. R. Acad. Sci.* **98**, 457.
Pasteur, L. (1885). *C. R. Acad. Sci.* **101**, 765.
Pawan, J. L. (1936). *Ann. Trop. Med.* **30**, 401.
Pottevin, H. (1898). *Ann. Inst. Pasteur, Paris* **12**, 301.
Raynaud, M. (1879). *C. R. Acad. Sci.* **89**, 714.
Remlinger, P. (1903). *C. R. Acad. Sci.* **55**, 1433.
Remlinger, P. (1905). *Ann. Inst. Pasteur, Paris* **19**, 625.
Remlinger, P. (1935). *Bull. Acad. Med., Paris* **113**, 836.
Rivers, T. M., Sprunt, D. H., and Berry, C. P. (1933). *J. Exp. Med.* **58**, 39.
Roux, E. (1887). *Ann. Inst. Pasteur, Paris* **1**, 87.
Roux, E. (1888). *Ann. Inst. Pasteur, Paris* **2**, 18.
Sellers, T. F. (1927). *Amer. J. Pub. Health* **17**, 1080.
Semple, D. (1919). *Brit. Med. J.* **2**, 333–371.
Smithcors, J. F. (1958a). *Vet. Med.* pp. 149–154.
Smithcors, J. F. (1958b). *Vet. Med.* pp. 267–273.
Smithcors, J. F. (1958c). *Outbreaks America* pp. 435–439.
Stuart, G., and Krikorian, K. S. (1928). *Ann. Trop. Med.* **22**, 326.
Tierkel, E. S., Graves, L. M., Tuggle, H. G., Wardley, S. L. (1950). *Am. J. Public Health* **40**, 1084–1088.
Trousseau, A. (1865). "Clinique médicale de l'Hotel-Dieu de Paris," 2nd ed., Vol. 2, p. 342. Bailliére et Fils, Paris.
Umeno, S., and Doi, Y. (1921). *Kitasato Arch. Exp. Med.* **4**, 89.
Webster, L. T. (1937). *New England J. Med.* **217**, 187.
Webster, L. T. (1939). *Am. J. Hyg.* **30**, 113–134.
Webster, L. T. (1942). "Rabies", Macmillan Co., New York.
Webster, L. T., and Clow, A. D. (1936). *Science* **84**, 487.
Webster, L. T., and Dawson, J. R. (1935). *Proc. Soc. Exp. Biol. Med.* **32**, 570.
Zinke, G. (1804). "Neue Ansichten der Hundswuth, ihrer Ursachen und Folgen, nebst einer sichern Behandlungsart der von tollen Thieren gebissenen Menschen." Gabler, Jena **16**, 212.

PART I
The Virus

CHAPTER 2

Morphology and Morphogenesis

Frederick A. Murphy

I. Morphology of Rabies Virus

The characterization of rabies virus has a complex and confusing history. Except for filtration and solvent sensitivity data which suggested myxoviruslike properties, very little information was available on the physical properties of the virus before 1962. In addition, the earliest negative contrast and thin section electron microscopy of the virus yielded confusing results; initially, in fact, no virus particles were found in association with typical inclusion bodies (Hottle *et al.*, 1951).

A. NEGATIVE CONTRAST ELECTRON MICROSCOPY

Almeida *et al.* (1962) used negative contrast microscopy to study cultured hamster kidney cells infected with a fixed rabies virus. In infected cells, but not in controls, they found irregularly shaped particles up to 400 nm in diameter. These were membranous, covered with fine surface projections 10 nm long and contained a long, wavy, ribbonlike filament with repeating sub-units at a 5-nm interval. Pin-

33

teric *et al.* (1963) used street, Flury, and fixed virus strains propagated in mouse brain to repeat these experiments; they found the same membranous sacs covered with projections and containing a wavy regular filament. It is now clear that only disrupted particles were present in these early preparations; uncoiling of the helical core and swelling of the membrane envelope yielded particles as described.

Bullet-shaped virus particles were first described in rabies virus-infected chicken embryo cell cultures by Davies *et al.* (1963) and in infected BHK-21 cells by Atanasiu *et al.* (1963b,c). Definite and exclusive association of these particles with infectivity was soon established (Pinteric and Fenje, 1966; Lépine *et al.*, 1966). Pinteric and Fenje (1966), in particular, elucidated the surface and internal detail of bullet-shaped rabies virus particles: they found mean dimensions of 140 by 100 nm, surface projections 6 nm long, a vesicular appendage from the planar end of particles, an axial channel, and the release of helical ribbon-like internal components from intact bullet-shaped particles. In addition a pyramidal or bell-shaped variation of some particles was described. The character of the internal helical component was contrasted with that of myxoviruses–paramyxoviruses (Almeida and Waterson, 1966), and the striking similarity to vesicular stomatitis virus noted.

Presently, rabies virus particles are described as cylindrical with one round or conical end and one planar or concave end (Fig. 1). From the surface inward they consist of (1) surface projections, (2) membrane envelope, and (3) helical ribonucleoprotein capsid (Fig. 2). The fine fringe of surface spikes or projections is 6 to 8 nm thick; this layer usually does not cover the planar end of particles. Individual projections, each with a knoblike distal end, are placed on the virus surface at 4- to 5-nm intervals. In most preparations the surface projections appear randomly spaced, but on occasion they are arrayed in rows giving a honeycomb appearance which likely reflects a symmetry in underlying layers (Figs. 3 and 4) (Hummeler *et al.*, 1967). Brown and his colleagues have strongly implied the presence of a symmetrical layer independent of the membrane envelope in vesicular stomatitis virus (F. Brown, personal communication, 1971; Cartwright *et al.*, 1969).

When negative contrast medium penetrates rabies virus particles beyond the surface projection layer, the envelope layer itself is resolved (Fig. 5). The dimensions of membranes viewed transversely in negative contrast are not a measure of their actual thickness, but the electron lucid unstructured zone is characteristic of typical unit membrane. Contiguity of this viral layer with fragments of host cell membrane has been observed in negative contrast preparations from

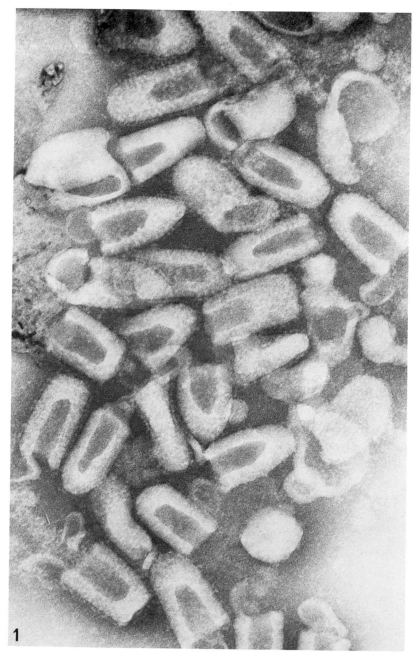

Fig. 1. Rabies virus (Flury HEP strain) propagated in BHK-21 cells, purified, and prepared for negative contrast electron microscopy. Axial channels are especially pronounced. ×180,000. (Micrograph courtesy of Joan Crick, C. J. Smale, and F. Brown.)

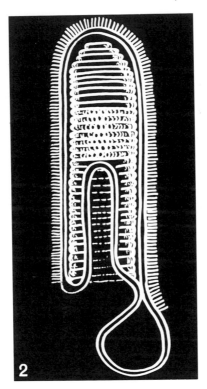

Fig. 2. Diagrammatic representation of rabies virus illustrating the surface projection layer, the unit membrane envelope (double lines) with invagination forming an axial channel and extra membrane forming a terminal bleb, and helical ribonucleoprotein capsid.

Fig. 3. Negatively stained rabies virus particle (Flury HEP strain) illustrating the symmetrical structural arrangement of surface projections and knoblike protrusion at distal end of projections. ×300,000. (Micrograph courtesy of K. Hummeler.)

Fig. 4. Rabies virus particle (Flury HEP strain) with honeycomb appearance of membrane envelope suggestive of symmetrical insertion of surface projections. ×300,000. (Micrograph courtesy of Joan Crick, C. J. Smale, and F. Brown.)

Fig. 5. Rabies virus particle (CVS strain) penetrated by negative contrast medium to delineate the unit membrane envelope beneath surface projections (arrows). ×400,000.

Fig. 6. End-on view of rabies virus particles (Flury HEP strain) in negative contrast preparation. Of the three rings discerned, the outer is likely the surface projection layer, the middle the membrane envelope and the inner the coiled nucleocapsid. ×300,000. (Micrograph courtesy of K. Hummeler.)

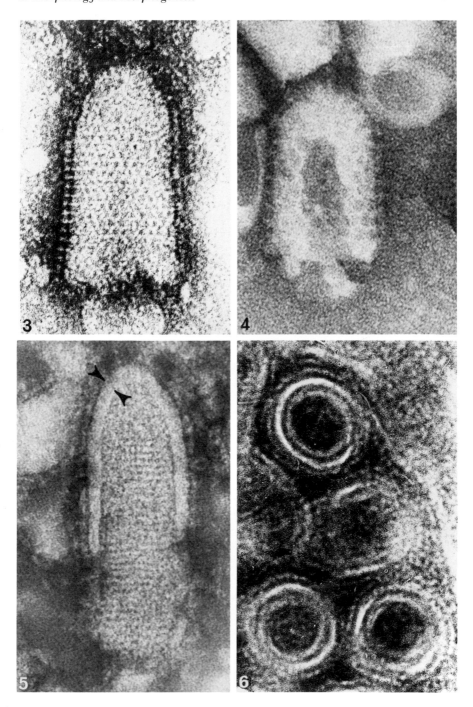

crude rabies infected cell cultures. The membrane envelope lies closely apposed to the internal constituent of the virus and at the planar end may be invaginated a variable distance, allowing the penetration of negative contrast material and the definition of an axial channel (Figs. 1 and 4). The avulsion of excess host cell membrane at the site of budding and pinching off explains the common presence of a membranous bleb at the planar end of many rabies virus particles (see Pinteric and Fenje, 1966).

Further penetration of negative contrast medium and delineation of the helical ribonucleocapsid in intact rabies virus particles has been difficult to effect in many laboratories. Nevertheless, transverse cross striations of the helix have been demonstrated by Hummeler and Atanasiu (cited in Howatson, 1970) and in our laboratory. The dimensions of the intact helical core of rabies virus are essentially the same as those of vesicular stomatitis virus (Nakai and Howatson, 1968); rabies virus has approximately 30–35 coils of a strand of ribonucleoprotein and these coils form a cylinder 50 nm wide and approximately 165 nm long. The cross-striation interval is 4.5 nm (Hummeler *et al.*, 1967). These measurements, especially those of the number of coils, have been made in our laboratory from few particles; significant numbers of particles of different rabies virus strains must be measured to establish mean values. The helical core is immediately beneath the membrane envelope as illustrated in Fig. 6, which gives an end-on view of particles. The inner lucent zone is the ribonucleoprotein helix, and the outer one is the membrane envelope.

When rabies virus particles are disrupted spontaneously or by means of detergents, the internal helix unwinds into a wavy ribbon as described in the first successful electron microscopic studies of rabies virus (Almeida *et al.*, 1962). The single-strand wavy ribbon varies in thickness with the plane of viewing; its dimensions are: length, 4.2 μm; thickness, 2 by 6.5 nm (ribbon); periodicity, 7.5 nm (Hummeler *et al.*, 1968; Sokol *et al.*, 1969; Fig. 7). The strand has a great tendency to recoil to a diameter of approximately 16 nm (Hummeler *et al.*, 1968; Sokol *et al.*, 1969; Fig. 8). Dimensional measurements have recently been used to construct a model of the rabies virion (Vernon *et al.*, 1972).

Fig. 7. Unwound nucleocapsid of rabies virus particles (Flury HEP strain) isolated by CsCL density gradient ultracentrifugation. The strands appear as twisted ribbons. ×300,000. (Micrograph courtesy of K. Hummeler.)

Fig. 8. Nucleocapsid strands of rabies virus (Flury HEP strain), isolated by sucrose gradient ultracentrifugation, have a strong propensity to recoil into a helix approximately 16 nm in diameter. ×200,000. (Micrograph courtesy of K. Hummeler.)

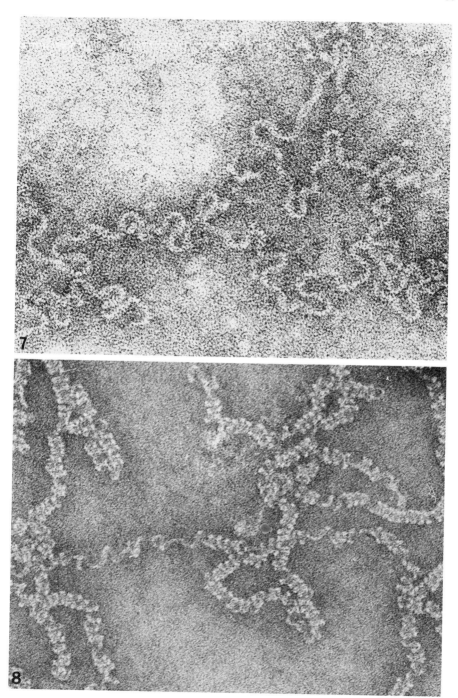

Mean rabies virus particle dimensions are 180 by 75 nm exclusive of surface projections (Hummeler *et al.*, 1967; Sokol *et al.*, 1968). Further testing is required to determine whether all rabies virus strains, including street viruses, have exactly the same dimensions as the four fixed viruses used by Hummeler and his colleagues.

Anomalous particles of several types are commonly seen in most rabies virus preparations observed by negative contrast electron microscopy. Short particles, analogous to the T (truncated) component of vesicular stomatitis virus cultures (Hackett, 1964; Hackett *et al.*, 1967), are common in preparations of several fixed rabies strains (street viruses have not been studied adequately). These T rabies particles vary from 70 to 100 nm in length but have all other dimensions and features of normal B (bullet) particles, namely round and flat end, surface projections, axial channel, and coiled nucleocapsid. Their capacity to act as interfering agents, as is the case with other rhabdoviruses, is under study in several laboratories. Excessively long rabies virus particles, up to 400 nm long, usually with two flat ends, are not uncommon in preparations from cell cultures, especially when virus is harvested late in the course of infection. Except for this variation in length such particles likewise have all the attributes of normal B particles; penetration of negative contrast medium reveals extra coils of nucleocapsid rather than stretching of a normal coil. Finally, envelopment of more than one nucleocapsid within a common envelope may produce the branched or multiple "polymers," which may be V-shaped (two capsids), Y-shaped (three capsids), or rectangular (two, three, or four capsids side by side).

B. Thin-Section Electron Microscopy

Although thin-section electron microscopy usually must be considered secondary to the negative contrast approach in elucidation of viral morphology per se, for rhabdoviruses each technique complements the other very well. Rabies virus particles were first described in thin section by Matsumoto (1962, 1963a,b), Atanasiu *et al.* (1963a,b,c), and Roots and Schultze (1963). These first observations weighed heavily in the association of infectivity with the bullet-shaped particles described at the same time in negative contrast preparations. The only quandary in these early thin-section electron microscopy studies concerned interpretation of the many anomalous tubular structures associated with the virus and the viral inclusion body; the exact nature of some of these tubules is still unknown.

In thin section, rabies virus appears to be bullet-shaped when cut longitudinally but has circular or elliptical profiles when cut transversely or obliquely. The surface projection layer is usually well preserved and appears thicker and denser than it does by negative contrast; individual spikes are not resolved, nor is the knoblike distal end of spikes indicated by any density variation. Surface projections do not extend beyond the junction of the budding virus particle with host cell membrane. The unit membrane structure of the viral envelope and its contiguity with host cell membrane are clear in favorably oriented and appropriately stained preparations. Depending upon the plane and thickness of the section the internal component, the nucleocapsid helix, has a varying appearance in longitudinally sectioned virus particles. In some particles the coils of the helix are clearly seen as cross striations either tightly or loosely wound (Figs. 9 and 10). In others, very thinly sectioned through their centers, the helix appears as a dense, beaded layer closely apposed to the inside of the envelope (Fig. 11). Such particles show an increased density of the outer and inner surfaces of the nucleocapsid layer and have an especially lucent center space. In the more commonly seen thicker sections (Fig. 12), both profiles of the nucleocapsid are superimposed so that a very dense, solid bullet-shaped core within the viral envelope or even a bullet-shaped whole particle with no substructure is observed. In any case, the nucleocapsid is never seen to project into the host cell cytoplasm at the site of budding. The same layers are evident in cross section: surface projections, membrane envelope, and closely adherent nucleocapsid with surfaces of greatest density. In addition, some free particles seen in cross section have a central density which may represent the collapsed membrane of an axial channel extending from the planar end.

Measurements of rabies virus particles in thin section were accumulated from studies of several virus strains in several host systems (all in epoxy embedment with polymerization shrinkage of 1%). The mean dimensions of particles are: length, 180 nm; diameter including surface projections, 75 nm; diameter excluding projections, 58 nm; diameter of inner margin of nucleocapsid coil, 38 nm; and length of surface projections, 9 nm.

Anomalously long and branched virus particles are observed in thin section, especially in late harvests of cultured cells and mouse central nervous system (Figs. 13 and 14). One other anomaly occurs when fixed rabies virus strains are propagated in cell cultures: a significant proportion of virus particles are attached to host cell membrane (budding sites) at both ends. In many such particles the contained nucleocapsid does not have a rounded end (Fig. 15).

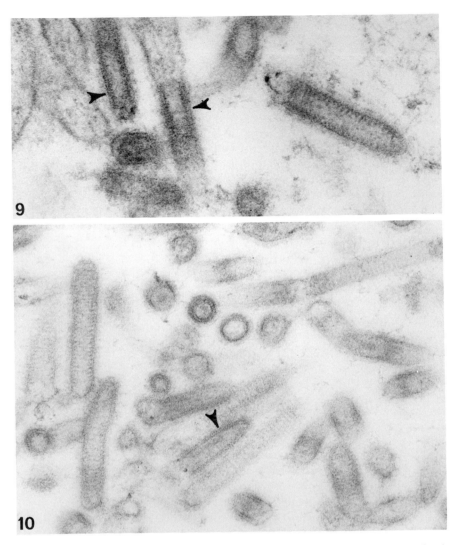

Fig. 9. Rabies virus (street strain) in ultrathin section from skunk salivary gland. Longitudinal sections showing either cross striations or double dense lines or beads (arrows) at margins. ×115,000.

Fig. 10. Rabies virus (street strain) in section; beaded marginal layer (arrow) and cross striations represent varying planes of section through longitudinally oriented particles. ×110,000.

Fig. 11. Rabies virus (street strain), especially thinly sectioned through particle centers, illustrating the absence of density central to the coiled nucleocapsid (arrows). ×95,000.

Fig. 12. Rabies virus (street virus) in fox salivary gland showing the common profile of double marginal density and central density varying with the plane of section. Axial channels (arrows) and terminal blebs (double arrow) are visible. ×95,000.

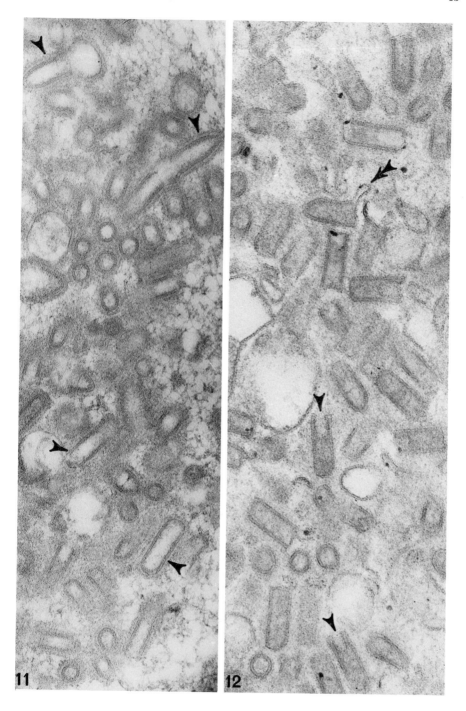

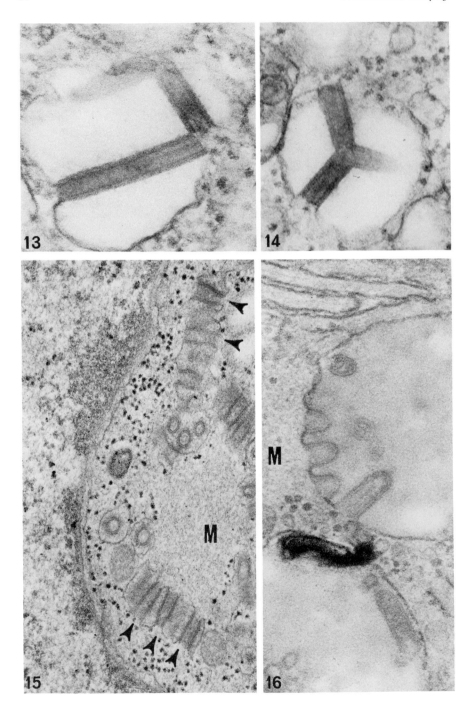

Obviously, the synthesis of enveloped, infectious virus from such progenitors must be inefficient; an instability of such particles would explain their absence from negative contrast preparations.

II. Morphogenesis of Rabies Virus

The development of rabies virus particles in association with intracytoplasmic inclusion bodies or matrix (the Negri body of light microscopy) was first demonstrated by Matsumoto (1962, 1963a,b) and later by Matsumoto and Miyamoto (1966). They associated rabies virus morphogenesis with three morphologic types of particles. The first type was cylindrical, 120–130 nm wide, and limited by a single membrane. The second was cylindrical, 100–110 nm wide, and limited by both a double membrane and a third internal membrane. The third type was cylindrical or bullet-shaped, 80–90 nm wide and limited by a double membrane. Type three particles always budded from and were enclosed within the lumen of endoplasmic reticulum close to matrix (see Matsumoto, 1970). This third type of particle is now considered the virus itself; type two reflects profiles of virus contained within closely apposed host cell membrane, and type one remains as unexplained organization within the viral matrix.

The presently accepted concept of the mode of rabies virus morphogenesis is that budding occurs upon host cell membrane with a concomitant coiling of the nucleocapsid from a less organized strand in the cytoplasm. Pinching off of a mature virus particle occurs after the coiling is complete (Figs. 16 and 17). The modification of host cell membrane at the site of budding must be highly synchronized with this process since surface projections are visible upon even the shortest budding particles and consistently reach only to the site where virus is contiguous with host membrane.

Fig. 13. Anomalously long rabies virus particles (street strain) in skunk brain. The longer particle is > 400 nm long and its envelope is attached to reticulum membrane at both ends. ×95,000.

Fig. 14. Anomalously branched rabies virus particle (street strain) in neuronal reticulum. Three nucleocapsids are likely contained in a common envelope. ×95,000.

Fig. 15. Rabies virus (CVS strain) in BHK-21 cell illustrating the anomalous yet common formation of particles with envelopes attached to reticulum membrane at both ends (arrows). M, matrix. ×55,000.

Fig. 16. Varying stages in the budding process of rabies virus (street strain) upon vacuolar membranes in skunk salivary gland. Coiling of the nucleocapsid is synchronous with growth of the viral bud. M, matrix. ×95,000.

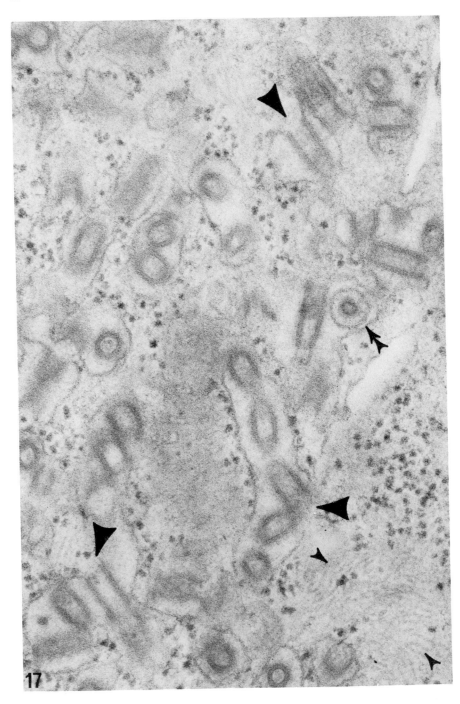

17

A. Morphogenetic Aspects of Infection in
Cultured Cells

The early events of rabies virus invasion of BHK-21 cells have been studied by Iwasaki *et al.* (1973). Within 5–30 minutes after addition of virus to cell cultures, particles approached cell surfaces and some were engulfed in phagocytic vacuoles. Viral envelope fusion occurred with plasma membrane and vacuolar membranes; fusion began with the planar end of particles. Thereafter no viral morphogenetic events were visible until 5 hours postinfection. Virus particle budding was initially observed upon plasma membranes at 6 hours.

In those cultured cells which have been studied most extensively by electron microscopy, rabies virus budding has not been restricted to any particular membrane system. Thus, Matsumoto and Kawai (1969) showed that significant virus assembly occurs upon plasma membranes of infected chick embryo fibroblasts. Hummeler *et al.* (1967) and Hummeler and Koprowski (1969) illustrated massive viral (Flury HEP strain) accumulations in BHK-21 cells within (1) cisternae of reticulum as a consequence of budding from internal membranes, (2) extracellular spaces after budding from plasma membranes, and (3) cytoplasm itself as a consequence of apparent *de novo* synthesis of membrane envelope constituents (Fig. 18). The latter is one of the only known examples of rhabdovirus assembly independent of preformed host membranes (also see Atanasiu *et al.*, 1969). In our laboratory, a challenge virus standard (CVS) rabies strain adapted to hamster kidney cells by 112 passages (Kissling and Reese, 1963) was used to infect BHK-21 cells grown in suspension (Halonen *et al.*, 1968; Murphy *et al.*, 1968). The same indiscriminate budding of virus particles from all membrane systems was noted, including the outer lamella of the nuclear envelope, but no particles were found free in the cytoplasm (Figs. 15 and 17). It must be concluded that the primary mode of rabies virus assembly requires an intimate association of preformed host cell membrane with viral nucleocapsid. Such association is the key influence for the coiling of nucleocapsid into its precise helix. Formed nucleocapsid helices have not been identified free in the cytoplasm of infected cells (Lepine and Gamet, 1969).

Fig. 17. High magnification of rabies virus (CVS strain) budding (large arrows) in BHK-21 cell. All viral morphogenesis is associated with endoplasmic reticulum membrane. Fibrillar nature of some areas of cytoplasm is likely due to replacement of normal content by viral nucleocapsid (arrow). The latent virus of hamster cells is indicated (double arrow). ×105,000.

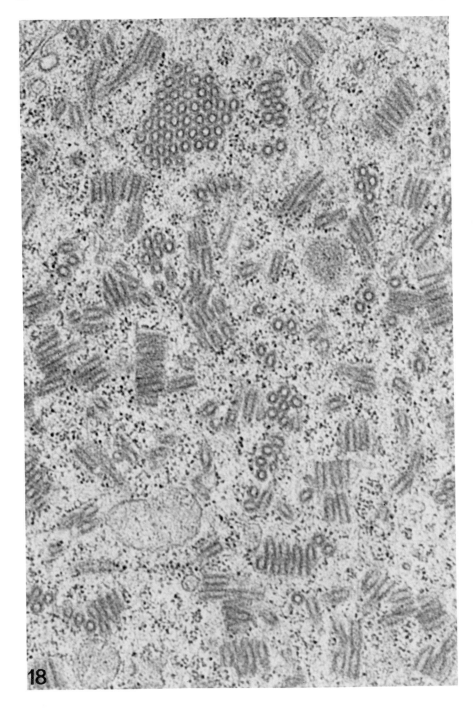

As a result of infection, cultured cells such as BHK-21 cells undergo progressive cytopathic changes including vacuolation, rarifaction or condensation, massive disruption of cytoplasmic organelles and lysis. Such changes apparently occur rather late after peak virus particle morphogenesis (e.g., 4 days versus 2 days). Many other cell cultures which support moderate amounts of viral growth show little or no cytopathic changes, but these have not been well studied ultrastructurally. All observations of rabies virus-induced cytopathology have been made in studies employing fixed or attenuated virus strains. Therefore, direct comparisons of *in vivo* changes with those in cultured cells suffer the criticism of dubious relevancy since the key observations of street viruses in cell cultures have not been made.

B. Morphogenetic Aspects of *In Vivo* Infection

The budding process of rabies virus is of the same character *in vivo* as in cultured cells. However, street rabies virus strains have extremely limited budding sites in cells of the central nervous system (primarily neurons) of all animals which have been studied; only membranes of the endoplasmic reticulum have clearly been shown to yield mature virus particles. In our laboratory, this generalization has held up through studies of at least seven street virus strains and in four host species. Street rabies virus strains have rarely been observed budding from plasma membranes of central nervous system cells or accumulating in extracellular spaces. Thus, the source of free virus for amplification of infection in the central nervous system remains obscure. In contrast, the one *in vivo* site where rabies virus maturation effectively results in the release of large quantities of extracellular virus is the salivary gland. In studies of this organ in infected foxes (Dierks *et al.*, 1969) and skunks (R. E. Dierks, A. K. Harrison, and F. A. Murphy, unpublished), street rabies virus was found budding from plasma membranes of mucous acinar cells and accumulating in salivary secretions in the massive numbers associated with transmission by bite (up to 10^7 LD$_{50}$/ml of saliva).

Although nearly all neurons of all areas of the brain and spinal cord of mice inoculated with street rabies virus strains are infected at the time of morbidity, most of these cells contain only a few virus

Fig. 18. Rabies virus particles (Flury HEP strain) within the cytoplasm of a BHK-21 cell. This massive accumulation of particles without relation to host cell membranes is the only evidence of a variation in rabies morphogenesis involving *de novo* synthesis of envelope constituents. ×48,000. (Micrograph courtesy of K. Hummeler.)

particles and/or a small amount of matrix per plane of section. Such cells are often normal in all other ultrastructural detail, an observation consistent with the minimal neuronal degeneration seen by light microscopy. Some neurons in mice, however, appear somewhat dense (moderate cytoplasmic condensation), and some appear to have retracted from their junctions; more drastic changes are not characteristic (Miyamoto and Matsumoto, 1967). Only a small number of infected neurons of mice become crowded with virus particles and associated matrix (Fig. 19); such cells may occur in all parts of the brain and cord. Similar changes, moreover, have been reported in the neural elements of mouse cranial nerves and their ganglia (trigeminal; Jenson *et al.*, 1969). The same spectrum of minimal neuronal damage with varying virion accumulation has been noted in limited studies of street virus strains in the hamster, fox, and skunk. These results are consistent with extensive light microscopic observations by many investigators over many years.

In contrast to the effects with street virus strains, there is considerable cytopathology in the central nervous system of experimental animals infected with fixed virus strains. Ultrastructural changes resemble those described in cultured cells; they range from cytoplasmic disorganization to frank neuronal necrosis and are consistent with parallel observations made by light microscopy (Johnson and Mercer, 1964). Many mouse neurons shown to be infected with fixed virus by the presence of matrix contain few or no mature virus particles; such would be uncommon with street viruses. Viral matrices in neurons infected with fixed viruses are small and usually are not visible by light microscopy. Although not frequently observed, fixed virus budding from neuronal plasma membranes does occur, with consequent accumulation of extracellular particles. Since fixed virus strains routinely yield much higher levels of infectivity in mouse brain than street viruses, it is probable that much of the intracellular virus seen in the latter is (1) physically defective anomalous forms; (2) permanently bound to intracytoplasmic membranes, and hence trapped; (3) thermally denatured after slow accumulation over a protracted course of central nervous system infection. The dramatic appearance of some neurons infected with *street* virus strains, as illustrated by Fig. 19, is not reflective of whole brain terminal infectivity. Infectious *fixed* virus, on the other hand, often reaching 10^7 LD_{50}/g (in newborn mice) and causing severe brain

Fig. 19. Neuron of mouse inoculated with rabies virus (human isolate, first passage). This cell is crowded with virus particles (arrows) and matrix (M), and its cytoplasm is denser than normal. ×25,000.

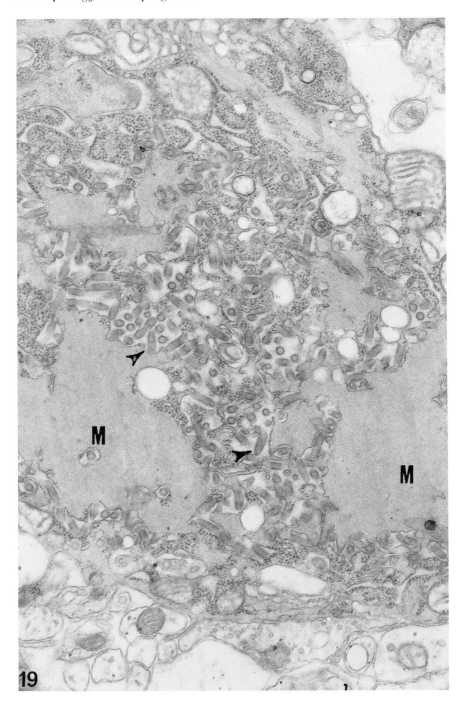

destruction, is associated with only subtle evidence of virion accumulation. A higher proportion of fixed strain particles must be infectious. Taken together, the characteristics of infection of individual
neurons by street and by fixed rabies viruses may be used to distinguish between strains (see Lépine and Gamet, 1969; Matsumoto,
1970).

C. RELATIONSHIP OF MATRIX TO VIRUS MORPHOGENESIS

The original ultrastructural studies of rabies by Matsumoto (1962,
1963a,b) made clear the intimate relationship of viral matrix to virus
particle production. However, considering the diverse nature of viral
inclusions associated with different viruses, some being excess constituents (e.g., myxoviruses), some complex "viroplasm" (pox-
viruses), some viral crystals (adenoviruses), some host cell debris
(herpesviruses), etc., it is no wonder that interpretation of the nature
of the rabies matrix varied among early investigators. This issue was
complicated by ambiguous findings in studies of the chemical con-
stituency of the matrix or Negri body, and by the simplicity of the ultrastructural appearance of the matrix.

Miyamoto and Matsumoto (1965) and Miyamoto (1965) demonstrated conclusively by serial thick (light microscopy) and thin (electron microscopy) sectioning that the rabies intracytoplasmic inclusion body (the Negri body) as seen by light microscopy and the viral
matrix as seen by electron microscopy are identical. Nevertheless, in
deference to the definition of the Negri body which includes aniline
dye staining properties, the term *matrix* remains preferable in electron microscopy. Although in early micrographs this matrix appeared
smoothly granular (with various inclusions), it is now clear that it
consists of randomly massed twisted filaments (Fig. 20). Hummeler
and his colleagues (1968) showed by ferritin-labeled antirabies antibody that the matrix consists of strands about 15 nm in diameter
and that these strands are randomly oriented viral nucleocapsid. At
sites of viral budding, labeled strands could be seen at the bases of
some particles and the same label delineated strands throughout
large matrices.

The rabies matrix is unbounded and lies free in the cytoplasm.

Fig. 20. Matrix (M) of rabies virus (street strain in skunk brain) as actually massed,
randomly twisted filaments—viral nucleocapsid strands accumulated in excess. The
virus particles in cross section (arrow) shows the triple ring profile of the closely apposed nucleocapsid and envelope. The rather lucent projection layer is also visible.
×126,000.

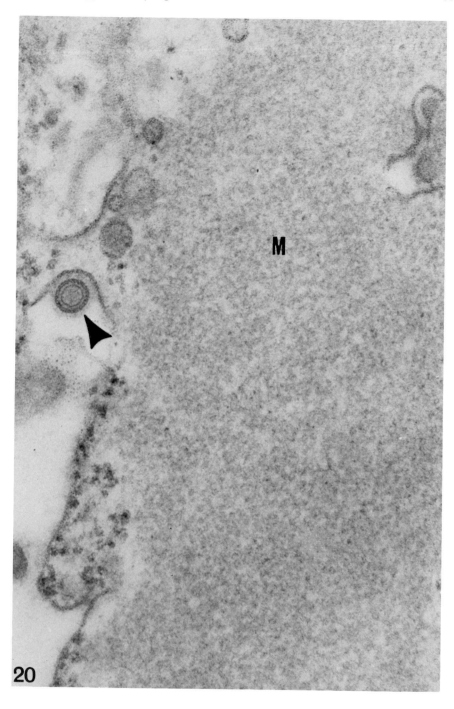

There is a progression of condensation of the strands making up the matrix as well as an increase in number, size, and complexity of matrices in individual cells throughout the course of infection. In infected cell cultures very delicate profiles with indistinct margins occur early and inclusions with increased density and precise edges occur more often in later harvests. Further variations in matrix appearance include linear arrays of strands (Fig. 21), which occur most often in cultured cells, and bizarre tubular inclusions within matrices (Fig. 22), which are most common *in vivo*. The latter are the type one structures of Matsumoto and Miyamoto (1966), the nature of which is unresolved. In addition, membrane proliferation occurs in association with viral morphogenesis; one such convoluted mem-

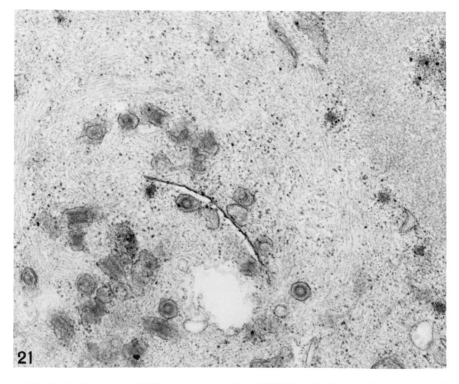

Fig. 21. Rabies virus (CVS strain) matrix in a BHK-21 cell of usual character (right) and variation consisting of parallel arrays of strands (left). ×35,000.

Fig. 22. Rabies virus matrix (street virus; first passage from deer isolate) in a thoracic spinal cord neuron of a mouse illustrating the complex tubular structures commonly found with street virus strains *in vivo*. The nature of these tubules is obscure. ×30,000.

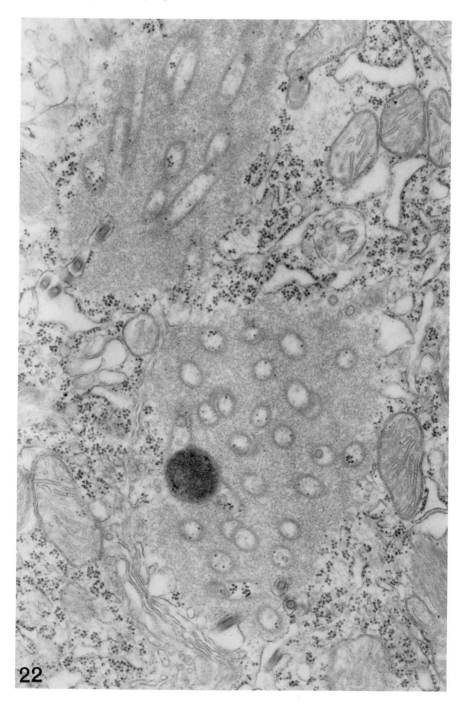

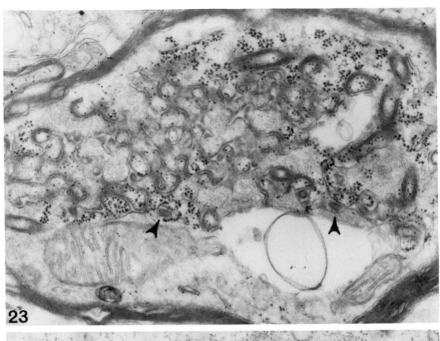

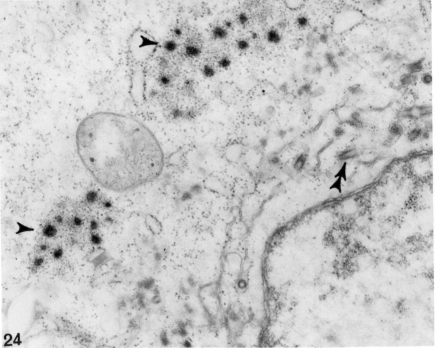

brane profile is illustrated in Fig. 23, and other variations are known (Jenson *et al.*, 1967). Finally, accumulations of abnormally large numbers of ribosomes and polyribosomes may form around viral matrices and infrequently these may aggregate and thus may be considered another kind of "inclusion" (Fig. 24). There is no explanation for this aggregative phenomenon. In summary, there is considerable evidence that the rabies matrix is actually a result of the synthesis of a great excess of viral ribonucleoprotein capsid strands within the cytoplasm of the infected cell and that various cell organelles trapped within this material account for the internal basophilia seen by light microscopy. This eventually highly condensed nucleocapsid material is probably not free for virion morphogenesis.

III. The Bearing of Morphology and Morphogenesis on the Placement of Rabies Virus in the Rhabdovirus Group

The rhabdoviruses (bullet-shaped viruses) of animals (Wildy, 1971; Melnick, 1972) may be subdivided on morphologic–morphogenetic, serologic, and physicochemical bases. Such subdivision is quite arbitrary, but may be of value in questioning the potential of new isolates as human or animal pathogens. In the list below of animal rhabdoviruses, capital letters A–M indicate serological subdivision (see Chapter 8, this volume) and horizonal lines indicate morphologic and/or morphogenetic subdivision (Murphy and Shope, 1972):

All of the morphologic–morphogenetic subdivisions differ from that including rabies virus. The most significant variance is that other viruses bud primarily or exclusively from the plasma membranes of mouse neurons, whereas rabies virus buds upon intracytoplasmic membranes as described above (Murphy *et al.*, 1969). Other variances have been described (Howatson, 1970). Of the viruses within the rabies subdivision, Lagos bat and Mokola viruses, which have recently been shown to be serologically related to rabies virus (Shope *et al.*, 1970), are indistinguishable from rabies by all ultra-

Fig. 23. Convoluted membranous structures in a myelinated axon in the thoracic spinal cord of an adult mouse inoculated with rabies virus (street strain; deer isolate). Virus particles (arrows) and uncondensed matrix are associated with these membranes. ×25,000.

Fig. 24. Unusual condensation of ribosomes into dense aggregates (arrows) in a BHK-21 cell infected with rabies virus (CVS strain). Similar "inclusions" have been noted infrequently in several host cell systems. Virus particles (double arrow). ×30,000.

Animal Rhabdoviruses[a]

A. 1. Vesicular stomatitis (VSV)—Indiana (Reczko, 1961)
   a. Prototype (Howatson and Whitmore, 1962)
   b. Cocal (VSV-Argentina) (Federer *et al.*, 1967; Ditchfield and Almeida, 1964)
   c. Alagoas (VSV-Brazil) (Federer *et al.*, 1967)
   2. Vesicular stomatitis—New Jersey (Bergold and Munz, 1967)
   3. Piry (Murphy and Shope, 1972)
   4. Chandipura (Murphy and Shope, 1972)

B. 1. Rabies (Matsumoto, 1962; Almeida *et al.*, 1962)
   2. Lagos bat (Shope *et al.*, 1970)
   3. Mokola (Shope *et al.*, 1970)
   4. Duvenhagé (Meredith *et al.*, 1971; R. E. Shope, G. H. Tignor, and F. A. Murphy, personal communication, 1973)

— — — — — — — — — — — — — — — — — — — —

   5. Kotonkan (Kemp *et al.*, 1973)
   6. Obodhiang (Schmidt *et al.*, 1965)
C. Klamath (Murphy *et al.*, 1972)

D. Bovine ephemeral fever (Lecatsas *et al.*, 1969; Ito *et al.*, 1969; Holmes and Doherty, 1970; Murphy *et al.*, 1972)

E. Kern Canyon (Murphy and Fields, 1967)

F. I 6235 (R. E. Shope, personal communication, 1972)

G. 1. Flanders (Murphy *et al.*, 1966)
   2. Hart Park (Murphy *et al.*, 1966)
H. Mount Elgon bat (Murphy *et al.*, 1970)
I. Joinjakaka (I. Marshall, personal communication, 1970)
J. Navarro (Karabatsos *et al.*, 1973)
K. Kwatta (Karabatsos *et al.*, 1973)
L. Mossuril (Karabatsos *et al.*, 1973)

M. Marburg (Kissling *et al.*, 1968; Murphy *et al.*, 1971)

[a] Division of the animal rhabdoviruses is made on the bases of serologic and morphologic-morphogenetic characteristics. Serologic division is indicated by letters A—M and members of each serogroup are indicated by numbers. There are no serologic cross-reactions between serogroups. Morphologic-morphogenetic division is indicated by horizontal lines. Several subgroups may be defined by both serologic and morphologic criteria (VSV, rabies subgroups). The dashed line in the rabies subgroup is to emphasize the serologic inclusion of Kotonkan and Obodhiang viruses, and at the same time to emphasize the morphologic distinction between these two viruses and rabies.

structural approaches. Only Klamath virus closely resembles rabies virus on a morphologic-morphogenetic basis by (1) budding from intracytoplasmic membranes of mouse neurons, (2) growing in association with large matrices, and (3) being rather noncytopathic in mouse brain (Murphy *et al.*, 1972), and yet is serologically unrelated to rabies or any other known virus. As new rhabdoviruses are isolated and characterized, ultrastructural comparison with rabies (street strains), especially in central nervous system cells, is certainly warranted.

Acknowledgment

The investigative work carried out in the author's laboratory was done in collaboration with Mrs. Alyne K. Harrison; her contribution to this review is gratefully acknowledged.

References

Almeida, J. D., and Waterson, A. P. (1966). *Symp. Ser. Immunobiol. Stand.* 1, 45.

Almeida, J. D., Howatson, A. F., Pinteric, L., and Fenje, P. (1962). *Virology* 18, 147.

Atanasiu, P., Lépine, P., and Gragonas, P. (1963a). *Ann Inst. Pasteur, Paris* 195, 813.

Atanasiu, P., Lépine, P., Sisman, J., Daugnet, J. C., and Witten, M. (1963b). *C. R. Acad. Sci.* 256, 3219.

Atanasiu, P., Orth, G., Sisman, J., and Barreau, C. (1963c). *C. R. Acad. Sci.* 257, 2204.

Atanasiu, P., Lepine, P., and Sisman, J. (1969). *C. R. Acad. Sci.* 269, 1226.

Bergold, G. H., and Munz, K. (1967). *J. Ultrastruct. Res.* 17, 233.

Cartwright, B., Smale, C. J., and Brown, F. (1969). *J. Gen Virol.* 5, 1.

Davies, M. C., Englert, M. E., Sharpless, G. R., and Cabasso, V. J. (1963). *Virology* 21, 51.

Dierks, R. E., Murphy, F. A., and Harrison, A. K. (1969). *Amer. J. Pathol.* 54, 251.

Ditchfield, J., and Almeida, J. D. (1964). *Virology* 24, 232.

Federer, K. E., Burrows, R., and Brooksby, J. B. (1967). *Res. Vet. Sci.* 8, 103.

Hackett, A. J. (1964). *Virology* 24, 51.

Hackett, A. J., Schaffer, F. L., and Madin, S. H. (1967). *Virology* 31, 114.

Halonen, P. E., Murphy, F. A., Fields, B. N., and Reese, D. R. (1968). *Proc. Soc. Exp. Biol. Med.* 127, 1037.

Holmes, J. H., and Doherty, R. L. (1970). *J. Virol.* 5, 91.

Hottle, G. A., Morgan, C., Peers, J. H., and Wyckoff, R. W. G. (1951). *Proc. Soc. Exp. Biol. Med.* 77, 721.

Howatson, A. F., and Whitmore, G. F. (1962). *Virology.* 16, 466.

Howatson, A. F. (1970). *Adv. Vir. Res.* 16, 195.

Hummeler, K., and Koprowski, H. (1969). *Nature* 221, 418.

Hummeler, K., Koprowski, H., and Wiktor, T. J. (1967). *J. Virol.* 1, 152.

Hummeler, K., Tomassini, N., Sokol, F., Kuwert, E., and Koprowski, H. (1968). *J. Virol.* 2, 1191.

Ito, Y., Tanaka, Y., Inaba, Y., and Omori, T. (1969). *Nat. Inst. Anim. Health Quart.* 9, 35.

Iwasaki, Y., Wiktor, T. J., and Koprowski, H. (1973). Lab. Invest. 28, 142.

Jenson, A. B., Rabin, E. R., Wende, R. D., and Melnick, J. L. (1967). Exp. Mol. Pathol. 7, 1.

Jenson, A. B., Rabin, E. R., Bentinck, D. C., and Melnick, J. L. (1969). J. Virol. 3, 265.

Johnson, R. T., and Mercer, E. M. (1964). Aust. J. Exp. Biol. Med. Sci. 42, 449.

Karabatsos, N., Lipman, M. B., Garrison, M. S., Mongillo, C. A. (1973). J. Gen. Virol. 21, 429.

Kemp, G. E., Lee, V. H., Moore, D. L., Shope, R. E., Causey, O. R., and Murphy, F. A. (1973). Amer. J. Epidemiol. 98, 43.

Kissling, R. E., and Reese, D. R. (1963). J. Immunol. 91, 362.

Kissling, R. E., Robinson, R. Q., Murphy, F. A., and Whitfield, S. G. (1968). Science 160, 888.

Lecatsas, C., Theodorides, A., and Erasmus, B. J. (1969). Arch. Gesamte Virusforsch. 28, 390.

Lépine, P., and Gamet, A. (1969). "La Rage." L' Expansion Scientifique Francaise, Paris.

Lépine, P., Atanasiu, P., and Sisman, J. (1966). Symp. Ser. Immunobiol. Stand. 1, 31.

Matsumoto, S. (1962). Virology 17, 198.

Matsumoto, S. (1963a). Annu. Rep. Inst. Virus Res., Kyoto Univ. 6, 57.

Matsumoto, S. (1963b). J. Cell Biol. 19, 565.

Matsumoto, S. (1970). Advan. Virus Res. 16, 257.

Matsumoto, S., and Kawai, A. (1969). Virology 39, 449.

Matsumoto, S., and Miyamoto, K. (1966). Symp. Ser. Immunobiol. Stand. 1, 45.

Melnick, J. L. (1972). Prog. Med. Virol. 14, 321.

Meredith, C. D., Rossouw, A. P., and VanPraagkoch, H. (1971). So. African Med. J. 45, 767.

Miyamoto, J. (1965). Annu. Rep. Inst. Virus Res., Kyoto Univ. 8, 10.

Miyamoto, K., and Matsumoto, S. (1965). J. Cell Biol. 27, 677.

Miyamoto, K., and Matsumoto, S. (1967). J. Exp. Med. 125, 447.

Murphy, F. A., and Fields, B. N. (1967). Virology 33, 625.

Murphy, F. A., and Shope, R. E. (1972). Int. Virol. 2, 261.

Murphy, F. A., Coleman, P. H., and Whitfield, S. G. (1966). Virology 30, 314.

Murphy, F. A., Halonen, P. E., Gary, G. W., Jr., and Reese, D. R. (1968). J. Gen. Virol. 3, 289.

Murphy, F. A., Harrison, A. K., and Whitfield, S. G. (1969). Proc. Electron Microsc. Soc. Amer. 27, 372.

Murphy, F. A., Shope, R. E., Metselaar, D., and Simpson, D. I. H. (1970). Virology 40, 288.

Murphy, F. A., Simpson, D. I. H., Whitfield, S. G., Zlotnik, I., and Carter, G. B. (1971). Lab. Invest. 24, 279.

Murphy, F. A., Johnson, H. N., Harrison, A. K., and Shope, R. E. (1972). Arch. Gesamte Virusforsch. 37, 323.

Murphy, F. A., Taylor, W. P., Mims, C. A., and Whitfield, S. G. (1972). Arch. Gesamte Virusforsch. 38, 234.

Nakai, T., and Howatson, A. F. (1968). Virology 35, 268.

Pinteric, L., and Fenje, P. (1966). Symp. Ser. Immunobiol. Stand. 1, 9.

Pinteric, L., Fenje, P., and Almeida, J. D. (1963). Virology 20, 208.

Reczko, E. (1961). Arch. Gesamte Virusforsch. 10, 588.

Roots, E., and Schultze, I. (1963). Zentralbl. Bakteriol., Parasitenk., Infektionskr. Hyg., Abt. 1: Orig. 188, 159.

Schmidt, J. R., Williams, M. C., Lulu, M., Mivule, A., and Mujomba, E. (1965). *East African Vir. Res. Inst. Rep.* **15**, 24.

Shope, R. E., Murphy, F. A., Harrison, A K., Causcy, O. R., Kemp, G. E., Simpson, D. I. H., and Moore, D. L. (1970). *J. Virol.* **6**, 690.

Sokol, F., Kuwert, E., Wiktor, T. J., Hummeler, K., and Koprowski, H. (1968). *J. Virol.* **2**, 836.

Sokol, F., Schlumberger, H. D., Wiktor, T. J., and Koprowski, H. (1969). *Virology* **38**, 651.

Vernon, S. K., Neurath, A. R., and Rubin, B. A. (1972). *J. Ultrastruct. Res.* **41**, 29.

Wildy, P. (1971). *Monogr. Virol.* **5**, 51.

CHAPTER 3

Antigenic Composition of Rabies Virus

H. G. Aaslestad

I. Introduction

A great many investigations into the antigenic character of the rabies virus have been made since Pasteur first applied antirabies therapy (Pasteur, 1885), possible applications of new biochemical findings to vaccine production have recently been reviewed (Sokol, 1971). But serologic assays have yet to give us a clear understanding of the structural and functional character of the structural components of the rabies virion. In the past two and a half decades, however, there has been a dramatic increase in our knowledge about virus purification and analysis (see Chapters 4 and 7, this volume). The time would appear to be ripe to exploit this information and construct a more complete picture of the antigenic composition of the rabies virion.

Rabies virus is a member of the characteristically bullet-shaped rhabdovirus group composed of members which are considered to be antigenically distinct (a discussion of the newly isolated rabies-related viruses is given in Chapter 8). The virion consists of a helical ribonucleoprotein capsid (NC) enclosed within a lipoprotein membrane or envelope which in turn appears to be covered with a fringe of short projections (see Chapter 2), probably a glycoprotein in nature. Theoretically each of these structural elements might behave as a unique antigen and each might carry one or more antigenic sites. In addition, nonstructural viral proteins, such as virus-specific enzymes, must also be considered as potential antigens.

This chapter summarizes investigations of rabies antigens present in the infected cell, the intact virion, the disrupted virion, and in the "soluble" antigen. As an integral part of such a summary, we attempt to indicate areas where knowledge is incomplete and the prospect for fruitful research exists.

II. Rabies Antigen in Infected Cells

Prior to the development of modern methods for rabies virus assay, rabies infection was defined by the demonstration of rabies inclusion bodies within the infected cell. Examination of infected neurons by specific staining procedures (see Chapter 10), revealed the characteristic rabies Negri body (Negri, 1903). Fluorescent antibody staining (Goldwasser and Kissling, 1958) gave further evidence of the rabies-specific nature of these bodies. Electron microscopy of thin sections of infected cells has shown that these cytoplasmic inclusions consist of a moderately electron-dense matrix in which rabies virus particles may occasionally be detected (Matsumoto and Miyamoto, 1966). Subsequent microscopic observations of thin sections of *in vitro*-infected non-neural cell cultures leave little doubt that the rabies cytoplasmic inclusion bodies are concentrations of rabies-specific structures (Hummeler *et al.*, 1967); such inclusions were not limited by membranes and appeared to contain fine granular material with some filamentous areas. These matrices are hypothesized to be concentrations of rabies NC by Hummeler *et al.* (1968) on the basis of morphology and the fact that they stained with ferritin-labeled hyperimmune antirabies antisera. Specific staining of such material with fluorescent antibody to rabies virus NC has been demonstrated recently (Wiktor, T. J., unpublished). The development of the viral matrix was paralleled by an increased intensity to which infected tissue culture cells stained with fluorescent antibody (Hummeler *et al.*, 1967). There is no evidence that these inclusions represent virus-specific enzymes. On the contrary, it is unlikely that concentrations of viral enzymes would ever attain sufficient mass to be visualized, and in any case they might not react immunologically with antisera prepared against virus structural protein. The recent development of a peroxidase-tagged antibody staining procedure (Atanasiu *et al.*, 1971) should add a tool equal in sensitivity to that of fluorescent antibody staining for the investigation of rabies antigen(s) in infected cells.

Since virus maturation occurs most commonly by release of the virion by a budding process, membranes of the infected cell, particularly the plasma membrane, should be specifically altered as a consequence of rabies infection. Hummeler *et al.* (1968) reported that rabies virus in the process of budding through the plasma membrane could be stained with ferritin-labeled antirabies antibody. Chronically rabies virus-infected cells in tissue culture have been shown to be susceptible to immune lysis only at those times when virus was actively being released from the cell membrane (Wiktor & Clark, 1972).

When tissue culture cells from such diverse species as hamster, rabbit, and human were infected, rabies antigen that stained with fluorescent antirabies serum was found to be present during several cell divisions (Fernandes *et al.*, 1963). Wiktor *et al.* (1968) reported that hyperimmune antirabies serum was able to effect lysis of infected human or hamster tissue culture cells; cytolysis was dependent upon the presence of serum complement. In addition, these workers observed that fluorescein-conjugated antibody stained the surface membrane of infected cells in the absence of complement, whereas in the presence of complement intracytoplasmic staining was observed. Both lytic and virus-neutralizing (N) antibodies were found in the γ-globulin fraction of hyperimmune antirabies serum. When monkeys were immunized with living or inactivated rabies vaccines, these two antibodies did not necessarily appear at the same time.

In recent experiments with cellular membranes prepared from homogenates of rabies-infected baby hamster kidney (BHK-21) cells and fractionated by centrifugation in a discontinuous sucrose density gradient by the method of Caliguiri and Tann (1970), a class of smooth membranes enriched in complement-fixing (CF) antigen was demonstrated (H. G. Aaslestad, unpublished data). These membranes have a buoyant density in sucrose of approximately 1.11 g/cm^3 and contain little or no infectious virus and no rabies-specific hemagglutination (HA). Further experiments may clarify the role of such membrane fractions in rabies envelopment.

In summary, it seems clear that both intracytoplasmic antigen(s), presumably NC, and membrane-bound antigen(s) capable of fixing complement and possibly serving as a cytolysis target, are present within the rabies-infected tissue culture cell. The relation of these antigens to the development of the disease is still uncertain.

III. Antigens of the Rabies Virion

Concentrated and purified viral antigen(s) must be available to induce formation of monospecific antibody if the antigenic analysis of
the rabies virion or the rabies-infected cell is to be made. The
methods summarized in Chapter 7 permit rabies virion suspensions
of a high degree of purity to be obtained. However, care must be
taken in evaluating an antiserum produced against a concentrated
suspension of rabies virions. NC antibody, antibody against "soluble
antigen," and antibody against virion surface structures may each be
present in the antiserum, and most hyperimmune sera are probably
mixtures of such antibodies. Care must be taken in the production
and treatment of the antigen and in the adsorption protocol to render
a given serum truly monospecific.

Sokol *et al.* (1968) analyzed a partially purified rabies virus suspension by sucrose density gradient centrifugation and found that the
virus infectivity, CF activity, HA activity, and the radioactivity incorporated in the viral ribonucleic acid (RNA) sedimented together.
When concentrated virus suspensions such as these were inactivated
with β-propiolactone, the resulting vaccine was 700 times more potent in protecting mice ("protective activity," Seligmann, 1966) than
unconcentrated virus (Wiktor *et al.*, 1969). Rabies antisera induced in
rabbits by such preparations were shown to be efficient in neutralizing rabies when assayed by the plaque reduction method (Sedwick and Wiktor, 1967; Wiktor *et al.*, 1968). These antigenic properties of purified rabies virus and similar data from other studies are
summarized in Table I.

An interesting aspect of the characterization of the rabies virion
reported by Sokol *et al.* (1968) was the finding that rabies HA is
bound exclusively to the virion. On the other hand, virion-free fluids
prepared from both infectious cell culture fluid and infected animal
tissues have been found by many workers to contain considerable
amounts of CF antigen(s) termed, most often, soluble antigen. Subsequent work by Kuwert *et al.* (1968) described the properties of
rabies HA and confirmed the absence of soluble HA material in
fluids decanted from rabies-infected BHK-21 cells. HA titration of
fluids containing rabies virus afford a direct measure of virion content since only the virion appears to carry the HA function; the CF
assay and other immunological assays, such as gel diffusion, are
complicated by the presence of subviral antigens.

Rabies HA was first demonstrated by Halonen *et al.* (1968) and its
antigenic character was established by the fact that hyperimmune an-

Table I

Antigenic Properties of Purified Rabies Virus

Virus strain/source	Purification[a]	Rabies antigenic property[b]				References
		CF	HA	N	Other	
HEP/BHK-21	Sucrose density gradient	+	+	n.t.	i. ppt.	Sokol *et al.*, 1968
CVS/BHK-21	CsCl density gradient	+	+	n.t.	i. ppt.	Murphy *et al.*, 1968
HEP/BHK-21	CsCl density gradient	+	+	+	i. ppt. vaccine	Schneider *et al.*, 1971a,b
PM/WI-38	Zinc acetate precipitation plus ultracentrifugation	+	n.t.	n.t.	Vaccine	Wiktor *et al.*, 1969
HEP/BHK-21		+	n.t.	n.t.	Vaccine	
PM/BHK-21	Zinc acetate precipitation plus ultracentrifugation	+	n.t.	+	Vaccine	Schlumberger *et al.*, 1970
ERA/BHK-21	Sucrose density gradient	+	n.t.	+	Vaccine	Wiktor *et al.*, 1973

[a] Each density gradient purified rabies suspension was reported to be homogeneous and essentially free of nonviral impurities.

[b] Complement fixation (CF), agglutination of goose erythrocytes (HA), and the induction of neutralizing antirabies antibody formation (N) are qualitatively summarized. Also shown are positive reactions in immunodiffusion precipitation trials (i. ppt.) and the ability of the virus suspension to protect experimental animals, "protective activity," from lethal rabies challenge (vaccine); n.t. denotes not tested.

tirabies serum inhibited its agglutination of erythrocytes. The pH requirements for HA by fixed rabies virus strains have been found to be strain dependent and may serve as useful strain markers (T. J. Wiktor, unpublished). Development of an HI test for rabies antibody has been hindered by the fact that the HA reaction is sensitive to non-specific inhibitors present in animal serum. However, successful removal of inhibitors with kaolin (human serum) or acetone extraction (rabbit and horse sera) has recently been demonstrated (T. J. Wiktor, unpublished). HI antibody titers obtained in tests of human sera were parallel to, but slightly lower than, those determined by serum-neutralization tests. Recently developed methods for the removal of inhibitors from sera used in arbovirus HI tests may also be applicable for rabies HI sera (Monath *et al.*, 1970; Altemeier *et al.*, 1970).

Numerous investigators have sedimented partially purified rabies virus to an equilibrium position in CsCl density gradients. In an early report the viral infectivity was found to band in a rather hetero-geneous pattern between 1.20 and 1.24 g/cm³ (Neurath *et al.*, 1966). Through equilibrium centrifugation, Murphy *et al.* (1968) found that both rabies HA and CF activity banded with viral infectivity at a density position of 1.22 g/cm³ in a CsCl density gradient (Table I), confirming the finding of Sokol *et al.* (1968) that these antigens were virion bound. A CF antigen, not associated with viral infectivity or HA activity, was detected at a density of 1.30 g/cm³. The CF antigen not bound to virions was found to react with hyperimmune rabies an-tiserum in gel diffusion studies and may be rabies NC.

Schneider *et al.* (1971a) performed a similar analysis and reported two peaks of infectivity following CsCl density gradient banding. The major infectious peak was in the density position 1.22 g/cm³ and the minor peak at 1.20 g/cm³. Rabies CF and HA activity were as-sociated with both infectious bands and, in agreement with Murphy *et al.* (1968), a CF antigen free of HA activity banded at 1.32 g/cm³. Electron microscopic observations of negatively stained particles revealed that virions taken from both the 1.20 and 1.22 g/cm³ posi-tions of the CsCl gradient were identical in morphology. Virus puri-fied by CsCl density gradient was shown to be a potent immunogen and mice injected with vaccine prepared from such a suspension were protected from a lethal rabies challenge (Schneider *et al.*, 1971b).

Differences in the buoyant densities of rabies virions were ana-lyzed by Sokol *et al.*(1972). When partially purified rabies virus was centrifuged to equilibrium in a sucrose density gradient, approxi-mately half of the virus particles lost phospholipid from the viral envelope. Partially "delipidized" rabies particles (density, 1.16 g/cm³) could be separated from intact virions (density, 1.14 g/cm³) and, while both fractions were infectious, the normal bullet-shape of the intact virions became bag-shaped in the phospholipid-depleted particle. Unfortunately no determination of HA or CF activity was performed on these fractions, and no correlation between these bio-logical properties and loss of membrane phospholipid can be made.

A partial definition of the common antigenic characteristics of rabies virus can now be made. Antigenic sites exist on the viral envelope of the rabies virion, and they may induce the synthesis of antibodies capable of neutralizing viral infectivity and binding com-plement. It is reasonable to assign the HA antigenic character to the virion surface. Purified and inactivated rabies virus is an effective immunogen.

IV. Antigens of Disrupted Virions

In order to explore the antigenic nature of the structural components of the rabies virion, a number of disruptive agents were used to solubilize or fragment purified virions (Table II).

The disruption of purified virions with an anionic detergent, sodium deoxycholate (DOC), resulted in the rapid inactivation of viral infectivity and the dramatic loss of most of the HA activity. On the other hand, CF activity remained unaltered (Sokol *et al.*, 1969). Examination of the disrupted virus by density gradient centrifugation and electron microscopy revealed strands of NC which had a sedimentation coefficient of approximately 200 S. The buoyant density of the rabies NC, as determined in CsCl, was that of a nucleoprotein, 1.32 g/cm³. The NC fraction was shown to contain the viral RNA and possessed CF activity but not HA activity (Table II).

CF activity which sedimented at a slower rate in a sucrose density gradient than the NC was also present in DOC-treated rabies suspensions, as well as a low level of rabies HA which sedimented slowly into the gradient (Sokol *et al.*, 1969). Thus envelope components, as well as rabies NC, could be accounted for after disruption with detergent. Such envelope components possessed the ability to interfere with the rabies HA reaction. A specific inhibition of HA resulted when dilutions of DOC-derived envelope components were mixed with a standard suspension of intact rabies virus prior to the addition of erythrocytes. This inhibition was probably the result of competition for erythrocyte receptor sites between the envelope components and the intact virus and indicates that the solubilized material originated from the virion surface.

The disruption of concentrated, partially purified rabies virions by the natural detergent saponin resulted in the disruption and inactivation of viral infectivity, whereas rabies HA, CF, and immunogenic capacity remained largely unaltered (Schneider *et al.*, 1971b). In fact, rabies HA activity was found to increase as much as fourfold after treatment with saponin under optimal conditions. Saponin-treated rabies virus was analyzed by equilibrium centrifugation in CsCl, and the viral HA activity was found to band at 1.29 g/cm³, the density position characteristic of free protein. Equal amounts of CF activity banded at 1.29 g/cm³ and 1.32 g/cm³, the latter density position being characteristic of rabies NC. When the saponin-solubilized HA material (HA antigen) was rebanded, all of the HA activity and about 90% of the CF activity was recovered at a density position of 1.29 g/cm³.

Table II

Antigenic Properties of Disrupted Purified Rabies Virus

| Disrupting agent | Antigenic[a] and physical[b] properties of | | | | | | | | | | References |
| | Soluble components | | | | | Particulate components | | | | | |
	CF	HA	N	Other	Physical properties	CF	HA	N	Other	Physical properties	
DOC	40	<5	<5	HA blocking activity vaccine	~10–20 S	60	0	<1	i. ppt.	Helical strands; 200 S; 1.32 g/cm³ density	Sokol et al., 1968; Wiktor et al., 1973
NP-40	n.t.	n.t.	30	Strong vaccine	Soluble glycoprotein and lipid	n.t.	n.t.	~5	Weak vaccine	"Core particle" <600 S; 1.17 g/cm³ density	György et al., 1971; Wiktor et al., 1972
Saponin	50	90–100	50–80	Strong vaccine	1.29 g/cm³ density	50	0	~5	Weak vaccine	1.32 g/cm³ density	Schneider et al., 1971a,b

[a] The values indicated for the various antigenic properties are defined by the author on the basis of activity relative to the intact virion taken at an arbitrary value of 100. These number values are given only for illustrative purposes. No attempt is made to evaluate activities with respect to different disrupting agents. See Table I footnotes and the text for the definition of abbreviations.

[b] Only those physical properties that serve to identify a given fraction are listed.

When this purified HA fraction was treated with DOC, the HA titer was abolished but the CF activity remained unaffected. Mice immunized with an equivalent mass of purified virus or isolated HA antigen formed high levels of N antibody and were protected to almost the same extent from a lethal rabies challenge. It was not reported whether the HA antigen was immunogenic after DOC treatment. Thus, for the first time, a noninfectious immunogen possessing multiple biologic properties characteristic of the surface of the rabies virion was obtained. Since DOC treatment of the HA antigen resulted in selective loss of HA activity, while CF activity remained unaffected, it may be concluded either that these two antigenic sites reside on different proteins, or that some conformational property of the antigen surface is critical for HA activity.

Immunogenicity of rabies virus suspensions is altered through treatment with various detergents (Crick and Brown, 1970). Tween 80–ether, the nonionic detergent Nonident-P40 (NP-40), and DOC, when used at rather low concentrations, yielded solubilized antigens that induced rabies neutralizing (N) antibody in mice. Resistance to infection was found to correlate with the N antibody level in the test animal but no determinations of CF or HA activity of the solubilized antigen were reported. Sodium dodecylsulfate, on the other hand, completely destroyed immunogenicity. These detergent-derived viral immunogens appeared quite dissimilar when examined by the electron microscope. The Tween–ether preparation contained virions that were largely intact with no apparent removal of surface spikes. Treatment with NP-40 produced skeleton-like structures with spikes removed, whereas DOC caused further disruption, resulting in the appearance of NC strands similar to those observed by Sokol *et al.* (1969).

The use of NP-40 to disrupt rabies virus and liberate surface proteins was also employed by György *et al.* (1971). They found that the envelope glycoprotein (Sokol *et al.*, 1971) and viral lipids were selectively solubilized when this detergent was added at a specific concentration relative to the mass of viral protein. The other viral proteins and RNA remained associated in the form of a structured "core" and were readily separated by sucrose density gradient centrifugation. Since it had been shown that the envelope glycoprotein of another rhabdovirus, vesicular stomatitis virus, was capable of binding N antibody (Kang and Prevec, 1970), intense interest centered on the immunogenic properties of NP-40-prepared rabies glycoprotein.

Recently Wiktor *et al.* (1973) determined that NP-40-solubilized rabies glycoprotein can induce N antibody in mice and that mice so treated can resist a lethal rabies challenge. On the other hand, "core" particles obtained after NP-40 treatment were found to induce a lower level of N antibody formation. The induction of N antibody was as much as 800-fold higher in mice injected with rabies glycoprotein than after injection of an equal mass of "core" particles. N antibody was induced by "core" particles only to the extent expected from the amount of contaminating glycoprotein present. Although the ability of the glycoprotein to react in HA assay has not been established, one might anticipate that it would possess HA-blocking activity, since its origin is the surface of the virion. DOC-derived envelope components were also found to stimulate N antibody formation in mice, whereas isolated NC was much less effective in antibody induction.

Schneider *et al.* (1973) characterized the antibodies elicited by ribonucleoprotein (RNA – synonymous to NC) and glycoprotein antigens isolated from rabies virus and the rabies serogroup Mokola and Lagos bat virus. RNP antigen was found to exhibit group specificity, being common to all of the rabies group viruses. The envelope glycoprotein antigens were found to elicit neutralizing antibodies of virus type specificity. Although the M proteins of rabies virus have not yet been obtained in pure form, comparative characterization of the M, G, and N proteins of the rhabdovirus VSV has recently been described (Dietzschold *et al.*, 1974). The M protein of VSV elicited CF and precipitating antibodies, but no neutralizing antibody.

Wiktor *et al.* (1973) compared partially purified rabies virus disrupted by DOC, NP-40 or saponin relative to the recovery of "protective activity." Their findings showed that saponin was superior to NP-40 in this regard, but they did not report biophysical studies which would have permitted a comparison of NP-40 treatment with that of saponin. Nevertheless, it seems clear that the envelope glycoprotein of rabies virus is responsible for the induction of N antibody formation and for the protection of animals against rabies infection.

The studies on the antigenic nature of the disrupted virion summarized in Table II permit some conclusions and open some avenues for further exploration. The surface of the rabies virion bears sites for HA, CF antigen activity, and for N antibody induction. The NC, likewise, can fix complement but does not possess HA activity. The presence of unique external and internal CF antigens could be verified by experimental tests in CF assays utilizing rabies antisera produced in response to immunization with purified NC or purified virions. The envelope glycoprotein appears to the principal determinant responsible for N antibody induction, whereas the NC and NP-40 derived "core" are inactive. The use of specific antisera directed against individual rabies virion components (both as reagents and in antibody blocking assays) is required before a definitive antigenic picture of the rabies virion can be constructed. In addition, specific antisera, such as specific NC or glycoprotein antiserum, would also be useful in judging the antigenic relation between rabies strains as well as between rabies virus and other rhabdoviruses.

V. Soluble Antigen

Rabies virus-infected cells produce complement-fixing soluble antigen(s) (SA) which may be separated from the intact virion by centrifugation. This naturally occurring noninfectious antigen was first reported by Polson and Wessels (1953) in preparations of rabies-infected suckling mouse brain. As a source of SA, these workers and most later investigators have used clarified tissue homogenates or cell culture fluids, freed of intact rabies virus by high-speed centrifugation. The particle diameter for this CF antigen was determined to be 12.4 nm and its approximate sedimentation coefficient was 25 S. Van den Ende *et al.* (1957) reported that SA was produced in suckling mouse brain in parallel with infectious virus and was partially purified by precipitation at pH 4.3. They also characterized the antigen as insensitive to pH variation over range 6–10, stable to heating at 56°C, and to treatment with dilute phenol or formaldehyde, but sensitive to trypsin digestion. Attempts to break up rabies virus by repeated freezing and thawing or by exposure to ultrasonic vibration failed to release significant amounts of SA. Kipps *et al.* (1957) determined that an increase in infectivity preceded the first appearance of SA in mice after intracerebral injection of rabies virus, and that SA continued to increase after the maximum level of infectivity had been reached. When mice were immunized with SA, high levels of CF antibody could be obtained, but no N antibody was induced.

Mead (1962a,b) continued the study of SA prepared from suckling mouse brain. He confirmed the utility of precipitation at acidic pH as a concentration device, but was unable to further purify SA by chromatographic and electrophoretic techniques. At least two, and perhaps four, antigenic entities were present in SA preparations, the largest being resistant to trypsin digestion (Mead, 1962b). This resistance permitted Katz *et al.* (1968) to utilize enzyme treatment and ultracentrifugation to concentrate and purify the largest rabies SA. The purified antigen sedimented at about 16 S and had a buoyant density of 1.34 g/cm³ in CsCl. It was found to contain appreciable amounts of pentose, in addition to protein, and was observed to be a ringlike particle of 10 nm diameter. Katz *et al.* (1968) speculated that this antigen may have arisen from disrupted segments of rabies NC. It would be reasonable to consider SA identical to fragmented NC since both of these CF antigens have equivalent buoyant densities. Now that NC has been isolated (Sokol *et al.*, 1969), a direct comparison of these two antigens is possible.

Culture fluids decanted from rabies-infected cell cultures have also been a source of SA. Neurath *et al.* (1966) reported that SA could be detected in fluids decanted from infected monolayers of BHK-21 cells. Sucrose density gradient centrifugation of a preparation of this antigen revealed two components with sedimentation coefficients of approximately 23 S and 10 S. This result finds support in the data of Atanasiu *et al.* (1963) who demonstrated two precipitin lines formed by soluble antigen(s) produced in cell cultures. Neurath *et al.* (1966) also reported that the antigen possessed a buoyant density of 1.26 g/cm³ in CsCl, which would cause one to question its identity with NC. Chromatography on Ecteola cellulose was used to indicate the complexity of the SA preparation; five separate antigenic components were isolated (Neurath and Rubin, 1967).

Wiktor *et al.* (1969) employed differential ultrafiltration to free the SA present in infectious tissue culture fluid from intact virions. The resulting virus-depleted filtrate was concentrated and, when compared with an equivalent concentrate of rabies virions plus SA, was found to contain only 0.005% of the viral infectivity and to be devoid of HA activity. On the other hand, complete recovery of CF activity was found in the concentrated SA fraction, and 21% of the "protective activity" remained. The authors concluded that SA was an immunogen for CF antibody formation as well as a vaccine which afforded protection against challenge with rabies.

The antigenic and immunogenic properties of SA were further studied by Crick and Brown (1969) and by Schlumberger *et al.*(1970). When centrifugation was used to deplete the culture fluid of infectious rabies virus, an SA of high CF titer remained in the supernatant (Schlumberger *et al.*, 1970). This antigen, however, showed poor "protective activity" in mice although it did induce the formation of N antibody in rabbits. In contrast to this, SA preparations obtained after the infectious virus was removed by zinc acetate precipitation (Sokol *et al.*, 1968), showed good "protective activity." Schlumberger *et al.* (1970) suggested that the formation of aggregates of SA during zinc acetate treatment may result in retention of "protective activity." The SA present in the supernatant fluid decanted from infected BHK-21 cells had a molecular weight of approximately 150,000 on the basis of exclusion chromatography (H. D. Schlumberger and T. J. Wiktor, personal communication). This is probably a minimum molecular weight since it would account for the presence of only two molecules of rabies glycoprotein and is not compatible with the data obtained through sedimentation analysis of SA. Gel immunodiffusion experiments using SA, purified by Sephadex G-150 chromatography, and antisera of different specificities have given qualitative indications that SA was not derived from NC but that it reacted to a high degree against antisera prepared against DOC-derived envelope proteins. These findings are obviously contradictory to the concept that SA was derived from NC.

The relationship of SA to the synthesis of infectious virus was recently studied in the human diploid cell line WI-38 (H. F. Clark and T. J. Wiktor, personal communication). High levels of CF antigen were found to be continually present in culture fluids decanted from chronically infected WI-38 cells. Such cultures displayed intensely positive staining with fluorescent antisera, but little or no infectious virus was detected either within the cells or in supernatant fluids. When culture fluids rich in CF antigen were concentrated and assayed for their ability to protect mice from rabies infection, only very low levels of protection were afforded.

It remains to be determined whether the rabies SA detected in suckling mouse brain are similar to the SA present in infected tissue culture fluid. Both preparations fix complement and seem to share some physical properties. The relationship of the soluble CF antigen (SA) to the viral NC or to protein present on the surface of the virion has yet to be determined. It also appears that more than one antigenic species may be present in the SA studied thus far, although the various antigens have not yet been biologically characterized. It is probable that both NC protein and viral proteins of envelope origin are present in SA. The possibility of using SA as a noninfectious immunogen for the protection of animals should be explored further; however, because the level of "protective activity" afforded by SA as compared to vaccine prepared from virions is low, the practical use of SA for immunization may be limited.

VI. Conclusion

Rather than conclude this chapter with a recital of the antigenic features of rabies virus thus far revealed, we would like to point out once more some of the areas open to experimental tests. Foremost in this regard is the requirement that monotypic antisera be prepared against purified components of the virion. Methodology is already at hand for the preparation of pure NC (Sokol *et al.*, 1969) and this subviral component should easily serve as a primary reagent. The NC antigen is the logical starting point for antigenic analysis because it is reasonably stable to the physical stress of purification, except for a tendency to fragment to short lengths, and because it is composed of only one major peptide (Sokol *et al.*, 1971). Monotypic NC antisera will be invaluable in confirming the nature of the rabies cytoplasmic inclusion bodies present in infected cells as NC concentrations, in establishing the identity of the envelope CF antigen and the saponin-derived HA antigen complex of Schneider *et al.* (1971b), and in defining the relationship of rabies SA antigen(s) to the virion.

Whereas NC and specific NC antisera can be prepared with methods now available, the production of pure glycoprotein may present problems. The use of NP-40 to solubilize this structural protein (György *et al.*, 1971) yields an adequate immunogen for the preparation of neutralizing antisera (Wiktor *et al.*, 1973); however, the glycoprotein itself must be free of detergent before it can be used in serologic assays.Other methods to dissect rabies structural proteins and protein complexes, perhaps involving variations in pH or salt concentration (alone or in addition to detergent treatment) may result in alternatives to the present dependence upon detergent solubilization. In addition, further work for the isolation of soluble antigens, such as ion exchange chromatography and polymer phase system separation, etc., may well provide alternatives to the density gradient centrifugation methods now in use. Questions which may be answered when specific glycoprotein reagents become available include: Does glycoprotein react in CF or HA assays? Does it bind to N antibody? Can glycoprotein block immune cytolysis? Is glycoprotein identical to or part of the HA complex obtained following the treatment of rabies virus with saponin? Answers to these questions and others not formulated here are fundamental to a full understanding of the antigenic composition of this virus.

The antigenic picture of rabies virus which emerges from this review is that of an image formed in adequate contrast but lacking in fine detail. Thus, we can see the outlines of the antigenic character of the virion, that it fixes complement, reacts as a hemagglutinin, and can induce N antibody formation. We can also see in considerable detail two of its components, the NC and glycoprotein. But the antigenic nature of all of the structural parts of the virion still remains shadowy. Present advances are providing insights into the antigenic composition of rabies virus, and give cause for an optimistic forecast for the creation of a more complete picture in the near future.

Acknowledgments

Supported, in part, by U. S. Public Health Service research grants AI-09706 from the National Institute of Allergy and Infectious Diseases, Contract No. NIH-71-2292 from the Department of Health, Education, and Welfare, and RR-05540 from the Division of Research Resources, and by funds from the World Health Organization.

References

Altemeier, W. A., Mudan, F. K., Top, F. H., and Russell, P. K. (1970). *Appl. Microbiol.* 19, 785.

Atanasiu, P., Lépine, P., and Dragonas, P. (1963). *Ann. Inst. Pasteur, Paris* 105, 813.

Atanasiu, P., Dragonas, P., Tsiang, H., and Harbi, A. (1971). *Ann. Inst. Pasteur, Paris* 121, 247.

Caliguiri, L. A., and Tann, I. (1970). *Virology* 42, 100.

Crick, J., and Brown, F. (1969). *Nature (London)* 222, 92.

Crick, J., and Brown, F. (1970). *In* "The Biology of Large RNA Viruses" (R. D. Barry and B. W. J. Mahy, eds.), pp. 130–140. Academic Press, New York.

Dietzschold, B., Schneider, L. G., and Cox, J. H. (1974). *J. Virol.* 14, 1.

Fernandes, M. V., Wiktor, T. J., and Koprowski, H. (1963). *Virology* 21, 128.

Goldwasser, R. A., and Kissling, R. E. (1958). *Proc. Soc. Exp. Biol. Med.* 98, 219.

György, E., Sheehan, M. C., and Sokol, F. (1971). *J. Virol.* 8, 649.

Halonen, P. E., Murphy, F. A., Fields, B. N., and Reese, D. R. (1968). *Proc. Soc. Exp. Biol. Med.* 127, 1037.

Hummeler, K., Koprowski, H., and Wiktor, T. J. (1967). *J. Virol.* 1, 152.

Hummeler, K., Tomassini, N., Sokol, F., Kuwert, E., and Koprowski, H. (1968). *J. Virol.* 2, 1191.

Kang, C. Y., and Prevec, L. (1970). *J. Virol.* 6, 20.

Katz, W., Larsson, K. M., and Mead, T. H. (1968) *J. Gen. Virol.* 2, 399.

Kipps, A., Naudé, W. Du T., Polson, A., and Selzer, G. (1957). *Nature of Viruses, CIBA Found. Symp., 1956,* p. 224.

Kuwert, E., Wiktor, T. J., Sokol, F., and Koprowski, H. (1968). *J. Virol.* 2, 1381.

Matsumoto, S., and Miyamoto, K. (1966). *Symp. Ser. Immunobiol. Stand.* 1, 45.

Mead, T. H. (1962a). *J. Gen. Microbiol.* 27, 397.

Mead, T. H. (1962b). *J. Gen. Microbiol.* 27, 415.

Monath, T. P. C., Lindsey, H. S., Nickolls, J. G., Chaprell, W. A., and Henderson, B. E. (1970). *Appl. Microbiol.* 20, 748.

Murphy, F. A., Halonen, P. E., Gary, G. W., Jr., and Reese, D. R. (1968). *J. Gen. Virol.* **3**, 289.

Negri, A. (1903). *Z. Hyg. Infektionskr.* **43**, 507.

Neurath, A. R., and Rubin, B. A. (1967). *Experientia* **23**, 872.

Neurath, A. R., Wiktor, T. J., and Koprowski, H. (1966). *J. Bacteriol.* **92**, 102.

Pasteur, L. (1885). *C. R. Acad. Sci.* **101**, 765.

Polson, A., and Wessels, P. (1953). *Proc. Soc. Exp. Biol. Med.* **84**, 317.

Schlumberger, H. D., Wiktor, T. J., and Koprowski, H. (1970). *J. Immunol.* **105**, 291.

Schneider, L. G., Dietzschold, B., Dierks, R. E., Matthaeus, W., Enzmann, P. J., and Strohmaier, K. (1973). *J. Virol.* **11**, 748.

Schneider, L. G., Horzinek, M., and Matheka, H. D. (1971a). *Arch. Gesamte Virusforsch.* **34**, 351.

Schneider, L. G., Horzinek, M., and Novicky, R. (1971b). *Arch. Gesamte Virusforsch.* **34**, 360.

Sedwick, W. D., and Wiktor, T. J. (1967). *J. Virol.* **1**, 1224.

Seligmann, E. B. (1966). *World Health Organ. Monogr. Ser.* **23**, 145.

Sokol, F., Kuwert, E., Wiktor, T. J., Hummeler, K., and Koprowski, H. (1968). *J. Virol.* **2**, 836.

Sokol, F., Schlumberger, H. D., Wiktor, T. J., Koprowski, H., and Hummeler, K. (1969). *Virology* **38**, 651.

Sokol, F., Stancek, D., and Koprowski, H. (1971). *J. Virol.* **7**, 241.

Sokol, F., Clark, H. F., György, E., and Tomassini, N. (1972). *J. Gen. Virol.* **16**, 173.

Sokol, F. (1971). *Recent Advances in Microbiology*, Xth Int. Congress Microbiology, pp. 551–562, Ed. A. Pérez-Miravete and Dionisio Pelaez, Mexico.

van den Ende, M., Polson, A., and Turner, G. S. (1957). *J. Hyg.* **55**, 361.

Wiktor, T. J., Kuwert, E., and Koprowski, H. (1968). *J. Immunol.* **101**, 1271.

Wiktor, T. J., Sokol, F., Kuwert, E., and Koprowski, H. (1969). *Proc. Soc. Exp. Biol. Med.* **131**, 799.

Wiktor, T. J., and Clark, H. F. (1972). *Infection and Immunity* **6**, 988.

Wiktor, T. J., György, E., Schlumberger, H. D., Sokol, F., and Koprowski, H. (1973). *J. Immunol.* **110**, 269.

CHAPTER 4

Chemical Composition and Structure of Rabies Virus

*Frantisek Sokol**

I. Introduction

It is remarkable that for several decades rabies investigators have claimed progress in their research while knowing virtually nothing about the basic properties of rabies virus itself. During the last few years several virus strains have been adapted for growth in tissue cultures, and in some virus-cell systems relatively high virion yields have been obtained (see Chapters 8 and 9). This breakthrough has been followed by improvement of techniques for *in vitro* assay of the virus and of viral antigens (see Chapters 3,5,6, and 9). With the necessary tools in hand, it was not too tedious to develop procedures for purification of the virus and to obtain several milligrams of virions sufficiently purified to allow study of their chemical composition and structure. These studies have been initiated and are currently being expanded. Since progress in this field is recent and has been motivated mainly by urgent need for an improved rabies vaccine, the reader should not be surprised that data justly considered as basic

* Because of the death of Dr. Sokol at the time the production of this volume was begun, the proofs of this chapter were read by Dr. Kong Beng Tan of The Wistar Institute, Philadelphia, Pennsylvania.

and elementary are still missing and that some of the work cited here is still in progress and, therefore, fragmentary.

Rabies virus infection does not generally cause the destruction of tissue culture cells. Virus-producing cells survive and multiply for several cell generations and can be serially passaged (see Chapter 9). Efficient purification procedures have been worked out only for virus released from the infected cell by budding through the plasma membrane. Thus, all data in this chapter, unless otherwise specified, are related to extracellular rabies virions.

II. Properties of the Virion

The lack of effect of different inhibitors of deoxyribonucleic acid (DNA) synthesis and DNA transcription on the replication of the virus in tissue cultures indicated that rabies virus contained ribonucleic acid (RNA; Hamparian *et al.*, 1963; Kissling and Reese, 1963; Defendi and Wiktor, 1966; Maes *et al.*, 1967). The fact that the core of the virus was surrounded by a membrane (envelope) (see Chapter 2) and the observation that the infectivity of the virus was sensitive to periodate (Kuwert *et al.*, 1968) suggested that carbohydrates were included in the architecture of the virion. Sensitivity of viral infectivity to organic solvents and to detergents (Remlinger, 1918; Kissling and Reese, 1963; Kuwert *et al.*, 1968) suggested that lipids were also constituents of the viral coat. The first two of these tentative conclusions were later confirmed by isolation of the viral RNA (Sokol *et al.*, 1969) and of the envelope glycoprotein (Sokol *et al.*, 1971; György *et al.*, 1971). Characterization of lipids extracted from purified virions is now in progress (Diringer *et al.*, 1973; H. A. Blough and H. G. Aaslestad, unpublished experiments).

The specific biological activities, the gross chemical composition, and some physical properties, other than morphological features, of purified rabies virus are summarized in Table I. Different populations of virions vary with respect to several properties, and therefore data presented in this table should be regarded as characteristic for a representative virus preparation. Virions appreciably shorter than 180 nm (truncated viruses) have been detected by electron microscopy in purified Flury HEP and PM virus preparations, whereas almost all the virus particles in preparations of ERA virions were 180 nm long (Sokol *et al.*, 1968; K. Hummeler, H F. Clark, and F. Sokol, unpublished data). The length distribution of Flury HEP virions is not continuous, the truncated virus particles being either 150 or 125 nm long. Although virions of the latter strain are apparently uniform

Table I

Specific Biological Activities, Gross Chemical Composition, and Some Physical Properties of Purified Rabies Virus[a]

Property	Virus strain	Observation	References
Specific infectivity	Flury HEP	10^{10} PFU/mg protein[b]	Sokol *et al.*, 1968
	ERA	5×10^{10} PFU/mg protein[c]	F. Sokol and H F. Clark, unpublished observation.
Specific hemagglutinating activity	Flury HEP	10^4 HAU/mg protein[d]	Sokol *et al.*, 1968
Specific complement-fixing activity	Flury HEP	5×10^3 CFU/mg protein[d]	Sokol *et al.*, 1968
Gross chemical composition	Flury HEP	~22% lipids[e]	H. A. Blough and H. G. Aaslestad, unpublished data.
		~3% carbohydrates[f]	F. Sokol, unpublished observation.
		~1% RNA[g]	Sokol *et al.*, 1968
		~74% protein[h]	
Sedimentation coefficient	PM	600 S	Neurath *et al.*, 1966
Buoyant density in sucrose solution	Flury HEP	1.17 g/cm³	Sokol *et al.*, 1968 Sokol *et al.*, 1972
	ERA	1.14 g/cm³ [i]	György *et al.*, 1971

[a] Abbreviations: HEP = high egg passage; PM = Pitman Moore; PFU = plaque-forming unit; HAU = hemagglutinating unit; CFU = complement-fixing unit.

[b] A representative value, which varies with the proportion of infectious to noninfectious virions in the preparation.

[c] The specific infectivity of ERA virus preparations is consistently higher than that of Flury HEP virus grown under identical conditions.

[d] Definitions of HAU and CFU are given in Sokol *et al.* (1968).

[e] Determined from the difference in the dry weight of intact and delipidized virus.

[f] Determined by color reaction with anthrone reagent with glucose as standard.

[g] This value is based on the observations that viral nucleocapsid contains 4% RNA (Sokol *et al.*, 1969) and that the nucleocapsid protein represents 33% of total viral proteins (Sokol *et al.*, 1971).

[h] Determined from the weight of delipidized virus, after correction for carbohydrate and RNA content.

[i] Purified ERA virions are heterogeneous with respect to phospholipid content (Sokol *et al.*, 1972). The buoyant density listed here refers to virions with the highest phospholipid content.

in buoyant density in sucrose solution (Sokol *et al.*, 1968), their sedimentation rates vary (Fig. 1) (Sokol *et al.*, 1968; Sokol, 1971). On the other hand, purified ERA virions are heterogeneous with respect to their phospholipid content (Sokol *et al.*, 1972). After centrifugation

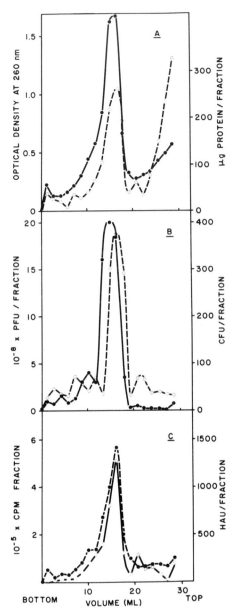

Fig. 1. Heterogeneity in sedimentation rate of Flury HEP rabies virions labeled with [³H] uridine. The virions were fractionated by velocity centrifugation for 20 min in a linear sucrose density gradient (5–22%, w/w) at 22,000 rev/min in the SW 25.1 head of a Spinco centrifuge. Symbols: (A) ○, protein content; ●, optical density at 260 nm; (B) ○, CFU; ●, PFU; (C) ○, radioactivity of [³H] uridine; ●, HAU. The three parts of the figure represent the same centrifugation experiment. Note that the peak of infectivity does not coincide with those of other viral activities. (Reprinted with permission from Sokol, 1971.)

82

in a sucrose density gradient, under conditions approaching equilibrium, ERA virions are recovered in two or three distinct bands (Figs. 2 and 3). The RNA content and size, as well as the proportions of various viral proteins (see Section V), were found to be similar, if not

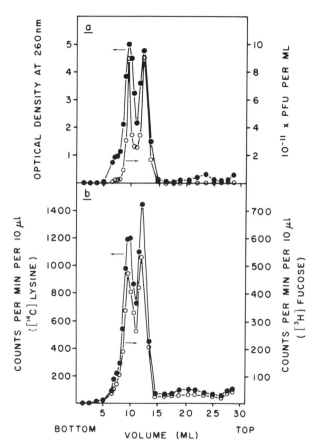

Fig. 2. Heterogeneity with respect to sedimentation properties of purified ERA virions. Extracellular ERA virus, labeled with [^{14}C]lysine and [^{3}H]L-fucose, was partially purified by precipitation with zinc acetate, filtration through a Sephadex column, and sedimentation by high-speed centrifugation. The partially purified and concentrated virus was then layered on 29 ml of linear sucrose density gradient (10 to 50%, w/w) and centrifuged for 90 min at 24,500 rev/min in the SW25.1 head of a Spinco centrifuge. The two parts of the figure represent the same centrifugation experiment. Symbols: (A) ●, optical density at 260 nm; ○, infectivity; (B) ●, [^{14}C]lysine radioactivity; ○, [^{3}H]fucose radioactivity. The peaks of the two bands were located at 1.165 and 1.150 g/cm^{3}, respectively. Under the conditions of centrifugation used in this experiment the equilibrium state is reached. Note that the specific infectivity of the two virus forms is similar. (Reprinted with permission from Sokol *et al.*, 1972.)

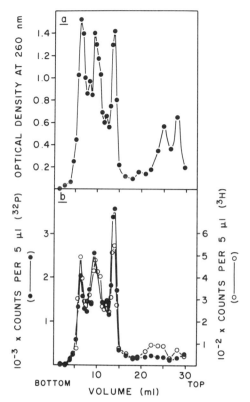

Fig. 3. Heterogeneity in phospholipid content of purified ERA virions. Extracellular ERA virus, labeled with [^{32}P]ortho-phosphate and [^{3}H]uridine, was partially purified and centrifuged in a sucrose density gradient as described in the legend
of Fig. 2. The two parts of the figure represent the same centrifugation experiment.
The ^{32}P/^{3}H ratios at the peaks of the three bands were 4.1, 5.4, and 6.5, respectively.
The peaks were located at 1.190, 1.170, and 1.135 g/cm^3, respectively. The over-
whelming majority of [^{32}P]phosphate is incorporated into the phospholipids of the
viral envelope, the amount incorporated into the viral RNA being negligible. The specific infectivities of the three viral forms (not shown here) were similar.

identical, for the different forms of ERA virus. The lipid-deficient
virus forms, however, were not bullet shaped, but were baglike in
morphology. Purified virions of the other fixed rabies virus strains
did not exhibit a similar heterogeneity.

Protein kinase is the only virion-associated enzyme which has
been detected in purified rabies virus preparations (Sokol and Clark,
1973). Treatments which activate the virion-associated RNA tran-
scriptase of vesicular stomatitis virus (VSV; Baltimore *et al.*, 1970) or
of Kern Canyon virus (Aaslestad *et al.*, 1971), failed to reveal similar

activity in rabies virions (H. G. Aaslestad, D. H. L. Bishop, and F. Sokol, unpublished data). Purified preparations of ERA or Flury HEP virions treated with phospholipase C exhibit DNA polymerase activity. However, a similar activity has been found in fluid of noninfected BHK-21 cell cultures, subjected to the same procedures as the infectious tissue culture fluid. Therefore, this enzyme is considered at present to be a host component (F. Sokol and H F. Clark, unpublished data).

III. Disruption of the Virus into Its Components

Treatment of enveloped, lipid-containing viruses with detergents or organic solvents effects the disruption of virions into subunits (Neurath and Rubin, 1971). The extent of disruption depends on the nature of the reagent used and the conditions of treatment. By investigation of the properties of the released components, some of the structure–function relationships in viruses can be elucidated.

Sodium deoxycholate (DOC), an ionic detergent, emulsifies the viral lipids and disrupts rabies virions into viral nucleocapsids and envelope components (Sokol et al., 1969). The latter can be separated from the nucleocapsid particles by velocity centrifugation in a sucrose density gradient. Nucleocapsid particles can then be further purified by equilibrium centrifugation in CsCl solution (Fig. 4). Many properties of rabies virus nucleocapsids (Table II) resemble those of paramyxovirus nucleocapsids (Compans and Choppin, 1971; Choppin et al., 1971). The envelope of the virus, which exhibits hemagglutinating activity before treatment, is disintegrated by DOC into relatively slowly sedimenting subunits. They possess hemagglutination-inhibition activity, but not hemagglutinating activity (Sokol et al., 1969; Sokol, 1971).

Treatment of purified rabies virus with a nonionic detergent, Nonidet P-40 (NP-40), results in emulsification of most of the lipids and preferential release of one of the envelope components, the viral glycoprotein (György et al., 1971; Sokol, et al., 1971). The delipidized "core" particles, from which the glycoprotein portion of the envelope has been removed, contain the viral RNA and the remaining protein components of the virus. The sedimentation rate of these particles is similar to that of virions, but their buoyant density in sucrose solution (1.20 g/cm^3) is higher. Results similar to those obtained after treatment of the virus with NP-40, were observed after exposure of the virions to tri-(n-butyl)phosphate in the presence of

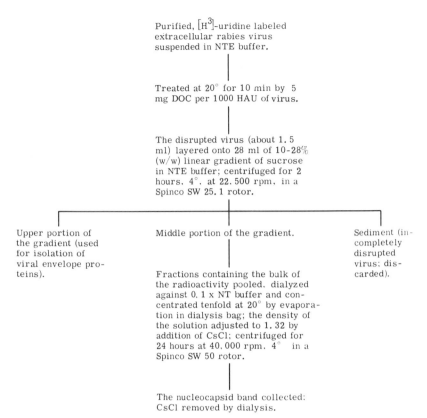

Fig. 4. A flow diagram of the procedure used for the disruption of [³H]uridine-labeled rabies virions by sodium deoxycholate and the purification of the released nucleocapsid.

Tween 80 (Neurath *et al.*, 1971). Viral proteins (glycoproteins), derived from DOC- or NP-40-treated virus, preserve at least a part of their immunogenic properties (Sokol *et al.*, 1969; Crick and Brown, 1970; Wiktor *et al.*, 1973).

When intact viruses, nucleocapsids, or "core" particles are treated with another ionic detergent, sodium dodecyl sulfate (SDS), the viral RNA is released and the protein components are dissociated to a large extent, although not completely (F. Sokol, unpublished results). Aggregates of protein molecules can be then fully dissociated into polypeptides by additional treatment with 2-mercaptoethanol (2-ME) and heating at 100°C for 1 min (Sokol *et al.*, 1971). Of course, treatment with SDS (Crick and Brown, 1970), as well as heating, causes complete or partial denaturation of viral proteins. The step-

Table II

Biological, Chemical, and Physical Properties of Viral
Nucleocapsid (Strain Flury HEP)

Property	Observation	References
Biological activities	Noninfectious,[a] exhibits complement-fixing, but not hemagglutinating activity.	Sokol *et al.*, 1969
Chemical composition	96% protein, 4% RNA; contains all the viral RNA; the nucleocapsid protein[b] consists of one major and one minor component (weight ratio 26.6).	Sokol *et al.*, 1969 Sokol *et al.*, 1971
Sedimentation coefficient	200 S	
Buoyant density in CsCl solution	1.32 g/cm^3	Sokol *et al.*, 1969
Molecular weight	1.15×10^8 daltons[c]	
Structure and size	Single-stranded, helix, 1 μm long, 100 Å in diameter, with a periodicity of 75 Å; 12 morphologically distinguishable protein units per one turn of the helix; the uncoiled helix is about 4.2 μm long and its width varies from 20 to 65 Å depending on the angle of viewing.	Sokol *et al.*, 1969 K. Hummeler and F. Sokol, unpublished observation.

[a] Determined at a concentration of 20 μg viral RNA per ml by plaque assay in suspended baby hamster kidney (BHK-21) cells (Sedwick and Wiktor, 1967), by inoculation of BHK-21 cell cultures, and by intracerebral inoculation of mice.

[b] A more detailed description of the properties of nucleocapsid proteins will be given later in this chapter.

[c] Calculated from the estimated molecular weight of viral RNA (see Table III) and the protein:RNA ratio in nucleocapsid particles.

wise disruption of rabies virus by the treatments mentioned is schematically presented in Fig. 5.

Recently, another reagent, saponin (Schneider *et al.*, 1971), was used to disrupt rabies virus for the purpose of producing an antirabies subunit vaccine. Treatment with saponin caused up to a fourfold increase in the hemagglutinating activity of the preparation. After equilibrium centrifugation in CsCl solution, the split products were recovered in two distinct bands. The component banding at 1.32 g/cm^3 had complement-fixing, but not hemagglutinating activity and most likely represented the viral nucleocapsid. The other component, with a buoyant density of 1.29 g/cm^3, contained all the hemagglutinating activity. The chemical nature and the protein composition of the two components were not characterized.

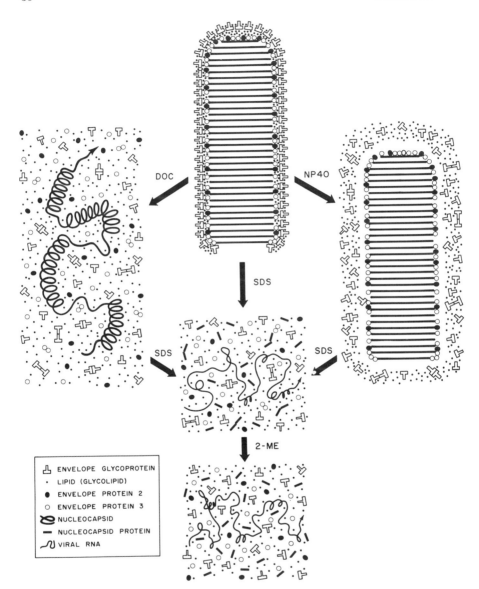

Fig. 5. Schematic representation of disruption of rabies virus and of its components by treatment with Nonidet P-40, sodium deoxycholate, sodium dodecyl sulfate, or 2-mercaptoethanol. The spikes on the surface of the virion are most likely of glycoprotein nature, because delipidized "core" particles obtained after treatment with NP-40 (Crick and Brown, 1970) or with tri-(*n*-butyl) phosphate and Tween 80 (Neurath *et al.*, 1971) lacked most of the surface projections.

IV. The Viral RNA

Viral RNA is released from rabies virions by treatment with 0.5–1.0% SDS. Dissociated protein components and solubilized lipids can then be separated from the viral RNA by phenol extraction of SDS-disrupted virions (Sokol et al., 1969) or by fractionation of disrupted virions by velocity centrifugation in a sucrose density gradient (F. Sokol, unpublished observation). The latter separation technique is based on the fact that the viral RNA sediments much faster than other SDS-dissociated virion components. The properties of naked Flury HEP rabies virus RNA are summarized in Table III. Some of the listed properties were also determined for RNA isolated

Table III

Biological, Physical, and Chemical Properties of RNA Isolated from Purified, Infectious Rabies Virions (Strain Flury HEP)

Property	Observation	References
Infectivity	Noninfectious[a]	
Sedimentation coefficient	45 S	
Secondary structure	Single-stranded (degraded to acid-soluble fragments by pancreatic ribonuclease; buoyant density in Cs_2SO_4 solution 1.66 g/cm³)	Sokol et al., 1969
Molecular weight	4.6×10^6 daltons[b]	Sokol et al., 1969
	4.4×10^6 daltons[c]	D. H. L. Bishop, H. G. Aaslestad, and H F. Clark, unpublished data
Length	4.6 μm[d]	Sokol et al., 1969
Nucleotide composition (moles/100 moles nucleotide)	26.4% adenylic acid, 29.4% uridylic acid, 21.1% guanylic acid, 23.1% cytidylic acid	Aaslestad and Urbano, 1971

[a] Determined at a concentration of 1 μg viral RNA per ml by plaque assay in suspended baby hamster kidney (BHK-21) cells (Sedwick and Wiktor, 1967), by inoculation of BHK-21 cell cultures, and by intracerebral inoculation of mice.

[b] Determined from the relationship between molecular weight and sedimentation coefficient of single-stranded RNAs (Spirin, 1963).

[c] Molecular weight of viral RNA determined from rate of migration in polyacrylamide gel, relative to that of ribosomal RNA markers (1.75×10^6 and 0.80×10^6 daltons molecular weight).

[d] Calculated from the estimated molecular weight of rabies virus RNA, the assumed internucleotide distance of 3.4 Å, and a mean molecular weight of 339 for a nucleotide.

from infectious virions of ERA or PM virus strains and were found to be similar, if not identical to those of Flury HEP virus RNA (Aaslestad and Urbano, 1971; D. H. L. Bishop, H. G. Aaslestad, and H. F. Clark, unpublished experiments; F. Sokol, unpublished observations). The properties of rabies RNA so far investigated, including the nucleotide composition, are very similar to those of RNA from the morphologically similar, infectious VSV (Huang and Wagner, 1966; Brown *et al.*, 1967; Huppert *et al.*, 1967; Nakai and Howatson, 1968; Stampfer *et al.*, 1969; Mudd and Summers, 1970; Schincariol and Howatson, 1970) and Kern Canyon (D. H. L. Bishop, H. G. Aaslestad, and H F. Clark, unpublished results) virus.

Although preparations of purified Flury HEP virus contain, as mentioned above, an appreciable proportion of virions shorter than 180 nm, RNA species sedimenting more slowly than 45 S were not detected, or were found only in very small amounts, in nucleic acid preparations derived from this virus strain (Sokol *et al.*, 1969; D. H. L. Bishop, H. G. Aaslestad, and H F. Clark, unpublished results). Apparently, even truncated forms of Flury HEP virus contain RNA of full length. Similarly, ERA virions were shown to contain only the 45 S RNA (Sokol *et al.*, 1972; D. H. L. Bishop, H. G. Aaslestad, and H. F. Clark, unpublished results) as was expected from the very rare occurrence of truncated virus particles in purified preparations of this strain (Fig. 6; K. Hummeler, H. F. Clark, and F. Sokol, unpublished observation). When RNA derived from purified PM virions was sized by velocity centrifugation in a sucrose density gradient, however, two distinct species of RNA, sedimenting at 45 S and 20 S, were detected (Aaslestad and Urbano, 1971). The 20 S RNA most likely represents the genome of defective PM virions, but the final proof of its viral origin will come either from the comparison of its nucleotide sequences with that of 45 S viral RNA or from the isolation of this RNA species from separated, defective PM virus.

V. Viral Structural Proteins

Electrophoretic fractionation in SDS-containing polyacrylamide gels of purified rabies virions, which have been previously dissociated by treatment with SDS and 2-ME, revealed that the protein moiety of rabies virus is composed of four major polypeptides and one minor one of different molecular sizes (Fig. 7) (Sokol *et al.*, 1971). The major nucleocapsid protein corresponds to the virion polypeptide with the second largest molecular weight (Fig. 8b). It is a

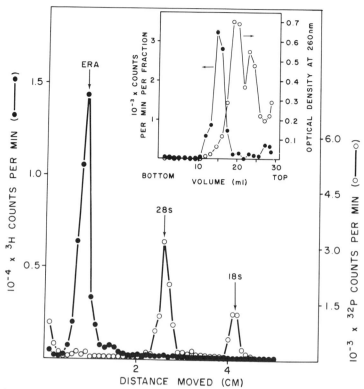

Fig. 6. Fractionation of rabies virus RNA by electrophoresis in polyacrylamide gel or velocity centrifugation in a sucrose density gradient. RNA was isolated from purified and [³H]uridine-labeled ERA virions by treatment with SDS, mixed with ³²P-labeled ribosomal RNA derived from hamster cells and electrophoresed in 2.2% polyacrylamide gel. *Inset:* Viral RNA was released from purified and [³H]uridine-labeled ERA virions by treatment at 20°C with 1% SDS, layered onto a sucrose gradient (5 to 20%, w/w) and centrifuged at 22,000 rev/min, 4°C, for 7 hours in the SW25.1 rotor of a Spinco centrifuge. The content of acid-insoluble radioactivity and the absorbance at 260 nm were then determined. The peak of the viral RNA band sedimented at 45 S.

phosphoprotein with phosphate groups concentrated at a terminal segment of the polypeptide chain (Sokol and Clark, 1973). The minor polypeptide could be clearly detected only when a relatively large amount of isolated nucleocapsid was fractionated by the same technique (Fig. 8a). It was recently identified as the nonphosphorylated fragment of the major nucleocapsid protein resulting from the cleavage of the nucleocapsid by proteolytic enzymes. The polypeptide with the largest molecular weight was found to be a glycoprotein, the glycopeptide portion of which contains D-glucosamine and L-fucose

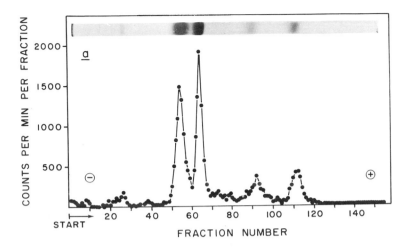

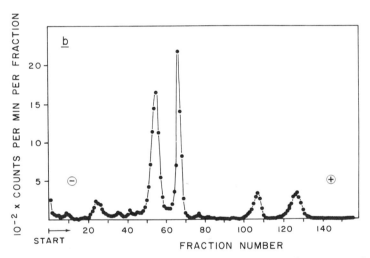

Fig. 7. Fractionation of rabies virus polypeptides by electrophoresis in polyacrylamide gel. a: Purified Flury HEP virus, labeled with a mixture of 16[³H]amino acids, was dissociated with SDS in a reducing environment and electrophoresed. The polypeptides were stained (inset) before the gel was sliced for determination of radioactivity. b: Same analysis carried out with ERA virions labeled with a mixture of [³H]amino acids. Under the conditions used in these experiments the polypeptides are separated on the basis of differences in molecular weight (Shapiro *et al.*, 1967). The low amount of polypeptides recovered in fractions 1 to 40 most likely corresponds to imperfectly dissociated aggregates. (Reprinted with permission from Sokol *et al.*, 1971.)

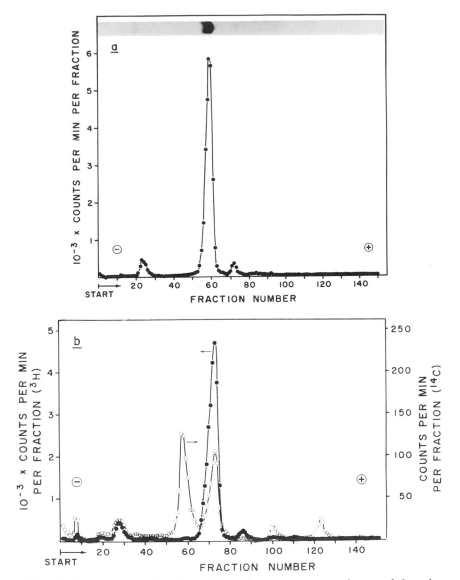

Fig. 8. Fractionation of polypeptides of rabies virus nucleocapsid by electrophoresis in polyacrylamide gel. a: Purified nucleocapsid, labeled with a mixture of
[³H]amino acids and isolated from DOC-treated virions (Flury HEP), was dissociated
by treatment with SDS and 2-ME and electrophoresed in 7% polyacrylamide gel for
13 hours. The gel was stained with Amido Black (inset) and then sliced for determination of the radioactivity. The component with the smallest molecular weight corresponds to the minor nucleocapsid polypeptide. The component closest to the top of
the gel is probably a dimer of the major nucleocapsid polypeptides. b: Nucleocapsids
labeled with a mixture of [³H]amino acids were mixed with purified virus labeled
with a mixture of [¹⁴C]amino acids, treated by SDS in a reducing environment and
electrophoresed. Note the coincidence of the major nucleocapsid polypeptide with the
virion polypeptide having the second largest molecular weight. (Reprinted with permission from Sokol *et al.*, 1971.)

94   *Frantisek Sokol*

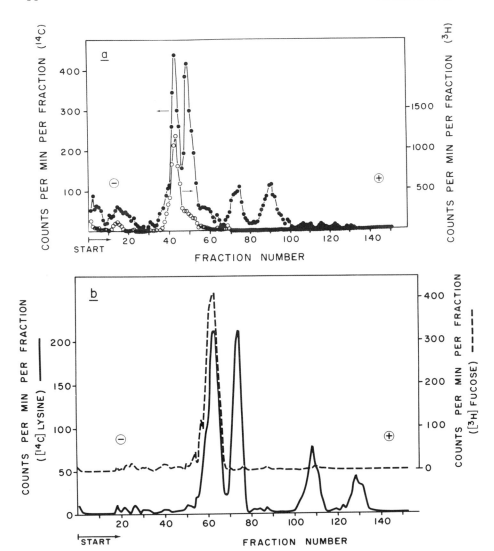

Fig. 9. Electrophoresis in polyacrylamide gel of polypeptides labeled with radioactive carbohydrates. a: Flury HEP virus labeled with [³H]D-glucosamine was mixed with virions labeled with a mixture of [¹⁴C]amino acids treated with SDS in a reducing environment and electrophoresed. b: ERA virus labeled with [³H]L-fucose was mixed with [¹⁴C]lysine-labeled virions, dissociated, and electrophoresed.

Note that in both experiments the component labeled with radioactive carbohydrate coincides with the virion polypeptide having the largest molecular weight. (Reprinted with permission from Sokol *et al.*, 1971, and György *et al.*, 1971.)

(Fig. 9), and probably other unidentified carbohydrates as well. The glycoprotein and the remaining two major polypeptides of relatively small molecular size are constituents of the viral envelope, if we define as envelope constituents those which are not contained in the viral nucleocapsid. The relative proportions of the four major polypeptides in virions of two different rabies virus strains are shown in Table IV, while the molecular weights of the five polypeptide components and the molecular composition of the protein moiety of the virus are given in Table V. The most important result of this analysis is that the glycoprotein, major nucleocapsid protein, and envelope protein 3 are present in the virions in approximately equimolar proportion, while the molecular ratio of any of these proteins to envelope protein 2 is close to 2. The implications of this finding in defining the arrangement of structural proteins in rabies virus are not yet recognized.

The envelope proteins 2 and 3 (membrane proteins) are more closely associated with the viral nucleocapsid than is the glycoprotein. When "core" particles isolated from NP-40-treated virus are dissociated into polypeptides and analyzed by polyacrylamide gel electrophoresis, only traces of glycoprotein can be detected, whereas the other three major polypeptides are present in a proportion similar to

Table IV

Relative Proportions of Major Rabies Virus Polypeptides[a]

Method	Virus strain	No. of determinations	Percent in component (average values)[b]			
			Glp	NCP	EP2	EP3
Optical density at 550 nm after staining with Amido Black	ERA	2	48.0	32.0	9.5	10.5
	Flury HEP	2	49.0	31.0	7.5	12.5
Labeling with [³H]amino acid mixture	ERA	2	47.0	34.0	8.5	10.5
	Flury HEP	6	43.5	32.5	10.5	13.5
Labeling with [¹⁴C]amino acid mixture	Flury HEP	5	43.0	34.5	10.0	12.5

[a] The relative proportions of the four major rabies virus polypeptides, separated by electrophoresis in SDS-containing polyacrylamide gel, was determined from the amount of dye bound by these components, as well as from the amount of ^{3}H or ^{14}C radioactivity recovered from them. A mixture of 16 [³H]amino acids or of 13 [¹⁴C]-amino acids was used for labeling the virions. (Reprinted with permission from Sokol *et al.*, 1971).

[b] Abbreviations: Glp, glycoprotein; NCP, nucleocapsid protein; EP2 and EP3, envelope proteins.

Table V

Protein Composition of Complete Rabies Virus[a]

Polypeptide[b]	Mol. wt.	No. of molecules per virion[c]
Glp	80,000	1,783
NCP	62,000	1,713
NCP-M[d]	55,000	76
EP2	40,000	789
EP3	25,000	1,661

[a] Reprinted with permission from Sokol *et al.*, 1971.

[b] Abbreviations as in footnote [b], Table IV.

[c] Average proportions of the four major polypeptides of Flury HEP virus used for the calculation (from Table IV): 44.3% Glp, 33.0% NCP, 9.8% EP2, 12.9% EP3.

[d] NCP-M, minor nucleocapsid protein; the number of NCP-M molecules per virion was calculated by using a weight ratio of NCP/NCP-M = 26.6.

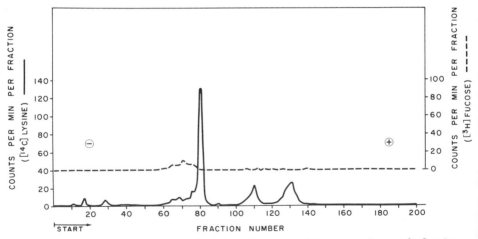

Fig. 10. Electrophoretogram of polypeptides derived from "core" particle fraction on Nonidet P-40-treated rabies virus (strain ERA). "Core" particles were isolated from [^{14}C]lysine- and [^{3}H]fucose-labeled and NP-40-treated (20 min at 22°C; ml detergent/g protein = 165) virus, dissociated into polypeptides, and fractionated by electrophoresis in SDS-polyacrylamide gel. The residual glycoprotein represents about 12% of total polypeptides. (Reprinted with permission from György *et al.*, 1971.)

that found in the whole virus (Fig. 10). On the other hand, the protein released from the virus by treatment with the nonionic detergent represents envelope glycoprotein contaminated with small
amounts of other structural proteins (Fig. 11). Thus, NP-40 treatment
effects a highly preferential, but not fully specific, release of the
envelope glycoprotein, leaving behind the other three major components and the viral RNA associated in the delipidized "core" particles. The specificity of the treatment depends on the ratio of NP-40
virus used (György et al., 1971). These results also demonstrate
that the glycoprotein is embedded in the envelope together with
the viral lipids (glycolipids). Thus, solubilization of lipids by NP-40
causes the detachment of the glycoprotein from the rest of the virion.

The amino acid composition of individual structural proteins of
rabies virus cannot be determined unless these components are
isolated in a pure form and in sufficiently large quantities. Electrophoretic fractionation of dissociated virion preparations, which

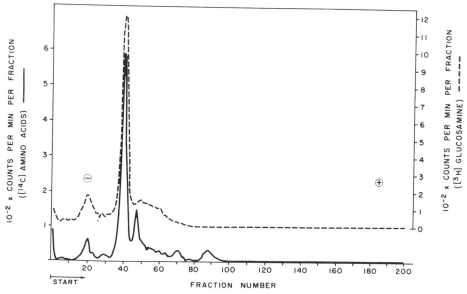

Fig. 11. Electrophoretogram of polypeptides derived from the glycoprotein fraction
of Nonidet P-40-treated rabies virus (strain ERA). Crude glycoprotein was isolated
from virus labeled with a mixture of [^{14}C]amino acids and [^{3}H]glucosamine treated
with NP-40 (20 min at 22°C; ml detergent/g protein = 33) virus, dissociated into
polypeptides and fractionated by electrophoresis in SDS-polyacrylamide gel. About
87% of the polypeptides correspond to glycoprotein. (Reprinted with permission from
György et al., 1971.)

Table VI

*Relative Proportions of Radioactivity Recovered in the Four Major Polypeptides
of Rabies Virions (Strain ERA) Labeled with Different Amino Acids*[a]

| | Percent of total radioactivity recovered in | | | |
Labeled precursor	Glp	NCP	EP2	EP3
[³H]Tryptophan	41.1	10.1	12.8	36.0
[³H]Serine	43.7	30.6	13.4	12.3
[³H]Leucine	39.4	28.7	16.5	15.4
[³H]Threonine	51.5	31.6	10.0	6.9
[¹⁴C]Lysine	44.0	32.2	14.8	9.0
[¹⁴C]Arginine	31.2	36.9	11.0	20.9

[a] All data are results from a single determination. Procedures and abbreviations are
similar to those given in Table IV.

have been labeled with different, single amino acids, has shown that
the nucleocapsid protein is rich in basic amino acids, that the envelope protein 3 is extremely rich in tryptophan and arginine, and that
the glycoprotein is rich in threonine (Table VI) (F. Sokol, unpublished results). These data also indicate that the envelope protein
3 is not a degradation product of envelope protein 2.

VI. Intracellular Virus and Viral Components

Rabies virus can be assembled either on the plasma membrane of
the infected cells or inside the cytoplasm, without any morphologically recognizable involvement of preexisting cell membranes (Hummeler *et al.*, 1967; Atanasiu *et al.*, 1969; Matsumoto and Kawai, 1969;
Matsumoto, 1970; Hummeler, 1971). In the latter type of maturation,
the whole viral envelope is most likely synthesized *de novo*. The
type of maturation depends on the virus strain used for infection, the
host cell, or both factors (see Chapter 2). The properties of intracellular virus, assembled in the cytoplasm, were not studied in detail, since methods for its purification have not been developed. Cell-
associated virus, released from disrupted cells, can be only partially
purified by the procedure used for purification of extracellular virus
(Sokol *et al.*, 1968). It often shows a much higher ratio of infectivity
to hemagglutinating activity than extracellular virus (Kuwert *et al.*,
1968; Sokol *et al.*, 1968), indicating a difference in the surface properties of these two virus forms. This ratio varies greatly from preparation to preparation, reflecting perhaps the proportion of truly in-

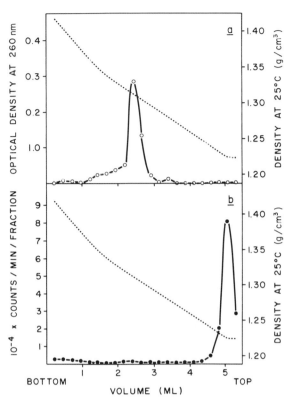

Fig. 12. Equilibrium centrifugation of intracellular, free nucleocapsid in CsCl solution. a: BHK-21 cells infected with the Flury HEP strain of rabies virus were disrupted by exposure to distilled water and mechanical homogenization. The cell extract was treated with deoxyribonuclease, mixed with CsCl and centrifuged to equilibrium. The viral nucleocapsid recovered at 1.32 g/cm³ density was further purified by repeated equilibrium centrifugation in CsCl solution. Symbols: ····, density; ○, optical density at 260 nm. b: Uninfected BHK-21 cells were mixed with [³H]uridine-labeled, purified Flury HEP virions and processed as described in the legend to Panel a. Note that nucleocapsid is not released from the virions during the purification procedure. Symbols: ····, density; ●, radioactivity.

tracellular virions to virus particles which have started to bud
through the plasma membrane.

Rabies virus-infected cells contain cytoplasmic inclusions composed mainly of free viral nucleocapsid particles (Hummeler *et al.*,
1968). Free viral nucleocapsids can be isolated from disrupted cells
and purified by a procedure (Sokol, 1973) similar to that used for the
purification of cell-associated nucleocapsids of a paramyxovirus
(Compans and Choppin, 1967) (Fig. 12). The properties of purified

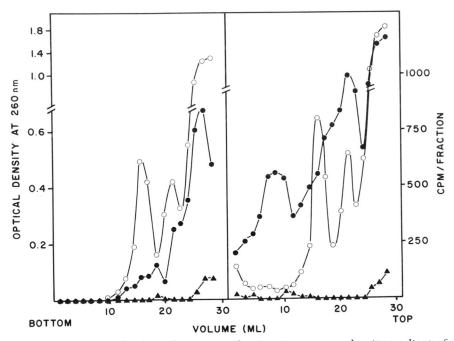

Fig. 13. Fractionation by velocity centrifugation in a sucrose density gradient of
rabies virus-specific RNA synthesized in infected hamster cells. *Right:* Confluent cultures of BHK-21 cells were infected with 100 PFU per cell of ERA virus. The virus
was allowed to absorb for 30 min at 33°C. After 1.5 hours, 1 μg/ml of actinomycin D
was added and the cultures were incubated at 33°C. The cells were labeled with 1
μCi/ml of [³H]uridine from 3 to 47 hours after virus absorption. Total RNA was then
isolated by treatment of the cells at 20°C with SDS and phenol, treated with deoxyribonuclease, extracted repeatedly with phenol, concentrated by precipitation with
ethanol, and layered onto 28 ml of linear sucrose gradient (5 to 23%, w/w). The content of the tube was centrifuged at 22,000 rev/min, at 4°C, for 8.5 hours in the SW 25.1
rotor of a Spinco centrifuge. Fractions were then assayed for absorbance at 260 nm (○)
and acid-insoluble radioactivity before (●) and after (▲) treatment at 33°C for 40 min
with 20 μg/ml of ribonuclease. *Left:* Similar experiments performed with mock-in-
fected cultures. The intrinsic 28 S and 18 S ribosomal RNAs served as sedimentation
markers.

intracellular nucleocapsid, including its helical structure, are similar to those of nucleocapsids derived from DOC-treated virions (see Table II; S. H. Fein and F. Sokol, unpublished data). RNA isolated from purified intracellular nucleocapsid, however, contains, in addition to the 45 S component, a more slowly sedimenting species, most likely derived from nucleocapsid particles fragmented during the purification procedure.

The infected cells contain several species of single-stranded, virus-specific RNA (Fig. 13). One of them, sedimenting at 45 S, is derived, at least in part, from mature virions and from free viral nucleocapsid. The function of the other RNA components, which sediment between 18 S and 38 S and are not found in uninfected cells, is not known. Rabies virus-infected cells do not seem to contain double-stranded virus-specific RNA (F. Sokol and H. F. Clark, unpublished data).

Acknowledgment

Supported, in part, by Public Health Service Research Grants CA-10815 from the National Cancer Institute and AI-09706 from the National Institute of Allergy and Infectious Diseases.

References

Aaslestad, H. G., and Urbano, C. (1971). *J. Virol.* 8, 922.

Aaslestad, H. G., Clark, H F., Bishop, D. H. L., and Koprowski, H. (1971). *J. Virol.* 7, 726.

Atanasiu, P., Lépine, P., and Sisman, J. (1969). *Acad. Sci.* 269, 1226.

Baltimore, D., Huang, A. S., and Stampfer, M. (1970). *Proc. Natl. Acad. Sci. USA* 66, 572.

Brown, F., Martin, S. J., Cartwright, B., and Crick, J. (1967). *J. Gen. Virol.* 1, 479.

Choppin, P. W., Klenk, H. D., Compans, R. W., and Caliguiri, L. A. (1971). *Perspect. Virol.* 7, 127–158.

Compans, R. W., and Choppin, P. W. (1967). *Proc. Natl. Acad. Sci. USA* 57, 949.

Compans, R. W., and Choppin, P. W. (1971). *In* "Comparative Virology" (K. Maramorosch and E. Kurstak, eds.), pp. 407–432. Academic Press, New York.

Crick, J., and Brown, F. (1970). *In* "The Biology of Large RNA Viruses" (R. D. Barry and B. W. J. Mahy, eds.), pp. 133–140. Academic Press, New York.

Defendi, V., and Wiktor, T. J. (1966). *Symp. Ser. Immunobiol. Stand.* 1, 119.

György, E., Sheehan, M. C., and Sokol, F. (1971). *J. Virol.* 8, 649.

Diringer, H., Kulas, H. P., Schneider, L. G., and Schlumberger, H. D. (1973). *Zeitschrift für Naturforschung* 28, 90.

Hamparian, V. V., Hilleman, M. R., and Ketler, A. (1963). *Proc. Soc. Exp. Biol. Med.* 112, 1040.

Huang, A. S., and Wagner, R. R. (1966). *J. Mol. Biol.* 22, 381.

Hummeler, K. (1971). *In* "Comparative Virology" (K. Maramorosch and E. Kurstak, eds.), pp. 361–386. Academic Press, New York.

Hummeler, K., Koprowski, H., and Wiktor, T. J. (1967). *J. Virol.* 1, 152.
Hummeler, K., Tomassini, N., Sokol, F., Kuwert, E., and Koprowski, H. (1968). *J. Virol.* 2, 1191.
Huppert, J., Rosenbergova, M., Gresland, L., and Harel, L. (1967). *In* "The Molecular Biology of Viruses" (S. J. Colter and W. Paranchych, eds.). pp. 463–468. Academic Press, New York.
Kissling, R. E., and Reese, D. R. (1963). *J. Immunol.* 91, 362.
Kuwert, E., Wiktor, T. J., Sokol, F., and Koprowski, H. (1968). *J. Virol.* 2, 1381.
Maes, R. F., Kaplan, M. M., Wiktor, T. J., Campbell, T. B., and Koprowski, H. (1967). *In* "The Molecular Biology of Viruses" (S. J. Colter and W. Paranchych, eds.). pp. 449–462. Academic Press, New York.
Matsumoto, S. (1970). *Advan. Virus Res.* 16, 257.
Matsumoto, S., and Kawai, A. (1969). *Virology* 39, 449.
Mudd, J. A., and Summers, D. F. (1970). *Virology* 42, 958.
Nakai, T., and Howatson, A. F. (1968). *Virology* 35, 268.
Neurath, A. R., and Rubin, B. A. (1971). "Viral Structural Components as Immunogens of Prophylactic Value." Karger, Basel.
Neurath, A. R., Wiktor, T. J., and Koprowski, H. (1966). *J. Bacteriol.* 92, 102.
Neurath, A. R., Vernon, S. K., Dobkin, M. B., and Rubin, B. A. (1971). *J. Gen. Virol.* 14, 33.
Remlinger, P. (1918). *C. R. Acad. Sci.* 166, 750.
Schincariol, A. L., and Howatson, A. F. (1970). *Virology* 42, 732.
Schneider, L. G., Horzinek, M., and Novicky, R. (1971). *Arch. Gesamte Virusforsch.* 34, 360.
Sedwick, W. D., and Wiktor, T. J. (1967). *J. Virol.* 1, 1224.
Shapiro, A. L., Viñuela, E., and Maizel, J. V., Jr. (1967). *Biochem. Biophys. Res. Commun.* 28, 815.
Sokol, F. (1971). *Proc. Int. Congr. Microbiol., 10th, 1970* pp. 551–562.
Sokol, F. (1973). *In* "Laboratory Techniques in Rabies" (M. M. Kaplan and H. Koprowski, eds.) pp. 165–178. Geneva. *World Health Organ. Monogr. Ser.*
Sokol, F., and Clark, H. F. (1973). *Virology* 52, 246.
Sokol, F., Kuwert, E., Wiktor, T. J., Hummeler, K., and Koprowski, H. (1968). *J. Virol.* 2, 836.
Sokol, F., Schlumberger, H. D., Wiktor, T. J., Koprowski, H., and Hummeler, K. (1969). *Virology* 38, 651.
Sokol, F., Stanček, D., and Koprowski, H. (1971). *J. Virol.* 7, 241.
Sokol, F., Clark, H. F., György, E., and Tomassini, N. (1972). *J. Gen. Virol.* 16, 173.
Spirin, A. S. (1963). *Progr. Nucleic Acid Res.* 1, 301.
Stampfer, M., Baltimore, D., and Huang, A. S. (1969). *J. Virol.* 4, 154.
Wiktor, T. J., György, E., Schlumberger, H. D., Sokol, F., and Koprowski, H. (1973). *J. Immunol.* 110, 269.

CHAPTER 5

Hemagglutinin of Rabies Virus

Pekka Halonen

I. Introduction

Rabies virus hemagglutination had been sought for in many laboratories, particularly since the virus was adapted to non-nervous tissue culture (Kissling, 1958), and the spiked surface projections found on virus particles (Hummeler *et al.*, 1967) are a property associated with hemagglutinating activity in other viruses. Late in 1966, a systematic series of experiments was carried out at the Center for Disease Control, Atlanta, Georgia, by a group of virologists working with rubella, rabies, and arboviruses, who finally revealed the unique requirements necessary for preparation and demonstration of rabies hemagglutinin (Halonen *et al.*, 1968). This was achieved after more than 200 experimental combinations of different cell culture media, incubation temperatures, pH levels, erythrocyte suspensions, etc., had been used. In several respects hemagglutination of rabies and

other bullet-shaped viruses was found to resemble that of arboviruses: avian erythrocytes are more sensitive than mammalian;
hemagglutination is pH dependent; hemagglutinin is extremely sensitive to nonspecific serum inhibitors of lipoprotein origin; hemagglutinin is labile at pH levels below 7.0. However, rabies hemagglutinin has properties which many arbovirus hemagglutinins do not
share, such as the strict requirement of low temperature (0°–4°C) for
incubation of erythrocytes, and inactivation of hemagglutinin by
Tween 80. The finding that viruses with a surface structure similar to
that of myxoviruses have an arbovirus-type hemagglutination was
unexpected.

The rabies hemagglutination test has been successfully used in
the purification and chemical analysis of virus (Sokol *et al.*, 1968;
Schneider *et al.*, 1971a), and has also been applied to vaccine improvement studies (Wiktor *et al.*, 1969; Schneider *et al.*, 1971b). A
great disappointment, however, has been the failure to develop the
hemagglutination inhibition test for assay of rabies antibody. The sensitivity of the hemagglutination inhibition test has not been sufficiently high, low antibody titers have resulted, and it has proved
difficult to remove nonspecific serum inhibitors without decreasing
antibody titers.

II. Optimal Conditions for Preparation and Demonstration of Hemagglutinin

A. Virus Strains

CVS 11 strain adapted to primary hamster kidney cell culture
(Kissling and Reese, 1963) was used in the development of the
hemagglutination test. However, hemagglutinating activity is not
strain dependent, and several other strains have been used later:
Pitman-Moore, Pasteur, Flury high egg passage strains, and ERA
(Sokol *et al.*, 1968; Kuwert *et al.*, 1968; Schneider *et al.*, 1971a).

B. Cell Cultures

Hemagglutinating activity has been demonstrated only with virus
grown in serum-free tissue cultures and not in tissue cultures with
fetal calf serum (Halonen *et al.*, 1968) or in mouse or hamster brain
material (Kuwert *et al.*, 1968). Nonspecific inhibitors in serum and in

brain material apparently inactivate the hemagglutinin but not the infectivity. Cell cultures of BHK-21 (Halonen *et al.*, 1968; Kuwert *et al.*, 1968; Schneider *et al.*, 1971a), Wl-38 and Nil-2 (Kuwert *et al.*, 1968) have been successfully used for hemagglutinin preparation, but in BHK-21 cells the highest titers have been consistently obtained in either suspension (Halonen *et al.*, 1968), monolayer (Kuwert *et al.*, 1968), or roller cultures (Schneider *et al.*, 1971a).

In cell culture maintenance media serum has been replaced by 0.1% to 0.4% bovine serum albumin, fraction V. However, if bovine serum albumin is necessary it is only to support the cells long enough for maximal yield of virus and not directly for the preparation of hemagglutinin. With vesicular stomatitis virus hemagglutinin titers after a 24-hour harvest period are at least as high in medium without bovine albumin as that obtained with 0.1–0.2% albumin (P. Halonen, unpublished observation).

In this connection it should be noted that not every lot of bovine serum albumin is necessarily completely inhibitor free. A single lot of rabies hemagglutinin varied in titer from 1:8 to 1:64 when various bovine albumin-borate saline solutions, pH 9.0, prepared from 7 batches of bovine serum albumin, fraction V (reagent for microbiological use, Armour Pharmaceutical Company, Kankakee, Illinois) were used in simultaneous titrations (P. Halonen, unpublished observation).

C. Erythrocytes

Erythrocytes of geese, adult chickens, 2-day-old chicks, guinea pigs, rats, sheep, human type O, vervet, and rhesus monkeys have been tested for sensitivity to rabies hemagglutinin (Halonen *et al.*, 1968). All are agglutinated but the highest titers have been obtained with an 0.25% suspension of goose erythrocytes. The sensitivity of different batches of goose erythrocytes varies considerably.

D. Optimal pH Level

The hemagglutination is strictly pH dependent. No hemagglutination has been observed with goose erythrocytes above pH 6.6 (Halonen *et al.*, 1968) or 6.8 (Kuwert *et al.*, 1968). The optimum pH may vary from 6.2 (Halonen *et al.*, 1968; Schneider *et al.*, 1971a) to 6.4 (Sokol *et al.*, 1968).

The hemagglutination of other bullet-shaped viruses is also pH dependent, each virus having its own optimum pH: VSV Indiana, pH 5.8; VSV New Jersey, pH 6.4; Cocal and Kern Canyon, pH 6.2 (Halonen et al., 1968).

E. OPTIMAL TEMPERATURE

With goose erythrocytes and a pH of 6.2 the optimal incubation temperature of rabies hemagglutination is 0°–4°C (Halonen et al., 1968; Kuwert et al., 1968). Once it is fully developed after incubation in an ice slurry, the hemagglutination pattern rapidly reverts to negative at room temperature (Halonen et al., 1968), and at the same time adsorbed virus elutes from the erythrocytes (Kuwert et al., 1968). Even at 4°C virus is quantitatively eluted after a 3-hour incubation (Kuwert et al., 1968).

III. Characteristics of Hemagglutinin

A linear relationship between virus infectivity and hemagglutinin titer was demonstrated by Kuwert et al. (1968), when the infectivity was 10^6 PFU/ml or higher.

In equilibrium sedimentation experiments of concentrated rabies virus grown in BHK-21 suspension cultures the hemagglutinating activity was localized exclusively in fractions containing infectious virus and truncated and aberrantly shaped particles exhibiting the spiked surface projections (Murphy et al., 1968). The density of the peak activity was 1.22 g/cm³. No hemagglutinating activity was found in the fractions with the major complement-fixing activity. These preliminary observations suggested that the hemagglutinating capacity is a surface function of the virus, and if truncated and aberrantly shaped particles have the characteristic surface structure they may also hemagglutinate.

Kuwert et al. (1968) concentrated virus grown in BHK-21 cells with dialysis against carboxymethylcellulose and in fractions collected after rate zonal centrifugation in sucrose gradient found only one peak of hemagglutinin associated with the peak of infectivity. No indication of a more slowly sedimenting "soluble" hemagglutinin was found in their experiments, neither in extracts of infected cells nor in virus preparations harvested from infectious cell culture media. The authors concluded that in this respect rabies virus differs from the myxoviruses that have noninfectious, slowly sedimenting hemagglutinin in addition to hemagglutinin associated with the virion. One of the crucial questions to be answered in the study of rabies hemagglutinin is whether a "soluble" hemagglutinating component is present in rabies virus preparations, and the possibility of releasing such a component from the virion, as can be done with lipid solvents in myxoviruses, paramyxoviruses, and arboviruses.

Recently, Arstila (1972) has demonstrated that hemagglutinin of vesicular stomatitis virus can be separated by sucrose gradient centrifugation into two components with different sedimenting properties corresponding to infectious B and noninfectious T particles. T particles appear to be significantly more potent in hemagglutination than infectious virions. In addition, indirect evidence suggests that some aggregated surface projections or small rosettes, in the same fractions as T particles, also have hemagglutinating activity. Preliminary findings (P. Arstila, personal communication) indicate that treatment of VSV virions with a nonionic detergent Nonidet P40 results in a hemagglutinating preparation with a single polypeptide as determined by polyacrylamide gel electrophoresis, and with aggregated spikes in electron micrographs.

Evidence of two hemagglutinating and infectious components of rabies virus with buoyant densities of 1.20 and 1.22 g/cm^3 has been reported by Schneider *et al.* (1971b). After two treatments with a low concentration of saponin at 4°C and pH 8.2 all rabies hemagglutinin banded at 1.29 g/cm^3 in CsCl equilibrium density gradient centrifugation, and the infectivity decreased 10,000 times or more. The effect of saponin depended on the treatment time and the temperature. At 37°C hemagglutinin titers increased up to 1 hour, at which time the titers were four times as high as in the nontreated preparations. Further treatment resulted in a twofold decrease from the starting level. At 37°C there first was a decrease and then an increase, with peak titers after 90–120 minutes. Electron microscopy of hemagglutinin treated twice with saponin showed uniformly coiled material.

Rabies hemagglutinin is heat labile. Heating at 56°C destroys its activity in 30–60 minutes (Halonen *et al.*, 1968; Kuwert *et al.*, 1968). Tween 80, with or without ether, inactivates rabies and VSV hemagglutinin completely (Halonen *et al.*, 1968; Kuwert *et al.*, 1968; Arstila *et al.*, 1969), distinguishing the nature of bullet-shaped virus hemagglutinins from that of myxoviruses, paramyxoviruses, rubella, and many arboviruses. Ether also inactivates rabies hemagglutinin, as does trypsin, pronase, and deoxycholate (Kuwert *et al.*, 1968; Schneider *et al.*, 1971b).

The effect of phospholipase C on rabies hemagglutinin is interesting, since it has been reported to remove the lipid envelope from

VSV particles while leaving the spikes unaffected (Cartwright *et al.*, 1969). In the experiments of Kuwert *et al.* (1968) phospholipase C inactivated rabies hemagglutinin completely. After sucrose gradient centrifugation at pH 9.0 hemagglutinin titer of a purified preparation of VSV treated with phospholipase C was the same as or higher than that of the nontreated control (P. Halonen, unpublished observation).

β-Propiolactone at 0.01–0.05% concentrations inactivated rabies infectivity but not hemagglutinin (Halonen *et al.*, 1968) when the method of Sever *et al.* (1964) was used and when the pH was frequently adjusted with NaOH during treatment. But Kuwert *et al.* (1968) and Wiktor *et al.* (1969) reported complete inactivation of rabies hemagglutinin with 0.025% β-propiolactone. At low pH levels rabies hemagglutinin is extremely labile. Even at the optimal pH level of 6.2 the hemagglutinating activity is slowly inactivated.

The nature of the hemagglutinin can be characterized further by identifying the specific receptors on the erythrocytes. RDE, proteolytic enzymes, and chemicals blocking sulfhydryl groups do not change the sensitivity of goose erythrocytes to rabies hemagglutinin (Kuwert *et al.*, 1968). Since the nonspecific serum inhibitors and the receptors on the erythrocytes are of identical or similar chemical nature, the receptors of rabies hemagglutinin on goose erythrocytes may be polar lipids attached to proteins (see Section V,A, below).

A. Salt-Dependent Hemagglutinin

A salt-dependent hemagglutinin like that reported by Schluederberg and Nakamura (1967) with measles virus can be demonstrated with rabies virus (P. Halonen, unpublished observation). In the test, $0.8\,M\,(NH_4)_2SO_4$ is added to the standard hemagglutination diluent of bovine albumin–borate saline solution, and this mixture is used as virus diluent. The phosphate saline solutions used as erythrocyte diluents must be changed slightly to obtain the correct final pH levels in hemagglutination. The optimal pH of the salt-dependent hemagglutinin is 5.8 when incubated at 0°–4°C with goose erythrocytes, and, contrary to the standard hemagglutinating activity, salt-dependent hemagglutinin can also be titrated at 37°C, as shown in Table I. Salt-dependent hemagglutinin titers are 2 to 8 times as high as hemagglutinin titers.

The nature of the salt-dependent hemagglutinin of rabies virus has not been studied and the possible advantages of the test are not known except in the hemagglutination inhibition test.

Table I

Effect of pH and Incubation Temperature on Hemagglutination and Salt-Dependent Hemagglutination of Rabies Virus with Goose Erythrocytes[a]

| | Hemagglutination | | | | | | | | | | | | | | | | Cell |
| | at 0°C | | | | | | | | at 37°C | | | | | | | | con- |
pH	4	8	16	32	64	128	256	512	4	8	16	32	64	128	256	512	trol
5.8	+	+	+	∓	−	−	−	−	−	−							
6.0	+	+	+	±	−	−	−	−	−	−							−
6.2	+	+	+	+	−	−	−	−	−	−							−
6.4	+	+	+	∓	−	−	−	−	−	−							−
6.6	+	±	−	−	−	−	−	−	−	−							−
6.8	−	−	−	−	−	−	−	−	−	−							−
	Salt-dependent hemagglutination																
5.8	+	+	+	+	+	±	∓	−	+	+	+	+	+	+	±	∓	∓
6.0	+	+	+	+	±	∓	∓	−	+	+	+	+	+	±	∓	∓	∓
6.2	+	+	+	+	±	∓	−	−	+	∓	∓	∓	∓	∓	∓	∓	∓
6.4	+	+	±	∓	−	−	−	−	+	∓	∓	∓	∓	∓	∓	∓	∓
6.6	−	∓	∓	∓	−	−	−	−	+	∓	∓	∓	∓	∓	∓	∓	∓
6.8	−	−	−	−	−	−	−	−	+	∓	∓	∓	∓	∓	∓	∓	∓

[a] + = complete agglutination of erythrocytes; ± and ∓ = partial agglutination; − = no agglutination.

IV. Relationship between Hemagglutinating and Immunizing Capacity of Rabies Virus Particles

As indicated by Murphy *et al.* (1968) the rabies virus hemagglutinin has a potential value in the hemagglutination inhibition test for assay of immunity to rabies, since the hemagglutinating antigen is separate from the complement-fixing and gel precipitating antigens, and would obviously measure almost identical antibodies as the neutralization test. A close relationship between the hemagglutinating antigen and immunizing potency of rabies virus was clearly demonstrated by Schneider *et al.* (1971b) when mice were immunized with gradient purified saponin-treated hemagglutinin. It was almost equally as immunogenic as gradient purified virion, and significantly more potent than the reference vaccine, in spite of the low protein concentration of the purified hemagglutinin.

Wiktor *et al.* (1969) were able to immunize mice against rabies with virion-free concentrated "soluble" antigen of high CF activity but no hemagglutinating activity. Before immunization the antigen was treated with β-propiolactone or UV irradiation. According to Schneider *et al.* (1971b) there is a direct relationship between the measurable complement-fixing and protective activities of rabies virus preparations as long as a certain structural conformation, especially the immunizing surface protein, remains unaltered. If the surface structure is disrupted beyond a critical level only CF activity can be measured. It should also be pointed out that, with the techniques used at the moment, hemagglutination is not as accurate a measure of viral antigen in rabies as in influenza and other viruses. Rabies hemagglutinin is rendered permanently nonmeasurable after a few minutes at low pH levels, or in a few seconds after contact with nonspecific serum inhibitors, yet the infectivity and all the other antigenicities may remain unaltered.

V. Hemagglutination Inhibition Test

After the development of the rabies hemagglutination test it was to be expected that the hemagglutination inhibition technique be developed as a simple and reliable test for assay of protective antibodies in rabies. Unfortunately, these expectations have not been realized to date.

The specificity of the hemagglutination inhibition test has been shown with antirabies hyperimmune sera from burros and goats (Halonen *et al.*, 1968). The hemagglutination inhibition titers of these sera were between 1:160 and 1:1280, and normal burro and goat sera produced no inhibition at a dilution of 1:20. A further indication of specificity was obtained from the observation that the hemagglutinins of other bullet-shaped viruses (VSV-Indiana, VSV-New Jersey, Cocal, Kern Canyon) did not cross react by hemagglutination inhibition with antirabies hyperimmune sera and had homologous titers of 1:80 to 1:160. However, the hemagglutination inhibition titers of rabies hyperimmune sera are 10–100 times lower than the neutralization titers. Another complication of the test is noted in tests with human sera collected after vaccination with duck embryo vaccine; the sera from these vaccines exhibit high titered hemagglutinin against goose erythrocytes, apparently produced by the duck tissue in the vaccine. This serum hemagglutinin activity can usually be adsorbed by two-cycle treatment with packed goose erythrocytes, or avoided by using chick erythrocytes in the test.

The presence of high-titered nonspecific inhibitors in all human and animal serum specimens makes it even more difficult to measure

Table II

Titers of Hemagglutination Inhibition and Inhibition of Salt-Dependent Hemagglutination in Antirabies Hyperimmune Burro Serum and in Normal Burro Serum

Serum	Hemagglutination inhibition	Inhibition of salt-dependent hemagglutination
Antirabies, adsorbed with kaolin	640	2560
Normal, adsorbed with kaolin	<20	<20
Antirabies, untreated	≥5120	≥5120
Normal, untreated	≥5120	≥5120

low antibody titers. To remove these inhibitors serum has to be diluted 1:10 for kaolin treatment at pH 9.0, resulting in a 1:20 dilution of serum to start with. Even at this dilution some sera from unvaccinated people are capable of inhibiting rabies hemagglutination, suggesting an incomplete removal of nonspecific inhibitors. The specific hemagglutination inhibition titers are so low that only two hemagglutinin units are required in the antibody assay, but such a small quantity of antigen again results in high titers (from 1:1000 to 1:40,000) of nonspecific inhibitors.

With salt-dependent hemagglutinin the specific antibody titers are two to four times as high as with standard hemagglutinin, but the nonspecific inhibition titers are equally high in each test, as indicated in Table II.

A. Nature of Nonspecific Serum Inhibitors

The identification of the chemical nature of nonspecific inhibitors of rabies hemagglutinin could make possible the development of specific techniques for removing these substances from serum without decreasing the antibody titers. Moreover, the receptors of the hemagglutinin on erythrocytes are most probably the same or similar compounds. This problem has been approached by Halonen *et al.* (1969) and Halonen *et al.* (1974).

Preliminary experiments with heparin-$CaCl_2$ precipitation indicated that about one-half of the total inhibitor activity of pooled normal human serum was associated with β-lipoproteins. After ultracentrifugation of serum at raised densities, inhibitor activity could be demonstrated in each of the fractions with density values at which either very low density, low density, or high density lipoproteins

Table III

Nonspecific Inhibitor Activities to Rabies Hemagglutinin
in Lipid Fractions of Pooled Normal Human Serum[a]

Fraction	Inhibitor titer
Untreated serum	4000
Total lipid extract	640
Neutral lipids	20
Polar lipids	1280
Phosphatidylethanolamine	320
Phosphatidylcholine	400
Sphingomyelin	320
Lysophosphatidylcholine	160
Buffer	10

[a] Lipids were extracted with chloroform–methanol (1:1) and fractioned with silicic acid chromatography followed by preparative thin-layer chromatography. Buffer was 0.13 M tris buffer, pH 8.3 with 1 mM EDTA and 2 mM sodium dodecyl sulfate (Halonen *et al.*, 1974).

float. The highest inhibitor activity was always found in the fractions in which low density lipoprotein was present. After delipidation of serum with diethyl ether–ethanol treatment no inhibitor activity was detected. When lipid extracts of the pooled serum were fractionated no activity was found in the neutral lipid fraction, virtually all the activity being in the polar lipids (Table III). All phospholipid fractions isolated from polar lipids possessed inhibitory activity. This finding was confirmed with commercial phospholipids which caused the same inhibition of rabies hemagglutinin as the serum phospholipids. The highest inhibition titers, 1:800 with a lipid concentration of 2.0 mg/ml, was obtained with phosphatidyl serine and phosphatidyl inositol. The low activity of phosphatidyl ethanolamine and cerebrocides may have been due to their inability to disperse as sufficiently fine particles in water.

Now that the chemical nature of the nonspecific inhibitors is known, it may be possible to develop efficient techniques for removing the inhibitors from serum without decreasing the antibody titer. Another possibility for improving the hemagglutination inhibition test is to increase the sensitivity of rabies hemagglutinin to antibody. Just as treatment with Tween 80 and ether increase the sensitivity of measles hemagglutinin, so rabies hemagglutinin treated with saponin, Nonidet P40 or other surface active chemicals may produce more suitable antigens than those presently available for the rabies hemagglutination inhibition test.

References

Arstila, P. (1972). *Acta Pathol. Microbiol. Scand., Sect. B* **80**, 33.

Arstila, P., Halonen, P. E., and Salmi, A. (1969). *Arch. Gesamte Virusforsch.* **27**, 198.

Cartwright, B., Smale, C. J., and Brown, F. (1969). *J. Gen. Virol.* **5**, 1.

Halonen, P. E., Murphy, F. A., Fields, B. N., and Reese, D. R. (1968). *Proc. Soc. Exp. Biol. Med.* **128**, 1037.

Halonen, P. E., Nikkari, T., and Toivanen, P. (1969). *Scand. J. Clin. Lab. Invest.* **23**, Suppl. 108, 59.

Halonen, P. E., Toivanen, P., and Nikkari, T. (1974). *J. Gen. Virol.* **22**, 309.

Hummeler, K., Koprowski, H., and Wiktor, T. J. (1967). *J. Virol.* **1**, 152.

Kissling, R. E. (1958). *Proc. Soc. Exp. Biol. Med.* **98**, 223.

Kissling, R. E., and Reese, D. R. (1963). *J. Immunol.* **91**, 362.

Kuwert, E., Wiktor, T. J., Sokol, F., and Koprowski, H. (1968). *J. Virol.* **2**, 1381.

Murphy, F. A., Halonen, P. E., Gary, G. W., Jr., and Reese, D. R. (1968). *J. Gen. Virol.* **3**, 289.

Norrby, E. (1962). *Proc. Soc. Exp. Biol. Med.* **127**, 1037.

Schluederberg, A., and Nakamura, M. (1967). *Virology* **33**, 297.

Schneider, L. G., Horzinek, M., and Matheka, H. D. (1971a). *Arch. Gesamte Virusforsch.* **34**, 351.

Schneider, L. G., Horzinek, M., and Novicky, R. (1971b). *Arch. Gesamte Virusforsch.* **34**, 360.

Sever, J. L., Castelland, G. A., Pelon, W., Huebner, R. J., and Wolman, F. J. (1964). *J. Lab. Clin. Med.* **64**, 983.

Sokol, F., Kuwert, E., Wiktor, T. J., Hummeler, K., and Koprowski, H. (1968). *J. Virol.* **2**, 836.

Wiktor, T. J., Sokol, F., Kuwert, E., and Koprowski, H. (1969). *Proc. Soc. Exp. Biol. Med.* **131**, 799.

CHAPTER 6

Passive Hemagglutination Test

Patricia M. Gough and Richard E. Dierks

The passive hemagglutination procedure (RPHA) has recently been adapted to the titration of antibodies against rabies virus in human sera. The test, as a means of determining the antibody titers, offers several advantages over other procedures available for this purpose.

This titration method involves the attachment of rabies virus to red blood cells by means of chromium chloride. Sera is diluted in microtiter plates and the virus–erythrocyte complex is added. After approximately an hour, reaction between rabies antibodies in the sera and the virus results in the passive agglutination of the red blood cells. The absence of antibodies in a serum is readily detected as a sharp button of unreacted erythrocytes in the bottom of the well in the microtiter plate.

I. Passive Hemagglutination Procedure

A. VIRAL ANTIGEN PRODUCTION AND CONCENTRATION

Rabies virus, CVS-11 (Kissling, 1958) is used for antigen production. This virus has been passaged 112 times in primary hamster kidney cell cultures and 13 times in baby hamster kidney cell cultures: BHK 21-clone 13 (MacPherson and Stoker, 1962) and BHK 21-clone 13 S (Vaheri *et al.*, 1965).

The cells used for antigen production are BHK 21-clone 13 cells. They are grown in roller bottles (654.5 cm^2 surface area) in BHK 21 medium (MacPherson and Stoker, 1962) containing 10% (v/v) heat-inactivated fetal calf sera, 10% (v/v) tryptose phosphate broth and antibiotics. A 48- to 72-hour stock culture of BHK 21-clone 13 cells is suspended in 100 ml of medium in each roller bottle. The bottles are pulsed 10 sec with CO_2 to enhance cell attachment and then incubated at 37°C until monolayers are formed at 48 hours. The growth medium is removed and the monolayers washed twice with phosphate buffered saline (Dulbecco and Vogt, 1954). Each roller bottle is infected with 10 ml of a 10^{-3} dilution of CVS-11 virus containing $10^{7.3}$ mouse intracerebral LD_{50}/ml. Diethylaminoethyl (DEAE) dextran, 50 μg/ml is added to the virus just prior to infecting the cell cultures. The inoculum is removed after 1 hour absorption at 34°C and replaced with 100 ml of BHK 21 medium containing 10% (v/v) tryptose phosphate broth, 0.4% (w/v) bovine serum albumin (fraction V, bovine albumin powder) and antibiotics. The roller cultures are then incubated for 96–120 hours at 34°C with adjustment of the pH as needed to maintain a pH of 7.2–7.4. The tissue culture fluids are harvested, centrifuged for 20 min at 1000 g to remove cellular debris, and either concentrated or frozen at -70°C for future use. Each lot of virus is routinely tested for mycoplasma contamination and assayed for virus titer at this point. A minimum titer of $10^{6.5}$ MLD_{50} as assayed by intracerebral inoculation of 3-week-old mice should be obtained if the lot is to be used for antigen production.

The virus is concentrated by zinc acetate precipitation of protein. Fifty parts of infectious tissue culture fluid are mixed with one part 1.0 *M* zinc acetate solution (pH 5.0). The mixture is allowed to stand at 4°C for 20–30 min with occasional agitation. It then is centrifuged at 1000 g for 20 min and the supernatant fluid discarded. The precipitate is resuspended to one-twentieth of the original volume of tissue culture fluids in a saturated solution of disodium ethylenediaminetetraacetate adjusted to pH 7.8 by the addition of solid tris-(hydroxymethyl)-aminomethane. The resulting virus suspension is clarified by centrifugation at 1000 g for 20 min and then dialyzed against 0.86% NaCl for 18 hours; the virus is stored at −70°C in small aliquots for future use. The recovery of virus from the precipitation procedure, based on intracerebral mouse titrations, averages from 90 to 100%.

Rabies virus (CVS-27) grown in suckling mouse brain and purified by chromatography on an ECTEOLA-cellulose column (Thomas *et al.*, 1965) has also been used as a RPHA antigen. It was just as satisfactory for this purpose but the purification procedure was less convenient than that with virus grown in tissue culture.

B. VIRUS–ERYTHROCYTE COUPLING

Rabies virus is coupled to goose erythrocytes for use in the test system. Human O, monkey, sheep, dog, guinea pig, hamster, mouse, chicken, and baby chick red blood cells also have been tested for use in the passive hemagglutination procedure, but results indicated that goose cells give the highest and most reproducible titers. The erythrocytes are collected in modified Alsevers solution (Kent *et al.*, 1946) and are aged at least 4 days before use. The erythrocytes are washed three times in 0.86% NaCl immediately before use.

Various buffers, including tris-(hydroxymethyl)-aminomethane, phosphate, borate, and acetate have been used for washing the red blood cells but, when they were substituted for 0.86% saline, precipitation of chromium salts accompanied by hemolysis of the erythrocytes often occurred during the coupling process.

A complex then is formed between rabies virus and the goose erythrocytes with hydrated chromium chloride, as described by Gold and Fudenberg (1967), using equal volumes of virus suspension, 0.1% chromium chloride solution in 0.86% NaCl, and packed saline-washed erythrocytes. The chromium chloride solution used as the complexing agent can be stored at 4°C for 1–2 weeks without any apparent adverse effects. There is a shift in the color spectrum from dark green to gray green on storage but this does not affect the coupling reaction. Increasing concentrations of chromium chloride greater than 0.1% caused increasing problems with agglutination of the red blood cells during the coupling process.

When the virus is combined with the red blood cells first, followed by the addition of the coupling agent, chromium chloride, the resulting antigen gives more reproducible results than when the reagents are added together in any other order. After 5 min of interaction at room temperature, the sensitized erythrocytes are washed three times with saline and are suspended at a concentration of 0.25% in 0.86% saline. The antigen complex is made as a fresh reagent each day it is to be used.

C. RABIES PASSIVE HEMAGGLUTINATION TEST

Sera to be tested are heat-inactivated at 56°C for 30 min and then absorbed with an equal volume of 1% washed normal goose erythrocytes. After 30 min of incubation at 37°C the red blood cells are sedimented from the sera by low speed centrifugation. Twofold serial dilutions of the sera are made in 0.4% bovine serum albumin–0.05 M sodium borate–0.86% sodium chloride, pH 9.0, diluent in V-shaped microtiter plates at volumes of 0.025 ml. Sensitized erythrocytes (0.05 ml) are added to each well and the plates are sealed with cellophane tape and held at 4°C for approximately 1 hour before examination for hemagglutination. A sharp button in the bottom of a well indicates a negative test; positive reactions appear as cells which failed to sediment, ring formation on the sides of the wells, or clumps of agglutinated cells.

II. Advantages of the Passive Hemagglutination Test

A. SPEED OF OBTAINING RESULTS

One of the major difficulties with the serum neutralization procedure, in tissue culture or in mice, for determining titers of rabies antibodies in serum is that at least 6–8 days are required before results can be estimated. The passive hemagglutination test overcomes this problem. A test can be completed within the same day the serum is received. Only approximately 1 hour is required for antibody to react with antigen and hemagglutination to occur. However, the agglutination is stable such that, if the situation demands, the tests may be left at 4°C for 24 hours or more before evaluation. Negative results have not been observed to convert to positive under these conditions. When very large numbers of sera have to be titrated this has been found to be a more practical procedure.

B. EFFICIENCY

The test is easy to perform. It requires no specialized equipment beyond the microtiter apparatus that has become standard equipment in most serology laboratories. No highly developed skills are required on the part of the technicians. A single technician can titrate more than a hundred sera to obtain an end point in a single day.

C. REPRODUCIBILITY

Titration of a given serum repeated at intervals over a period of 2 years have always given the same end point, within an error of one dilution. There is no biological variance to be considered, as observed when animals as mice are used in the titration procedure. Results obtained by various technicians with different levels of experience in performing serologic analyses have shown little difference in titers.

D. ECONOMY

The only laboratory equipment required for the passive hemagglutination test are the inexpensive microtiter diluters, droppers, and plates. While the serum neutralization test in mice needs large numbers of inbred animals of a specific age, with facilities for housing and care for these for several days during the test, no such demands are made by the passive hemagglutination procedure. Goose red blood cells are available from commercial sources.

E. CORRELATION WITH THE SERUM NEUTRALIZATION TEST IN MICE

Since the serum neutralization test in mice has been accepted as the standard procedure for evaluation of antibodies against rabies virus in serum, it is desirable that the titers measured by any new serologic test have some predictable relationship to those obtained by this method. Correlation between titers obtained by the passive hemagglutination and the serum neutralization procedures is very good for sera obtained late in the immune response when most of the specific antibody is immunoglobulin G. Sera from 347 individuals, following preexposure vaccination or postexposure prophylaxis for rabies were titrated by both procedures (Gough and Dierks, 1971). The relationship between the titers measured by both methods was analyzed by a scattergram (Fig. 1). Only eight points disagreed by more than one $\log_2$ dilution. Some discrepancy must occur between the values obtained by the two procedures because the serum neutralization method obtains titers on a continuous scale and the passive hemagglutination test obtains titers on a discontinuous scale. In spite of this, a correlation coefficient was calculated to be 0.81.

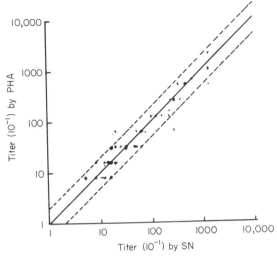

Fig. 1. Correlation between rabies virus antibodies titrated by SN and RPHA procedures. Solid line represents exact correlation; dotted lines are the limits of deviation permitted for agreement within $\pm 1 \log_2$ dilution.

F. Ability to Detect All Classes of Antibodies

The ability of the passive hemagglutination procedure to measure different classes of immunoglobulins has been determined by using this technique to titrate the antibodies in sera collected at several intervals postimmunization with rabies vaccine (Gough and Dierks, 1971). Antibodies with disulfide groups susceptible to reduction (im-

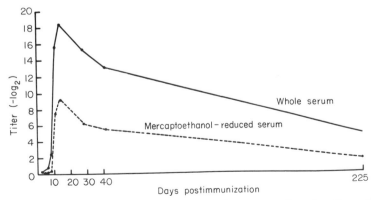

Fig. 2. Titers of mercaptoethanol-sensitive and mercaptoethanol-stable antibodies by the RPHA, following immunization with rabies vaccine. Each point represents the median value calculated from 63 samples.

munoglobulins M or A) were inactivated by treatment of serum with 0.1 *M* (final concentration) 2-mercaptoethanol at 37°C for 18 hours. In order to prevent the gelatinization that frequently occurs when this concentration of 2-mercaptoethanol is added to sera, 0.3 ml of each serum was diluted with 0.78 ml of 0.4% bovine serum albumin in saline before reduction with 0.12 ml of 1 *M* ME. Sera drawn from 63 persons were analyzed in this manner and the median titer was calculated for each of 9 days postvaccination (2, 4, 6, 8, 11, 14, 28, 42, and 225 days) (Fig. 2). Antibodies sensitive to reduction with 2-mercaptoethanol (immunoglobulin M) were detected soon after immunization and antibodies resistant to reduction were observed later in the immune response.

III. Disadvantages of the Test

A. High Titers Measured for Immunoglobulin M

Because antibodies of the immunoglobulin M class are generally many times more efficient in agglutination reactions than are those of the immunoglobulin G class, the amount of rabies antibodies are magnified when they are of this type, as early in the immune response. On the other hand, immunoglobulin M antibody may be less efficient in neutralizing viruses than is immunoglobulin G. If this is not considered in the evaluation of available antibody, and if the titer of the serum is assumed to be an indication of amount of protection, errors may be made in interpretations. This high sensitivity to early antibody, immunoglobulin M, may have an advantage in indicating that the recipient of the vaccine is responding to the antigenic stimulation. In a study in which the immune response of 63 individuals to rabies vaccine was followed for 7 months, high titers of antibody were observed initially by the passive hemagglutination procedure, while titers observed by the serum neutralization test remained low (Gough and Dierks, 1971). Later, when antibody was due to immunoglobulin G, rather than immunoglobulin M, titers by the passive hemagglutination and serum neutralization tests were nearly the same (Fig. 2).

B. Useful in Limited Serologic Systems

The conditions of the passive hemagglutination were developed for the maximum sensitivity in titration of rabies antibodies in human sera. It has been used with canine sera, with good correlation to results obtained with the serum neutralization procedure. Limited titrations of horse and goat antibodies have suggested it may be useful for these also.

The procedure has been very insensitive in the detection of rabies antibodies in rabbit sera. Titers in the thousands by the serum neutralization test are not at all detected by this procedure. The use of newborn calf serum, diluted 1:1000 with saline as the diluent, has resulted in the observation of titers, although still relatively low, with the rabbit serum while not affecting titers of antibodies in human serum.

C. ANTIGEN PREPARATION

Rabies virus obtained from mouse brain or tissue culture for use as antigen must be partially purified in order to remove other proteins against which the sera may contain antibodies. As contrasted with a neutralization test in which only antigens with the specific biologic activity of viral infectivity are measured, an agglutination test will react in the same manner with any antigen for which there are antibodies in the serum. No difference has been observed with the virus grown in fetal calf serum or in bovine serum albumin, although the latter has been reported to hemagglutinate. Virus grown in fetal calf serum has generally been used.

D. RED BLOOD CELL DONORS

The red blood cells of all geese are not equally appropriate for the test. Gander cells are more stable than those from hens and therefore are preferred; hen cells frequently hemolyze during the washing procedure and also more readily hemagglutinate spontaneously when exposed to the divalent chromium chloride coupling agent. The cells of some geese, obtained as adults, have been observed to agglutinate during the process of sensitization with rabies virus; perhaps these geese have been sensitized by previous infections with other viruses. No problems have been observed with geese hatched and raised under controlled conditions.

References

Dulbecco, R., and Vogt, M. (1954). *J. Exp. Med.* 99, 167–182.
Gold, E. R., and Fudenberg, H. H. (1967). *J. Immunol.* 99, 859–866.

Gough, P. M., and Dierks, R. E. (1971). *Bull. W.H.O.* **45**, 741–745.
Kent, J. F., Bukantz, S. C., and Rein, C. R. (1946). *J. Immunol.* **53**, 37
Kissling, R. E. (1958). *Proc. Soc. Exp. Biol. Med.* **98**, 223–225.
MacPherson, I., and Stoker, M. (1962). *Virology* **16**, 147–151.
Thomas, J. B., Ricker, A. S., Baer, G. M., and Sikes, R. K. (1965). *Virology* **25**, 271–275.
Valieri, A., Sedwick, W. D., Plotkin, S. A., and Mares, R. (1965). *Virology* **27**, 239–241.

CHAPTER 7

Concentration and Purification

Lothar G. Schneider

I. Introduction

During the last decade important data have been obtained concerning the structural, physical, chemical, and antigenic composition of rabies virus. These studies required large amounts of homogeneous virus preparations free from nonviral, cellular impurities. Characterization of virus properties depends on several factors: (1) available facilities for the large-scale production of the virus, (2) precise assay methods for virus-specific activities, and (3) reasonable concentration and purification procedures.

The advent of cell culture and the successful propagation of rabies virus in non-nervous mammalian cells has made possible the large-scale production of the virus. Rabies virus may be grown in various tissue culture substrates (Kuwert, 1970) with virus yields between 10^4 to 10^8 infectious units (PFU or LD_{50}) per milliliter tissue culture fluid. BHK-21 cells (Stoker and McPherson, 1964) in roller cultures are presently considered to be optimal for the large-scale production

125

of the virus (Sokol *et al.*, 1971). Virus yields averaging 10^8-10^9 LD_{50}/ml are often noted (Schneider *et al.*, 1971a). Since rabies virus multiplies without considerable cytopathic effect, the infectious fluid from roller cultures may be considered as an excellent starting material for subsequent purification work, containing the greatest possible concentration of virus and a minimum of nonviral impurities.

Assay methods for measuring virus activity should be rapid, accurate, and reproducible in order to follow the effectiveness of each step of purification. Successive purification steps should be judged by the number of units of virus-specific activities per unit mass of protein. An example for a stepwise purity control of a typical experiment (Sokol *et al.*, 1968) is given in Table I. Recovery of infectivity is an often-used criterion for purification. However, one should bear in mind that disruption or partial inactivation of rabies virus may occur by sudden changes in pH or molarity, for instance through dialysis or density centrifugation in the presence of high salt concentrations. The assay of rabies virus infectivity by means of the plaque test (Sedwick and Wiktor, 1967) gives results comparable to mouse inoculation (Koprowski, 1966); the choice of the test system depends on available facilities. The hemagglutinating (HA) activity of rabies virus assayed with goose erythrocytes as described by Halonen *et al.*, (1968) shows a linear correlation with infectivity (Kuwert *et al.*, 1968). The ease and rapidity of the HA test makes it a valuable tool in purification work, provided the starting material is free from HA-inhibiting substances. Unfortunately, the HA activity of rabies virus is rapidly destroyed by most detergents and lipid solvents; only saponin has been shown to disrupt the virus but to keep the HA activity intact (Schneider *et al.*, 1971b). The complement-fixation (CF) test is a sensitive assay method which requires minimal amounts of reagents if the microtechnique is employed (Casey, 1965; Kuwert *et al.*, 1968). The removal of impurities may be controlled quantitatively by using selective antisera against purified virus and cellular antigens. The CF test is mandatory for the isolation and purification of virus subcomponents because disrupted virus loses infectivity and HA activity, but usually retains CF activity.

Several purification steps are necessary in order to achieve purification. The primary step usually involves a reduction of the bulk of the material and results in concentration of the virus. Concentrated virus in a small volume is easily handled and reasonably stable against inactivation or spontaneous disruption, but further steps are necessary to effect greater purity. Purification procedures are not specific for a given virus or protein, but are selective procedures with regard

Table I

Virus Activity/Protein Ratios during Stepwise Concentration and Purification of Rabies Virus by Zinc Acetate Precipitation[a]

Sample	Vol (ml)	Amt. of protein per ml (mg)	PFU/ml ($\times 10^7$)	HAU/ml	CFU/ml	Rabies active counts per min per ml ($\times 10^4$)	PFU per mg of protein ($\times 10^6$)	Recovery rate (%)			
								PFU	HAU	CFU	Counts/min
Infective tissue culture fluid	550.0	3.55	1.9	32	16	1.60	5.3	100	100	100	100.0
Precipitate dissolved in EDTA solution	11.2	4.30	110	768	224	19.6	260	120	49	28	25.0
Pooled fractions after filtration through Sephadex column	30.0	1.90	480	326	85	6.36	250	144	56	29	21.7
Resuspended pellet after high-speed centrifugation	0.57	1.20	1700	8192	6144	80.1	14,000	110	31	47	9.1
Band after centrifugation in sucrose density gradient	4.75	0.12	80	768	640	9.98	6,600	38	21	35	5.3

[a] After Sokol et al., 1968 (reproduced by permission of Journal of Virology, 1968).

to differences in size, density, and surface properties between viral and nonviral cellular components. The methods involved are either chemical or physical. For concentration and partial purification of rabies virus various methods have been successfully used, including precipitation, ultracentrifugation, ultrafiltration and batch- or column-type chromatography; these are detailed below. Modern analytic methods such as preparative ultracentrifugation, electrophoresis, and chromatography have proven to be of value as final purification steps.

The degree of purity achieved is measured by biologic, and physical, and chemical properties of the purified virus. For example, highly purified preparations of virus had a high infectivity and high CF and HA activities in relation to protein content (Sokol *et al.*, 1968), while inoculation into animals produced little or no formation of antibodies against host cell components. On isopycnic centrifugation the virus gave a single sharp peak but it was less homogeneous in respect to size and shape as revealed by zonal centrifugation or by electron microscopy (Schneider *et al.*, 1971b). These criteria do not completely satisfy the requirements for absolute purity: There may also be impurities not detected serologically; The CF- and HA-activity/protein ratios may be misleading due to aggregation or disintegration of virus particles; the infectivity of highly purified rabies virus preparations is known to decrease rapidly due to the lack of stabilizing proteins. Nonetheless, many important properties of purified rabies virus became known during the last few years. The data from different laboratories have shown close correlation though different purification techniques were employed.

The following paragraphs describe different procedures which have been applied to the concentration and purification of rabies virus. The list of procedures and experiments is not complete, but rather special emphasis is given to those methods which have been shown to be reasonable in their performance and to provide highly purified preparations of virus from large volumes of starting material.

II. Methods for Concentration

A. PRECIPITATION

For many years infected animal brains were the main source for obtaining large quantities of rabies virus. The purpose of purification was primarily the improvement of brain tissue vaccines. Most early attempts were unsuccessful in separating virus from cellular material of tissue homogenates by means of precipitation with alcohol (Tagaya *et al.*, 1953; Sawai and Nakino, 1954), protamine sulfate (Warren *et al.*, 1949), or acid (Behrens *et al.*, 1939); the virus either coprecipitated with cell components or was rapidly inactivated. The protein content of the resulting preparations was high. Turner and Kaplan (1967) compared precipitation by methanol, ethanol, and acetone with the treatment of brain homogenates by arcton, diethyl ether, and chloroform. With the exception of arcton all organic solvents drastically reduced infectivity, and were not recommended for purification. Following treatment by 10% (v/v) arcton (trichlorotrifluoroethane), the infectivity was recovered quantitatively in the aqueous phase. It was shown later (Kaplan and Turner, 1968) that fluorocarbon treatment effectively separated the virus from the encephalitogenic substance of brain material which remained in the arcton phase. Fluorocarbon treatment should therefore be taken into consideration as a method for the partial purification of brain tissue vaccines for human use. Those countries with much human rabies and with limited facilities for the production of potent tissue culture vaccines will probably still be forced to use such type of vaccines during the coming decades.

Precipitation by acid at pH 4.5 has been successfully applied to isolate structural complement-fixing antigens (commonly referred to as soluble antigens) of rabies virus from infected mouse brains (Van den Ende *et al.*, 1957; Mead, 1962; Katz *et al.*, 1968).

Precipitation methods are definitely advantageous when used for the reduction of large volumes of infectious tissue culture fluid. The supernatant fluids from monolayer or suspension cell cultures contain considerably less protein and other extraneous material than brain homogenates, especially if the virus has been grown in the presence of 0.1–0.3% (w/v) bovine serum albumin instead of serum. Precipitation of rabies virus by zinc acetate has been reported by Neurath *et al.* (1966). The procedure was slightly modified by Sokol *et al.* (1968) and successfully applied to the purification of rabies virus as a primary concentration step. Crude tissue culture fluid, pH 7.4–7.8, was freed of cell debris by low-speed centrifugation and mixed with 1 M zinc acetate, pH 5.0, at a ratio of 50:1. The resulting precipitate was collected by low-speed centrifugation and the sediment was suspended in a volume of at least 1.25% of the original tissue culture fluid. On the average, 30- to 50-fold concentrations were achieved. The concentrated virus contained almost all of the infectious virus, variable amounts of bovine serum albumin, cellular components, and low molecular weight impurities which had been trapped in the precipitate. Filtration of the concentrated and partially purified virus through a Sephadex G-75 column effectively removed zinc ions and EDTA.

Precipitation by ammonium sulfate (30% w/v) required the addition of 2% (v/v) calf serum to the tissue culture supernatant fluid which acted as coprecipitant for the virus (Aaslestad and Wiktor, 1972). The pH was maintained at pH 7.5 by the addition of 1 M Tris, pH 8.0. The protective activity of rabies virus preparations concentrated by ammonium sulfate was compared to those concentrated by zinc acetate precipitation, ultrafiltration and adsorption to aluminum phosphate. After ammonium sulfate precipitation about 50% of the protective activity was recovered, compared to 32–35% by the other methods. The purity of the preparations as measured by the protein/activity ratios was highest with the adsorption and precipitation methods, but proved to be considerably less by ultrafiltration. Due to the nature of the filter membranes the ultrafiltrate contained all particulate material and macromolecules of greater than 20,000 molecular weight.

Precipitation of rabies virus from tissue culture fluid by polyethylene glycol (PEG) 6000 molecular weight was achieved at 4°C using a 5% (w/v) concentration of PEG at pH 8.0 (Mikhailovsky *et al.*, 1971). After mixing, the virus was agitated for 60 min and the resulting precipitate was sedimented at 2500 rpm for another 60 min. The recovery of infectivity was about 70% with a 100-fold reduction in volume. No data were reported concerning the purity of the concentrated preparation. From the author's own experience such preparations still contain considerable amounts of foreign protein coprecipitated with the virus.

B. SEDIMENTATION

Sedimentation of rabies virus by high-speed centrifugation represents the least difficult means of concentration. In addition to the virus, however, all particulate materials of the same size, or larger than the virus particles, will be deposited. High-speed centrifugation is usually restricted to smaller volumes (Atanasiu *et al.*, 1963), although the capacity of modern rotors of ultracentrifuges enables the handling of up to several liters of tissue culture fluid when used in consecutive runs. Concentration by centrifugation with a high-speed continuous flow device has not been evaluated yet for rabies virus, but might be of use for commerical purposes in the future.

The sedimentation conditions reported in the rabies literature are generally much higher than actually required. Based on a sedimentation coefficient $s_{20,w}$ of 600 S of the rabies virion (Neurath et al., 1966), approximately 12,000 g for 60 min would suffice to sediment the virus under most conditions. In fact, Schlumberger et al. (1970) sedimented more than 95% of the infectivity in the type rotor 30 of a Beckman Instruments Spinco model ultracentrifuge using 13,600 g for 60 min. Alternatively, the same effect would be obtained if gravitational forces of 78,000 g were employed for 10.2 min. Under the reported conditions, however, only 24% of the total complement-fixing activity were cosedimented with the virus. The majority of virus-specific, small molecular weight particles remained in the supernatant even after sedimentation for 64,000 g for 60 min. Sedimentation procedures, therefore, are of great value in separating virus particles from smaller sized viral and nonviral components, but concentration procedures other than sedimentation are necessary if efforts are directed toward the concentration of specific virus activities such as the protective activity, which may be associated with intact virions and smaller breakdown products as well.

The pellet resulting from high-speed sedimentation of crude tissue culture fluids is usually hard to dissolve and requires homogenization by vigorous pipetting, by sonic treatment for 1–2 min at 10 Kc and 0°C, or by the use of a saturated solution of disodium ethylene-diaminetetra-acetate (EDTA) to bring the virus back into suspension. Care should be taken to avoid excessive disruption of virus particles since further purification steps are very much dependent on the homogeneity of the virus preparation. In order to avoid pelleting of the virus together with cellular materials at the bottom of the centrifuge tube, sedimentation on a cushion of a concentrated salt solution is often preferred. If the buoyant density of the cushion is higher than that of the virus, the latter is prevented from entering the cushion but accumulates on top of it and is separated from cellular material of higher density. Neurath et al. (1966) used 2 ml CsCl of a 1.29 g/ml density, pH 7.0, as a cushion which they overlaid with 2 ml of a buffered CsCl solution of 1.145 g/ml density. Twenty ml of virus were placed on top of this cushion, and after sedimentation at 49,500 g for 4 hours, 96% of the infectivity was recovered in the interphase, i.e., on top of the cushion. If preconcentrated virus is used, this step represents further concentration and a partial purification already. For electron microscopic studies Pinteric and Fenje (1966) used a similar approach. From crude tissue culture fluids they sedimented rabies virus on a cushion of 3% (v/v) phosphotungstic acid and claimed to recover most of the virus in a drop of water laid on top of the virus/PTA pellet.

For the sedimentation of concentrated and partially purified rabies virus the following procedure has been recommended (Sokol, 1973): three 30 ml portions of a clear virus preparation are centrifuged in a swinging-bucket type SW25.1 rotor of a Spinco centrifuge at 20,000–22,000 rpm for 60 min at 4°C; the transparent virus pellet is overlaid with a small volume of buffer and the tubes kept for 3–4 hours at 4°C; gentle pipetting is sufficient to redissolve the pellet. Nonresuspendable material is removed by low-speed centrifugation.

C. ULTRAFILTRATION

One of the oldest methods for isolation and characterization of viruses is ultrafiltration through filter membranes of known porosity. Depending on the pore diameter, submicroscopic particles of different sizes are either separated or held back completely. The vertical flow exerted by pressure usually results in very fast clogging of the filter membranes since the nonfilterable particles are precipitated on the filter surface or become adhered in the pores. With a new method of virus concentration as described by Strohmaier (1967a,b) the suspension containing the virus is repeatedly recirculated from a supply vessel and passed continuously over the filter surface in tangential direction at a constant flow rate. Due to a pressure gradient on the filter layer the solvent passes through the filter membrane while nonfilterable material containing the virus is retained in the flowing solution. Since the volume of the solvent from the supply vessel is continuously decreasing, the concentration of virus is accordingly increased. Depending on the number of filter units used in the ultrafiltration apparatus, very large volumes may easily be concentrated.

The ultrafiltration apparatus constructed by Strohmaier (Fig. 1) has been used with nitrocellulose membranes with a porosity of 50 nm to separate virus from "soluble antigens" (Wiktor *et al.*, 1969). By using filter membranes with 10–20 nm porosity all virus-specific activities are concentrated, resulting in a total recovery of infectivity, hemagglutinating, complement-fixing, and protective activity of the starting material (Wiktor *et al.*, 1969; Schlumberger *et al.*, 1970). A fluid volume of 2 liters was concentrated 15- to 20-fold within 4–5 hours by using an effective filtration area of 1100 cm^2 and a filtration speed of 360–440 ml/hour. By increasing the number of filter units, Stroh-

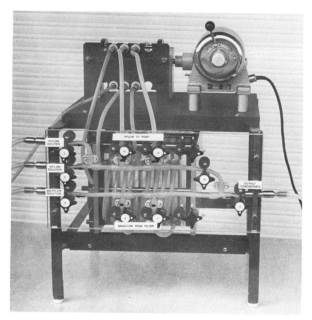

Fig. 1. Ultrafiltration apparatus as used for concentrating rabies virus (by courtesy of Dr. K. Strohmaier, Tübingen, W-Germany).

maier (1967b) concentrated 150 liters of virus-containing tissue culture fluid to 150 ml in 5 days.

The purity of rabies virus concentrated by ultrafiltration or high-speed centrifugation was found less satisfactory than of preparations obtained by adsorption or precipitation techniques (Aaslestad and Wiktor, 1972). However, ultrafiltration was found to be a suitable procedure for the rapid concentration of the immunogenic property of infectious tissue culture fluids. Sikes *et al.* (1971a) used β-propiolactone-inactivated experimental antirabies vaccine from various tissue culture sources, concentrated by ultrafiltration with or without further purification, for pre- and postexposure treatment of monkeys. The experimental vaccines had much higher potencies than conventional duck embryo or suckling mouse brain vaccines. In one trial it was shown for the first time that a single injection of vaccine given after a street virus challenge protected seven out of eight monkeys from rabies. Antirabies vaccines for human use, prepared in a similar way, are under field study now. Preliminary data, indicating a high response of neutralizing antibody in humans after one single dose of vaccine, are very promising for the use of potent tissue culture-origin antirabies vaccines in the near future.

D. ADSORPTION AND CHROMATOGRAPHY

Methods involving adsorption of rabies virus to selective adsorbents, or ion exchange resins, have been used for concentration and purification purposes as well. The solid adsorbent is usually packed into columns and the virus is allowed to flow through and adsorb to the column. When using batch-type procedures instead of columns the adsorbent is suspended in the virus suspension itself. In either case the virus is recovered by selective elution from the adsorbent with buffers of suitable pH and ionic strength.

For the separation of rabies virus from brain tissue components Muller (1950) and Sawai *et al.* (1954) used Amberlite cation exchange resin, XE-64, between 140 and 180 mesh. A reduction of total protein of 74–80% was accompanied, however, by some loss of infectivity. Thomas *et al.* (1965), employing ion exchange celluloses, found standard grade ECTEOLA to be a suitable adsorbent for rabies virus. Elution of the virus was optimal with 0.3 M KCl in 0.01 M potassium phosphate buffer, pH 7.0. At a purification rate of at least 1:240 almost all of the infectivity was recovered. As a vaccine the purified product was of good potency and was apparently free of encephalitogenic activity and of the tissue components that had caused local reactions (Sikes and Larghi, 1967). After a 3-years' immunity duration study in dogs, purified and inactivated vaccine (PRV) proved to be superior to several commercial inactivated or attenuated animal vaccines (Sikes *et al.*, 1971b).

While also aiming at the development of a purified brain tissue vaccine, Shokeir (1968) used calcium phosphate column chromatography. Though 98% of total proteins were removed effectively, the virus that eluted in 0.25–0.3 M phosphate buffer showed only little protective activity. Somewhat better results were obtained by Atanasiu and Tsiang (personal communication) who adsorbed rabies virus from a homogenate of brain tissue to a gel of calcium phosphate in a bath-type procedure. After several washings the virus was inactivated with β-propiolactone while still adhering to the calcium phosphate which, without being removed, served as an adjuvant for the final vaccine.

Schneider *et al.* (1971a) has described the concentration of rabies virus from large volumes of infected tissue culture supernatant fluids by batch adsorption to aluminum phosphate. Following adsorption to aluminum phosphate gel equilibrated with 0.05 M phosphate buffer at pH 7.1–7.4, the virus was eluted from the gel with 0.3 M phosphate buffer, pH 8.0, and pelleted by high-speed centrifugation at 22,000 rpm for 1 hour in a Spinco rotor type 30. The final product contained high virus activity/protein ratios, on the average of 10^{11} LD_{50}, $10^{5.3}$ hemagglutinating units and $10^{4.4}$ complement-fixing units per milligram of protein.

Virus/protein ratios were improved several thousand times over those of the initial tissue culture fluids, thus indicating a high degree of purity. Antisera prepared against rabies virus purified by aluminum phosphate had high virus-specific activities but little or no activity against nonviral proteins. The advantage of this method is the convenience of handling large volumes of virus and a final preparation having small volume but a considerable degree of purity.

Rabies virus concentrated by aluminum phosphate was shown by the standard mouse potency test to be a potent vaccine (Schneider *et al.*, 1971b). This was also demonstrated by Aaslestad and Wiktor (1972) who compared the recovery and protective activities of rabies vaccines made from virus concentrated by four different methods, including the batch adsorption to aluminum phosphate gel.

III. Methods of Purification

Many of the concentration procedures mentioned in the previous paragraphs have been applied successfully to concentrate or partially purify rabies virus for vaccination purposes. For physicochemical analyses or for studies of the antigenic structure, partially concentrated virus has to be further purified. Almost invariably such concentrated preparations still contain cellular or other nonviral, high molecular weight impurities which have to be removed by appropriate techniques. Chromatography has been used to separate a part of nonvirus proteins from the virus. The most efficient and usual last step in purification work, however, is density-gradient centrifugation.

A. Filtration and Chromatography

Filtration of preconcentrated rabies virus through Sephadex G-75 has been used prior to density-gradient centrifugation in order to remove low molecular weight impurities (zinc ions, EDTA) and a part of the serum components of the tissue culture medium (Sokol *et al.*, 1968). For this purpose, columns (33 by 3 cm) of Sephadex G-75 (particle size 40–120 μm) were equilibrated with tris buffer, pH 7.8, which also served as elution buffer. The capacity of the column allowed the filtration of about 10 ml of virus.

Diethylaminoethyl (DEAE) cellulose chromatography was used as intermediate purification step in order to remove serum albumin or proteins from serum (Aaslestad and Wiktor, 1972). These substances were quantitatively eluted when the column of DEAE cellulose was developed with 0.15 M NaCl, yet all the virus was retained on the column.

B. DENSITY-GRADIENT CENTRIFUGATION

The principle of density-gradient procedures is based on sedimenting particles through a liquid column of a salt or sucrose gradient in which the particles are separated into zones according to their size, shape, and density. The concentrated virus is either layered on top of a preformed gradient or is mixed with the solute, and the gradient is allowed to form during centrifugation. After varying centrifugation times the particles are resolved in zones and are made visible as light-scattering bands in a beam of light. Fractions of the gradient or individual zones are collected by puncturing the bottom of the tube with a hypodermic needle or other sampling device.

When the particles are sedimented in sucrose or glycerol and are separated according to their sedimentation rates, the process is called rate zonal centrifugation. In isopycnic or buoyant density centrifugation the particles are separated strictly on the basis of their own density. During centrifugation they reach equilibrium with the respective densities of the salt solution of the gradient, usually containing CsCl or other heavy metal salts.

For rate zonal centrifugation, 0.5–2 ml of concentrated rabies virus are layered on top of 28 ml of a preformed sucrose gradient. A 10% to 60% (w/v) gradient is centrifuged in a swinging bucket rotor for 90 min at 61,000 g (Sokol *et al.*, 1968). With 5–25% (w/v) gradients, centrifugation at 49,000 g for 20 min was used. This period of time is enough to band the virus particles in the middle of the gradient. A two- to threefold decrease in infectivity is usually encountered due to the fact that many virus particles are disrupted during removal of the sucrose by dialysis. Sokol (1973) recommends a stepwise dialysis of the purified virus against solutions of decreasing concentrations in order to hold inactivation to a minimum.

For buoyant density centrifugations, CsCl, either in substance or as a saturated solution in 0.01 M phosphate buffer, is mixed with the preconcentrated virus until an initial density of 1.20–1.22 g/ml is reached. The mixture is centrifuged in the Spinco SW39 rotor at

100,000 g for 16–20 hours. The virus has been reported to band in a single broad peak at a CsCl density of 1.20 (Neurath *et al.*, 1966) or 1.22 (Murphy *et al.*, 1968). Two distinct and separate virus bands at 1.20 and 1.22 have been repeatedly observed (Schneider *et al.*, 1971a). A considerable loss of infectivity is usually experienced with this procedure, even prior to dialysis, probably due to the action of the heavy inorganic salts on the virus. The resulting preparation, however, is extremely pure, making the method most useful as a final step in concentration and purification procedures.

C. Purification of Virus Subunits

The purification of subunits of rabies virus may be achieved by procedures similar to those described for the complete virus particle. Sokol *et al.* (1969) reported on the disintegration of the rabies virion by the action of sodium deoxycholate (DOC). After that treatment, the ribonucleoprotein (RNP) components were separated from incompletely disrupted virus and from membrane proteins and lipids by rate zonal centrifugation in a sucrose gradient (10–28% w/w) centrifuged at 22,500 rpm for 2 hours, 4°C, in a Spinco type SW25.1 rotor. Consequently, the band containing RNP particles was subjected to buoyant density centrifugation at 40,000 rpm for 25 hours in a Spinco SW50 rotor. The RNP purified from virus particles had a sedimentation coefficient $s_{20,w}$ of about 200 S, its buoyant density in CsCl was 1.32, and it contained 96% protein and 4% RNA.

The isolation and purification of the RNP of rabies and several other rhabdoviruses from infected tissue culture cells was achieved by chromatography on Sepharose 4B by Schneider *et al.* (1973). After treatment of infected cells with 1% (v/v) Nonidet P_{40}, 30% (v/v) trichlorotrifluoroethane, and sedimentation on a cushion of CsCl, the preconcentrated RNP was layered on a Sepharose 4B column (55 by 5 cm) and eluted with 0.15 M NaCl, 0.01 M tris-HCl and 0.001 M EDTA buffer, pH 7.4. The RNP was recovered in the exclusion peak of the column and sedimented at 80,000 g for 3 hours. The clear pellet was easily redissolved in a small volume of Tris-EDTA buffer, and banded by buoyant density centrifugation in CsCl at 145,000 g for 36 hours, 4°C, in a Spinco SW65 rotor. The RNP obtained from infected cells was indistinguishable from the RNP obtained from disrupted virions as determined by chemical, physical, and serologic analysis. The RNP proved to be free of virus membrane material and cellular contaminants. This method has the advantage that RNP can be isolated in milligram amounts from infected tissue culture cells which otherwise are of not much use, since concentration procedures almost exclusively involve extracellular rabies virus.

No procedures have yet been described for the isolation of purified rabies virus membrane components. By dissociating rabies virus with DOC the lipids are solubilized and, after separation in sucrose gradient, a mixture of disintegrated virus membranes was obtained which exhibited hemagglutination-inhibiting activity but no hemagglutinating activity (Sokol *et al.*, 1969).

In contrast, rabies virus membranes, stripped off the internal RNP core by the action of saponin, contained the total hemagglutinating and protective activity of the untreated sample (Schneider *et al.*, 1971b). The preparation had a density of 1.29 in CsCl, and contained lipids and a major protein of 80,000 daltons molecular weight. The membrane preparation was free of RNA and of residual RNP (L. G. Schneider and B. Dietzschold, unpublished data).

IV. Summary

Much information has accumulated during the past few years regarding the nature of the rabies virus. This has only been possible through the concentration and purification of rabies virus of tissue culture origin by the combined use of several of the aforementioned techniques. The availability of highly purified preparations of rabies virus enabled (1) morphological studies of the virus particle (Hummeler *et al.*, 1967) and of its subunits (Hummeler *et al.*, 1968), (2) chemical and physical analyses of the complete virus (Schlumberger *et al.*, 1973), of the nucleocapsid and the RNA (Sokol *et al.*, 1969), of the virus proteins (Sokol *et al.*, 1971; Neurath *et al.*, 1972), and of the virus lipids (Diringer *et al.*, 1973), and, finally (3) studies of the antigenic composition of the virus and its structural components (Kuwert *et al.*, 1968; Wiktor *et al.*, 1969; Crick and Brown, 1969; Schlumberger *et al.*, 1970; Schneider *et al.*, 1971b, 1973).

References

Aaslestad, H. G., and Wiktor, T. J. (1972). *Appl. Microbiol.* **24**, 37.
Atanasiu, P., Lépine, P., and Dighe, P. (1963). *C. R. Acad. Sci.* **256**, 1415.
Behrens, C. A., Schweiger, L. B., Barker, J. F., and Reeves, J. L. (1939). *J. Infec. Dis.* **64**, 252.
Casey, H. (1965). *U. S. Pub. Health Serv., Pub. Health Monogr.* **74**, Complete Monograph.

Crick, J., and Brown, F. (1969). *Nature (London)* **222**, 92.

Diringer, H., Kulas, H. P., Schneider, L. G., and Schlumberger, H. D. (1973). *Z. Naturforsch.* **28c**, 90.

Halonen, P. E., Murphy, F. A., Fields, B. N., and Reese, D. R. (1968). *Proc. Soc. Exp. Biol. Med.* **127**, 1037.

Hummeler, K., Koprowski, H., and Wiktor, T. J. (1967). *J. Virol.* **1**, 152.

Hummeler, K., Tomassini, N., Sokol, F., Kuwert, E., and Koprowski, H. (1968). *J. Virol.* **2**, 1191.

Kaplan, C., and Turner, G. S. (1968). *Nature (London)* **219**, 445.

Katz, W., Larsson, K. M., and Mead, T. H. (1968). *J. Gen. Virol.* **2**, 399.

Koprowski, H. (1966). *World Health Organ., Monogr. Ser.* **23**, 69–80.

Kuwert, E. (1970). *Zentralbl. Bakteriol., Parasitenk., Infektionskr. Hyg., Abt. 1, Supplementh.* **3**, 1.

Kuwert, E., Wiktor, T. J., Sokol, F., and Koprowski, H. (1968). *J. Virol.* **2**, 1381.

Mead, T. H. (1962). *J. Gen. Microbiol.* **27**, 397.

Mikhailovskii, E. M., Tsiang, H., and Atanasiu, P. (1971). *Ann. Inst. Pasteur, Paris* **121**, 563.

Muller, R. H. (1950). *Proc. Soc. Exp. Biol. Med.* **73**, 239.

Murphy, F. A., Halonen, P. E., Gary, G. W., Jr., and Reese, D. R. (1968). *J. Gen. Virol.* **3**, 289.

Neurath, A. R., Wiktor, T. J., and Koprowski, H. (1966). *J. Bacteriol.* **92**, 102.

Neurath, A. R., Vernon, S. K., Dobkin, M. B., and Rubin, B. A. (1972). *J. Gen. Virol.* **14**, 33.

Pinteric, L., and Fenje, P. (1966). *Symp. Ser. Immunbiol. Stand.* **1**, 9.

Sawai, Y., and Nakino, M. (1954). *Jap. J. Exp. Med.* **24**, 229.

Sawai, Y., Yanaka, H., Makino, M. A., and Kikuchi, K. (1954). *Jap. J. Bacteriol.* **9**, 509.

Schlumberger, H. D., Wiktor, T. J., and Koprowski, H. (1970). *J. Immunol.* **105**, 291.

Schlumberger, H. D., Schneider, L. G., Kulas, H. P., and Diringer, H. (1973). *Z. Naturforsch.* **28c**, 103.

Schneider, L. G., Horzinek, M., and Matheka, H. D. (1971a). *Arch. Gesamte Virusforsch.* **34**, 351.

Schneider, L. G., Horzinek, M., and Novicky, R. (1971b). *Arch. Gesamte Virusforsch.* **34**, 360.

Schneider, L. G., Dietzschold, B., Dierks, R. E., Matthaeus, W., Enzmann, P. J., and Strohmaier, K. (1973). *J. Virol.* **11**, 748.

Sedwick, W. D., and Wiktor, T. J. (1967). *J. Virol.* **1**, 1224.

Shokeir, A. A. (1968). *Ann. Soc. Belg. Med. Trop.* **48**, 613.

Sikes, R. K., and Larghi, O. P. (1967). *J. Immunol.* **99**, 545.

Sikes, R. K., Cleary, W. F., Koprowski, H., Wiktor, T. J., and Kaplan, M. M. (1971a). *Bull. W. H. O.* **45**, 1.

Sikes, R. K., Peacock, G. V., Acha, P., Arko, R. J., and Dierks, R. E. (1971b). *J. Amer. Vet. Med. Ass.* **159**, 1491.

Sokol, F. (1973). *World Health Organ., Monogr. Ser.* **23**, 165.

Sokol, F., Kuwert, E., Wiktor, T. J., Hummeler, K., and Koprowski, H. (1968). *J. Virol.* **2**, 836.

Sokol, F., Schlumberger, H. D., Wiktor, T. J., and Koprowski, H. (1969). *Virology* **38**, 651.

Sokol, F., Stanček, D., and Koprowski, H. (1971). *J. Virol.* **7**, 241.

Stoker, M., and McPherson, I. (1964). *Nature (London)* **203**, 1355.

Strohmaier, K. (1967a). "Methods in Virology" (K. Maramorosch and H. Koprowski, eds.) Vol. 2, pp. 245–274. Academic Press, New York.

Strohmaier, K. (1967b). *Zentralbl. Bakteriol., Parasitenk., Infektionskr. Hyg., Abt. 1, Orig.* **205**, 170.

Tagaya, I., Ozawa, Y., and Kondo, A. (1953). *Yokohama Med. Bull.* **4**, 78.

Thomas, J. B., Ricker, A. S., Baer, G. M., and Sikes, R. K. (1965). *Virology* **25**, 271.

Turner, G. S., and Kaplan, C. (1967). *J. Gen. Virol.* **1**, 537.

Warren, J., Weil, M. L., Russ, S. B., and Jeffries, H. (1949). *Proc. Soc. Exp. Biol. Med.* **72**, 662.

Wiktor, T. J., Sokol, F., Kuwert, E., and Koprowski, H. (1969). *Proc. Soc. Exp. Biol. Med.* **131**, 799.

van den Ende, M., Polson, A., and Turner, G. S. (1957). *J. Hyg.* **55**, 361.

CHAPTER 8

Rabies Virus Antigenic Relationships

R. Shope

I. Introduction

Rabies virus has been considered a single antigenic "species" by nearly all who have studied it with modern scientific methods. This concept of antigenic unity has been challenged by Shope *et al.* (1970), who have shown that rabies virus is a member of a group of serologically related viruses which are readily distinguishable *inter se*. It should here be emphasized that this concept of plurality of antigenic types in no way detracts from the usefulness of the older concept (one rabies virus) in formulating public health measures. Such measures include the reliance on a single type of vaccine for dogs and man, control of stray dogs, and prophylaxis with classical rabies virus vaccine for veterinarians and high-risk personnel. As of 1974 there is no indication that the newly recognized rabies-related

141

viruses have widespread distribution outside of sub-Saharan Africa and, even there, their epidemiologic and clinical significance is only incompletely known. It is in this perspective that the following description of the rabies-related viruses is given, with details of the antigenic interrelationships.

II. Antigenic Distinction between the Viruses of the Rabies Sero Group and Other Rhabdoviruses

We have been unable to demonstrate any cross reaction between classic rabies virus and 13 other rhabdoviruses (including the Marburg agent which shares certain morphologic features) by neutralization (N) and complement-fixation (CF) test (Tables I and II). The rabies-related viruses have also been tested by CF with most of these same rhabdoviruses and found to be unrelated.

III. Rabies-Related Viruses

There are four rabies-related viruses now recognized.

A. Lagos Bat Virus

Lagos bat virus was isolated in 1956 from pooled brains of frugivorous bats, *Eidolon helvum,* in Lagos Island, Nigeria (Boulger and Porterfield, 1958). Negri bodies were not seen in infected mouse brain or dog brain preparations, but have been detected in infected monkey brains (Percy *et al.,* 1973). The virus was pathogenic for infant and weanling mice by intracerebral (i.c.) inoculation, but not for weanling mice by intraperitoneal (i.p.) inoculation, or for guinea pigs or rabbits after intramuscular (i.m.) inoculation. Rhesus monkeys and dogs inoculated i.c. died with a rabieslike illness (Tignor *et al.,* 1973). There is at present only one existing strain of Lagos bat virus.

B. Mokola Virus

Mokola virus (IbAn 27377 strain) was isolated in 1968 from the viscera of shrews (*Crocidura* sp.) captured near Ibadan, Nigeria (Shope *et al.,* 1970; Kemp *et al.,* 1972). It has also been isolated on two occasions in Nigeria from patients with central nervous system disease (Familusi and Moore, 1972; Familusi *et al.,* 1972). The virus has a

Table I

Summary of Neutralization Test Results with Various Rhabdoviruses

Virus	Titer-log LD_{50}	Mouse hyperimmune sera										Guinea pig serum Marburg
		VS-Indiana	Cocal	VS-New Jersey	Piry	Chandipura	Hart Park	Flanders	Rabies	Kern Canyon	Mt. Elgon	
VS-Indiana	7.1	≥6.2ᵃ	4.2	1.9	0	2.6	0	0	0	0	0	0
Cocal	7.7	4.2	≥7.0	2.7	1.7	1.8	0	0	0	0	0	0
VS-New Jersey	5.5	2.2	0	≥5.0	0	0	0	0	0	0	0	0
Piry	7.9	2.3	2.6	2.5	5.7	3.4	0	0	0	0	0	0
Chandipura	7.3	2.5	2.7	0	4.6	≥5.7	0	0	0	0	0	0
Hart Park	4.6	0	0	0	0	0	≥4.1	4.1	0	0	0	0
Flanders	4.4	0	0	0	0	0	≥3.9	≥3.9	0	0	0	0
Rabies	5.9	0	0	0	0	0	0	0	≥5.4	0	0	0
Kern Canyon	5.4	0	0	0	0	2.2	0	0	0	≥4.9	0	0
Mt. Elgon	5.8	0	0	0	0	0	0	0	0	0	≥5.3	0

ᵃ Log neutralization index; 0 = ≤ 1.5.

Table II

Summary of Results of Complement-Fixation Tests with Various Rhabdoviruses

Antigen	Hyperimmune mouse sera or ascitic fluid													Guinea pig serum Marburg
	VS-New Jersey	VS-Indiana	Cocal	Piry	Chandi-pura	Flanders	Hart Park	Mokola	Rabies	Lagos bat	Mt. Elgon	Kern Canyon	Klamath	Marburg
VS-New Jersey	256/512[a]	0	0	0	0	0	0	0	0	0	0	0	0	0
VS-Indiana	0	256/512	32/128	0	0	0	0	0	0	0	0	0	0	0
Cocal	0	32/512	256/512	0	0	0	0	0	0	0	0	0	0	0
Piry	0	0	0	128/32	8/4	0	0	0	0	0	0	0	0	0
Chandipura	0	0	0	0	128/64	0	0	0	0	0	0	0	0	0
Flanders	0	0	0	0	0	64/16	32/4	0	0	0	0	0	0	0
Hart Park	0	0	0	0	0	32/16	256/64	0	0	0	0	0	0	0
Mokola	0	0	0	0	0	0	0	256/512	32/32	0	0	0	0	—
Rabies	0	0	0	0	0	0	0	32/128	1024/512	0	0	0	0	0
Lagos bat	0	0	0	0	0	0	0	64/128	64/128	8/128	0	0	0	—
Mt. Elgon	0	0	0	0	0	0	0	0	0	0	64/64	0	0	0
Kern Canyon	0	0	0	0	0	0	0	0	0	0	0	256/512	0	0
Klamath	0	0	0	0	0	0	0	0	0	0	0	0	256/64	—
Marburg[b]	0	0	0	0	0	0	0	—	0	—	0	0	—	64/32
Normal	0	0	0	0	0	0	0	0	0	0	0	0	0	0

[a] Reciprocal of serum/antigen titers; 0 = no reaction at 1:4 serum dilution; composite of 2 CF tests.

[b] The Marburg agent was included for comparison (probably not a rhabdovirus); reagents supplied by Drs. R. Kissling and F. M. Murphy of The Center for Disease Control, Atlanta, Georgia.

pathogenicity for mice similar to Lagos bat virus, and kills rhesus monkeys and dogs following i.c. injection (Tignor *et al.*, 1973). Negri bodies were found in infected monkey brains, but not in mouse or dog brains (Percy *et al.*, 1973).

C. Obodhiang Virus*

Obodhiang virus (Sudan Ar 1275-64 strain, Ar 1154-64 strain) was isolated in baby mice in 1963 on three separate occasions from pools of nonengorged *Mansonia uniformis* mosquitoes near Malakal, Sudan (Schmidt *et al.*, 1965). This virus and kotonkan virus (described below) have the unusual—for rabies-related viruses—potential of being arthropod-borne. In addition to having been isolated repeatedly from mosquitoes, Obodhiang virus multiplies in monolayer cultures of insect cells without prior adaptation (Buckley, 1973).

D. Kotonkan Virus

Kotonkan virus (Ib Ar23380 strain) was isolated in 1967 by infant mouse inoculation from *Culicoides* midges in Ibadan, Nigeria (Kemp *et al.*, 1973). Neutralizing substances for kotonkan virus were demonstrated in a high percentage of cattle sera and also of rodents, sheep, horses, and insectivores in Nigeria. The virus multiplies in insect cells (Buckley, 1973).

IV. Antigenic Relationships in the Rabies Group

The techniques used to characterize the relationship of these four viruses to classical rabies virus are the N, CF, fluorescent antibody, and vaccination-challenge tests.

A. Neutralization Tests

Boulger and Porterfield (1958), in their original description of Lagos bat virus, noted the failure of a potent rabies antiserum to neutralize the virus. Subsequent studies (Shope *et al.*, 1970; Trefzger and Dierks, 1971) indicated that the relationship of Lagos bat, Mo-

---

* Obodhiang is a virus name which has been proposed by Dr. J. R. Schmidt. The name is not yet published and its mention here is not intended to constitute priority.

Table III

Serum-Dilution Neutralization Test of Rabies-Related Viruses[a]

Virus	Inoculum: mouse LD_{50}	Serum (S) or mouse ascitic fluid (MAF)			
		Rabies burro S	Lagos bat MAF	Mokola MAF	Control MAF (M-1056)
Rabies, strain CVS	160	15,625[b]	11	0[c]	0
Rabies, vampire bat	200	15,625	11	1	0
Lagos bat	50	5	280	18	0
Mokola	100	3	15	320	0
Control (M-1056)	125	0	0	0	25

[a] Shope *et al.* (1970).

[b] Reciprocal of 50% neutralization endpoint of serum or ascitic fluid; fivefold serum dilutions versus constant virus dilution.

[c] No survivors.

kola, and rabies viruses was distant when tested by the serum dilution technique in mice (Table III), whereas the relationship was closer and readily demonstrable when undiluted hyperimmune sera were used in a constant serum-varying virus dilution test. Table IV shows representative test results, including comparison with Obodhiang and kotonkan viruses, which by this technique are at best distant relatives of rabies virus.

Studies with sera of monkeys and dogs inoculated experimentally with either Mokola or Lagos bat virus show that N antibody appears between the seventh and twenty-eighth days after inoculation. Cross-reacting antibody was regularly detected in dog sera, but rarely in the monkey sera (Table V).

Table IV

Neutralization[a] of Rabies Virus by Mouse Hyperimmune Ascitic Fluid to Rabies and to Four Other Related Viruses

Hyperimmune mouse ascitic fluid to		Log neutralization index
Rabies		≥5.3
Mokola		3.1
Lagos bat	Fluid #1	0.4
	Fluid #2	4.1
Obodhiang		0.3
Kotonkan		1.4

[a] i.e., infant mice; constant-serum, varying-virus technique.

Table V

Neutralizing Antibody in Monkeys and Dogs Inoculated
Intramuscularly with Mokola or Lagos Bat Virus[a]

Virus inoculated	Days post inoculation	Mean log neutralizing index					
		Dogs[b]			Monkeys[b]		
		Lagos bat	Mokola	Rabies	Lagos bat	Mokola	Rabies
Lagos bat	0	0[c]	0	0	0	0	—
	7	0.3	0	0	0.3	0.4	0
	14	1.3	0	0	1.2	0.4	0
	21	≥2.0	1.5	0	—	—	—
	28	≥2.7	≥2.6	0	1.6	0.4	0
	32–39	≥2.7	≥2.6	0	1.9	0.5	0
	42–46	≥2.7	≥2.6	1.8	2.2	1.3	0
Mokola	0	0	0	0	—	0	—
	7	0	0.4	0	—	0	—
	14	0.6	0.8	0	0	0.7	—
	21	1.3	1.8	2.0	0.6	1.9	0
	28	2.7	3.2	1.6	0.7	2.1	0
	32–42	3.8	—	1.8	0.6	2.3	0
	46	—	—	—	0	2.1	0

[a] Tignor *et al.* (1973).
[b] Number of animals: Lagos bat virus, two dogs and six monkeys; Mokola virus, two dogs and five monkeys.
[c] Mean log neutralizing index of undiluted serum tested intracerebrally in infant mice.

B. COMPLEMENT-FIXATION TESTS

By the use of hyperimmune mouse ascitic fluids, cross reaction among the rabies-related viruses is shown most readily with rabies, Mokola, and Lagos bat viruses; Obodhiang and kotonkan viruses are related to rabies virus only through Mokola and Lagos bat (Table VI).

Dogs and monkeys inoculated i.m. with Mokola and Lagos bat viruses usually did not form CF antibody. When antibody was found, it cross reacted with rabies, Mokola, and Lagos bat virus antigens.

C. FLUORESCENT ANTIBODY TESTS

Mouse brain impressions of Mokola and Lagos bat viruses tested with the conventional direct FA test (using a fluorescein-conjugated hyperimmune hamster antirabies serum) reacted strongly and were diagnosed as rabies virus. Inhibition of the staining reaction by prior

Table VI

Complement-Fixation of the Rabies Group of Viruses

	Mouse hyperimmune ascitic fluids				
Antigens	Rabies	Mokola	Lagos bat	Obodhiang	Kotonkan
Rabies	256[a]	64	0	0	0
Mokola	32	256	4	16	0
Lagos bat	16	128	32	8	0
Obodhiang	0	4	0	128	0
Kotonkan	0	32	0	0	64
Other mouse brain antigens[b]	0	0	0	0	0

[a] Reciprocal of ascitic fluid titer; 0 is <4.
[b] One hundred ninety-two antigens to arboviruses and other viruses of vertebrates did not react with the 1:4 ascitic fluid dilution.

absorption of the conjugate by rabies-infected mouse brain suspension confirmed the specificity of the staining reaction (E. H. Lennette, personal communication, 1970). Obodhiang virus when thus tested was negative.

When frozen sections of Mokola and Lagos bat virus-infected monkey brain were stained after addition of hyperimmune mouse ascitic fluids in the indirect technique, there was almost complete cross reactivity with Mokola, Lagos bat, and rabies fluids, but only slight cross reaction with Obodhiang fluid. Similar cross reactivity was noted when the same technique was used with Mokola and Lagos bat virus-infected dog brains; a specific diagnosis, however, could usually be achieved by diluting the mouse ascitic fluids (Tignor *et al.*, 1973).

Table VII

Intensity of Fluorescent Antibody Reactions of Rabies, Mokola, and Lagos Bat Viruses[a]

	Mouse brain impression smears		
Conjugates	Rabies CVS-11	Mokola	Lagos bat
CVS-11, Rabies	4+	2+	1+
Mokola	Negative	4+	1+
Lagos bat	Negative	Negative	3+

[a] J. A. Trefzger and R. E. Dierks (personal communication, 1971).

J. A. Trefzger and R. E. Dierks (personal communication, 1971) compared rabies, Mokola, and Lagos bat viruses using mouse brain impression smears and conjugates of a goat antirabies serum, and rabbit anti-Mokola and anti-Lagos bat sera. Brain impression slides of all three viruses reacted with the rabies conjugate and were specifically inhibited by rabies virus. The heterologous systems gave less intense fluorescence than the homologous (Table VII).

D. VACCINATION-CHALLENGE TESTS

Immunization of 12-week-old mice by the i.p. route with Mokola and Lagos bat viruses did not protect against rabies virus (Pasteur strain) challenge i.c., nor did immunization with Lagos bat virus protect against Mokola virus challenge. Immunization with Mokola virus, however, protected against both homologous and Lagos bat virus challenge (Table VIII).

In the above experiments the mice which survived sequential inoculations with Mokola–Lagos bat virus were challenged i.c. with $10^{4.4}$ suckling mouse i.c. LD_{50} of rabies virus. As shown in Table IX, numerous mice survived challenge after these sequential immunizations, although interference cannot be ruled out as playing a role in this survival.

Tignor and Shope (1972) have carried out quantitative vaccination challenge tests in mice. Mice immunized i.c. with rabies HEP Flury

Table VIII

Mice Surviving Challenge with Rabies or Rabies-Related Virus 23–27 Days after Immunization with Lagos Bat or Mokola Virus

Mouse group	i.p. Immunization	i.c. Challenge	log LD_{50}[a]	Survivors
1	Normal mouse brain	Rabies	2.8; 4.4	0/43
2	Normal mouse brain	Lagos bat	4.2; 3.8	16/49
3	Normal mouse brain	Mokola	3.6; 2.8	0/41
4	Normal mouse brain	Normal mouse brain	—	92/92
5	Mokola	Rabies	2.8	0/24
6	Lagos bat	Rabies	4.4	0/23
7	Mokola	Lagos bat	4.2	44/46
8	Lagos bat	Mokola	2.8	0/48
9	Lagos bat	Lagos bat	3.8	47/47
10	Mokola	Mokola	3.6	44/46

[a] Two values represent results of two separate experiments.

Table IX

*Mice Surviving Rabies Virus Challenge 12 Days after Completion
of Sequential Intraperitoneal–Intracerebral Immunization with Two Related Viruses*

Mouse group	i.p.–i.c. Immunization	i.c. Challenge	LD_{50}	Survivors
7	Mokola–Lagos bat	Rabies	$10^{4.4}$	14/21
10	Mokola–Mokola	Rabies	$10^{4.4}$	7/21
1	Normal–none	Rabies	$10^{4.4}$	0/23

vaccine resisted challenge with Lagos bat virus, and to a lesser extent with Mokola virus. Vaccination i.p. with Mokola, rabies, or Lagos bat viruses did not usually protect mice against a heterologous challenge; an exception was the resistance of rabies-vaccinated mice to Lagos bat challenge (Table X).

Limited experience with experimentally inoculated rhesus monkeys indicates that Mokola and Lagos bat viruses may not protect against an i.m. challenge of 10^5 suckling mouse i.c. LD_{50} of rabies virus (NYC/GA strain). Two of five controls died, two of four Lagos bat virus immune monkeys, and two of five Mokola virus immune monkeys. The challenge was 3–4 months after immunization and the animals which died all had homologous N antibody prior to challenge. The average survival time for monkeys dying after rabies challenge was 25 days for controls, 44 days for Lagos bat virus immunes, and 18 days for Mokola virus immunes.

Table X

*Summary of Log Protective Indices in Mice Vaccinated and Challenged
with Rabies, Lagos Bat, and Mokola Viruses[a]*

	i.c. Challenge		
i.p. Vaccine	Rabies	Mokola	Lagos bat
Rabies	>3.2	0.1	2.1
Mokola	0.3	1.9	0
Lagos bat	0.4[b]	0.6	>3.6

[a] Tignor and Shope (1972).
[b] Approximate value. (There were some deaths at the endpoint of the control rabies titration, and only an approximate value could be calculated.)

V. Other Antigenic Variants of Rabies Virus

Comparison of other strains of rabies virus including *Derriengue* from vampire bats (Johnson, 1948), arctic rabies (Crandell, 1966), and standard laboratory strains (J. A. Trefzger and R. E. Dierks, personal communication, 1971) has shown minor antigenic variation among rabies strains. In none of these studies were the differences as great as those described between classic rabies and Lagos bat or Mokola virus.

Three other viruses, *Oulou Fato*, Bolívar, and a virus from rodents in Czechoslovakia, may represent rabies-related viruses. Remlinger and Curasson (1924) described cross-challenge tests in rabbits with *Oulou Fato* virus of West Africa and a street rabies strain. Although concluding that the two viruses were antigenically the same, they reported that a rabbit immunized with *Oulou Fato* virus succumbed to rabies challenge while rabies immunization protected against *Oulou Fato* virus challenge. Bolívar virus from cattle in Venezuela has been extensively compared with the Pasteur strain of rabies by neutralization and vaccination-challenge tests (Kubes and Gallia, 1942). Immunization with the Pasteur strain of rabies virus did not protect against Bolivar virus challenge. Sodja *et al.* (1971) report 14 isolates of a rabies-like virus from rodents in Czechoslovakia. These are serologically related to rabies, but it has not yet been reported whether they are also antigenically distinct from classic rabies virus.

VI. Significance of Rabies-Related Viruses

What is the significance of the rabies group of viruses? Dog rabies in North America no longer represents a threat of virus transmission to man, and the effectiveness in North America of the single-type live virus vaccine for rabies prophylaxis in dogs is unquestioned. It is not so certain, however, that wildlife rabies in North America is of one type. It is now clear that multiple types exist in Africa and, most important, that human disease is associated with a rabies-related virus (Mokola). Are the reported rabies vaccine failures in Africa (Segonne, 1965) and South America (World Health Organization Expert Committee on Rabies, 1966) related to infection with heterologous viruses?

The currently practiced FA technique does not distinguish rabies from Mokola and Lagos bat viruses, yet these differ by N test and in cross-challenge experiments. Should not virus isolation and sero-identification by N test be used in suspect wildlife cases in addition to the FA? How may the presence of a rabies-related virus in a given geographic area affect the epidemiology of classical rabies? These are some of the unanswered questions about the significance of the rabies-related viruses.

References

Boulger, L. R., and Porterfield, J. S. (1958). *Trans. Roy. Soc. Trop. Med. Hyg.* **52**, 421.

Buckley, S. M. (1973). *Appl. Micro.* **25**, 695.

Crandell, R. A. (1966). *Proc. Nat. Rabies Symp. 1966* p. 37.

Familusi, J. B., and Moore, D. L. (1972). *African J. Med. Sci.* **3**, 93.

Familusi, J. B., Osunkoya, B. O., Moore, D. L., Kemp, G. E., and Fabiyi, A. (1972). *Amer. J. Trop. Med. Hyg.* **21**, 959.

Johnson, H. N. (1948). *Amer. J. Hyg.* **47**, 189.

Kemp, G. E., Causey, O. R., Moore, D. L., Odelola, F., and Fabiyi, A. (1972). *Amer. J. Trop. Med. Hyg.* **21**, 356.

Kemp, G. E., Lee, V. H., Moore, D. L., Shope, R. E. Causey, O. R., and Murphy, F. A. (1973). *Amer. J. Epid.* **98**, 43.

Kubes, V., and Gallia, F. (1942). *Bol. Inst. Invest. Vet., Maracay, Venez.* **1**, 3.

Percy, D. H., Bhatt, P. N., Tignor, G. H., and Shope, R. E. (1973). *Vet. Path.* **10**, 534.

Remlinger, P., and Curasson, M. (1924). *Bull. Acad. Med., Paris* **92**, 1112.

Schmidt, J. R., Williams, M. C., Lule, M., Mivule, A., and Mujomba, E. (1965). *East Afr. Virus Res. Inst. Rep.* **15**, 24.

Segonne, J. (1965). *Med. Trop. (Marseilles)* **25**, 67.

Shope, R. E., Murphy, F. A., Harrison, A. K., Causey, O. R., Kemp, G. E., Simpson, D. I. H., and Moore, D. L. (1970). *J. Virol.* **6**, 690.

Sodja, I., Lim, D., and Matouch, O. (1971). *J. Hyg. Epidemiol., Microbiol., Immunol.* **15**, 229.

Tignor, G. H., and Shope, R. E. (1972). *J. Infec. Dis.* **125**, 322.

Tignor, G. H., Shope, R. E., Bhatt, P. N., and Percy, D. H. (1973). *J. Infec. Dis.* **128**, 471.

Trefzger, J. A., and Dierks, R. E. (1971). *Bacteriol. Proc.* **71**, 183.

World Health Organization Expert Committee on Rabies (1966). *World Health Organ. Tech. Rep. Ser.* **321**, 23.

PART II

Pathogenesis and Pathology

CHAPTER 9

Growth of Rabies Virus in Cell Culture

T. J. Wiktor and H F. Clark

I. Introduction

The cultivation of rabies virus in tissue culture is not only an essential adjunct to an understanding of the basic structure of the virion, but also an important method for obtaining large quantities of virus in the production of vaccine.

During the past decade the immunofluorescent antibody staining method for the detection of viral antigen within infected cells and the plaque assay technique for testing infectivity have made it possible to explore the mechanisms by which cells are infected by rabies virus. With the adaptation of several virus strains to different tissue culture systems, opportunities were provided for a series of investigations on the relationship between cells and rabies virus, including nonlytic, chronic, and endosymbiotic types of infection. These investigations have provided new information on the role of interferon in rabies virus infection, the chemical composition of virus-induced cytoplasmic inclusions, and the fine structural features of rabies virus replication as revealed by electron microscopy.

This growth in knowledge about rabies replication in tissue culture systems has made possible the large-scale preparation of homogeneous cloned populations of the virus which, after concentration and purification, yield higher titers of pure virus than can be obtained from the brains of infected animals. By disruption of tissue culture-propagated virions, separate components, such as the virus envelope proteins, nucleocapsids, and a single-stranded, noninfectious viral RNA, have been obtained for analytic study.

The cultivation of rabies virus in tissue culture has made possible the demonstration of a cytolytic antibody, mediated by complement, in infected animals. Concentrated, purified, and inactivated virions of tissue culture origin have been used experimentally for the immunization of animals. These preparations are several hundred times more antigenic than a standard reference vaccine and induce extremely high levels of neutralizing antibody in animals. A single dose of vaccine, administered after a challenge with a street rabies virus, has been shown to protect experimental animals. A new method for determining the antigenicity of inactivated rabies vaccine by its antibody-binding capacity has been developed by employing plaque assay methods in cell culture.

II. Historical Review

Tissue culture techniques were first described early in this century, and attempts were made to propagate rabies virus in various *in vitro* systems. Noguchi (1913) and Levaditi (1913, 1914) reported independently that rabies virus could be maintained, and that it probably replicated *in vitro*, in fragments of brain, medulla oblongata, and spinal ganglia from experimentally infected animals. In Levaditi's experiments, transplanted cells were kept in coagulated monkey plasma. A continuous release of infectious virus was noted for up to 2 months after the initiation of the cultures. By this time, the original nerve cells had completely disappeared and the cultures were composed of fibroblastic cells. It was not possible, however, to transfer the infection to new cultures established from uninfected animals.

Stoel (1930) infected cultures of embryonic chicken brains and hearts (explanted in rabbit plasma clots) with rabies virus of mammalian brain origin; infection was maintained for five consecutive passages.

Successful serial cultivation of rabies virus in rabbit embryo brains suspended in Tyrode solution was reported by Kanazawa (1936, 1937). Subsequently, virus was also propagated in cultures of mouse or rat embryo brain (Bernkopf and Kligler, 1937; Schultz and Williams, 1937; Webster and Clow, 1936, 1937; Kligler and Bernkopf, 1941). Parker and Hollender (1945) demonstrated that rabies virus will multiply more efficiently in tissue cultures derived from embryonic mouse brain than in those established from the brains of newborn or adult animals. Similar observations were made by Bequignon *et al.* (1954), Vieuchange (1956), and Vieuchange *et al.* (1956a). Plotz and Reagan (1942) were the first to isolate street rabies virus directly in cell culture; they infected tissue cultures with material taken directly from the brain of a human patient with rabies and from the brain of a rabid dog. These strains were maintained for 11 and 9 passages, respectively. All other investigators have used fixed virus or virus from early passage in animals.

Following the observations of Levaditi and Schoen (1936), Levaditi *et al.* (1937), Schoen (1937), and Pearson *et al.* (1958), that rabies virus multiplies particularly efficiently *in vivo* in cells of serially propagated tumors (Pearce carcinoma of rabbits and mouse astrocytoma), Atanasiu and his co-workers (Atanasiu and Laurent, 1957; Atanasiu and Lépine, 1959; Atanasiu *et al.*, 1961) cultivated street and fixed strains of virus in a mouse ependymoma tumor cell line. After several passages, an inconsistent cytopathic effect was observed and intracytoplasmic inclusions resembling Negri bodies were seen for the first time in a cell culture system.

The susceptibility of mouse kidney cell cultures to infection with rabies virus was described by Vieuchange *et al.* (1956a,b). Kissling (1958) subsequently reported the serial passage of both fixed and street rabies viruses in primary hamster kidney tissue cultures. Further observations with this same system were made by Fenje (1960a,b), Martos and Atanasiu (1961), Ver *et al.* (1964), and Ver (1965).

Kissling and Reese (1963) first demonstrated the potential usefulness of fixed virus cultivated in cell culture for the preparation of a vaccine with demonstrable efficacy in experimental animals.

The susceptibility of chicken fibroblasts to rabies virus infection was first demonstrated by K. Habel (unpublished results). Kondo (1965) reported that, after several passages in chicken embryo cell cultures, the HEP Flury strain of virus produced a marked cyto-pathic effect which could be used as a means for the titration of viral infectivity. The production of interferon by rabies virus in chick embryo fibroblasts was suggested by the fact that rabies infection prevents plaque formation by Western equine encephalitis virus in this system (Kaplan *et al.*, 1960a). LEP and HEP Flury virus grown in chicken fibroblast cultures have been used for the immunization of animals (Koprowski, 1954), and the HEP vaccine has been used for the immunization of man (Fox *et al.*, 1957). A plaque assay system employing chick embryo cells was described by Yoshino *et al.* (1966).

Other primary cell culture systems used for rabies virus propaga-tion have been derived from dog salivary glands (Depoux, 1963, 1964, 1965a), bat adipose tissue (Allen *et al.*, 1964a,b), dog kidneys (Hronovský *et al.*, 1966; Mikhailovskii, 1966), pig kidneys (Abelseth, 1964a,b), and rhesus monkey kidneys (Lang *et al.*, 1969). Aksenova *et al.* (1966) reported the successful propagation of fixed strains of rabies virus in several primary and serially propagated cell cultures, including hamster kidney, sheep embryo kidney, and intestine, rabbit kidney, dog kidney, and human embryonic kidney, skin, muscle, and lung.

The adaptation of rabies virus to several established cell lines and strains has made a systematized approach to the study of rabies virus and its interaction with host cells especially practicable. Baby ham-ster kidney (BHK/21) cells (MacPherson and Stoker, 1962) have become the favorite substrate for rabies virus investigations *in vitro* because of their extreme susceptibility to the virus. BHK/21 cells have been used for the production of virus employed in concentra-tion and purification studies (Sokol *et al.*, 1968), electron microscopic investigations (Atanasiu *et al.*, 1963; Hummeler *et al.*, 1967), and the production of concentrated and purified vaccines (Wiktor *et al.*, 1969). The first reliable plaque assay system for rabies virus was developed with a subline of BHK/21 cells adapted to growth in sus-pension (Sedwick and Wiktor, 1967). The hamster cell line, Nil-2 (Diamond, 1967), also supports rabies replication to high titer and is used as substrate for vaccine production.

Human diploid cell strains (HDCS) (Hayflick and Moorhead, 1961) were extensively investigated as a potential cell substrate for the production of rabies antigens for human vaccine use. Various strains of rabies virus have been adapted to growth in this cell system by the serial subcultivation of infected cells and by a cell-mixing technique (Wiktor *et al.*, 1964). Both live and inactivated vaccines from virus grown in HDCS have been shown to be highly antigenic for experimental animals (Wiktor and Koprowski, 1965; Wiktor *et al.*, 1969; Wiktor, 1971; Sikes *et al.*, 1971). In human trials, inactivated HDCS vaccine demonstrated a high degree of immunogenicity (Wiktor *et al.*, 1973; Cabasso *et al.*, 1974) and it is hoped that a concentrated, purified, and inactivated rabies vaccine propagated in HDCS cells may replace the presently used animal tissue vaccines for human rabies immunization (see Vol. II, Chapter 21).

A rabbit endothelium cell line (Fernandes *et al.*, 1964) was shown to support the replication of rabies virus for at least 93 passages, accomplished by the subculture of viable, infected cells. The infection did not interfere with the mechanism of cellular replication, despite the fact that rabies antigen could be demonstrated in all dividing cells during the mitotic process. The complement-dependent lytic action of antirabies serum on rabies virus-infected cells was first demonstrated in this system (Fernandes *et al.*, 1964; Wiktor and Koprowski, 1967).

Rabies virus has been successfully propagated in cells of several established cell lines of poikilothermic vertebrate origin derived from fish (Solis and Mora, 1970), snakes, turtles, and lizards (Clark, 1972). Both a freshwater fish cell line, FHM, and a Russell's viper cell line, VSW, supported the replication of fixed rabies virus strains to high titer, without adaptation. The infection was successfully maintained in serially subcultivated VSW cells for more than 100 passages, and in serially subcultivated cells of a lizard cell line, GL1, for more than 60 passages.

III. Adaptation of Rabies Virus to Growth in Cell Culture

In most tissue culture systems the adsorption and penetration of virus can be enhanced by the addition of the polyions, diethylaminoethyl (DEAE) dextran (50 μg/ml) or protamine sulfate (1 mg/ml), to the infecting medium (Kaplan *et al.*, 1967).

The infection of HDCS and several other cell lines (Wiktor *et al.*, 1964) with the virus of brain or salivary gland origin was first noted by fluorescent (FA) staining in a very small number of cells, but serial transfer of either the supernatant medium or cell extracts in the homologous tissue culture system often resulted in a gradual decrease in the level of infection. The virus was lost after a few such passages in HDCS cells. Infected cultures maintained in an actively growing state by regular dispersal with trypsin and division every

3–4 days as cell sheets became confluent, however, showed a gradual increase in the number of infected cells. After a few such divisions (from four to ten, depending on the cell system and the virus strain), all the cells contained fluorescent antigen and intracytoplasmic inclusions.

With some infected cell systems, such as HDCS, cells stop dividing after a certain number of subcultures, but virus can be passaged by mixing a portion of the infected cells with a noninfected homologous cell population at each transfer passage. In most cases the virus is sufficiently adapted to growth in a given cell system after about 40 passages, and thereafter can be serially propagated by inoculation of either the supernatant medium or the cell extracts.

IV. Chronic Infection of Cell Culture Systems

Rabies virus-infected cells can generally be maintained in tissue cultures for extensive periods of time without showing any noticeable cytopathic effect. Different types of chronic infection take place, depending upon the cell system used.

Endosymbiotic infection, as found in rabbit endothelial cells infected with the CVS strain of virus (Fernandes et al., 1964), is characterized by the accumulation of only small intracytoplasmic inclusions in the cells. During a prolonged cultivation — more than 2 years — no interference with the mechanism of cellular replication appears to have occurred in these infected cultures. The growth rate, plating efficiency, and morphology of infected and uninfected control cultures were identical, although viral antigen was present in the cytoplasm of each cell of the infected cultures. Enhanced synthesis of DNA or RNA in infected cell populations could not be distinguished by studies of the rate of incorporation of tritiated thymidine or uridine. The presence of antirabies serum in the endosymbiotic system did not prevent the persistence of infection, unless complement was added to mediate cell lysis.

In carrier-type infections of fibroblasts of the hamster cell line, Nil-2 (Fig. 1; Wiktor and Koprowski, 1967; Wiktor and Clark, 1972), the production of new virus was observed to reach its peak in 3–4 days, and then to fall off sharply during the next six to seven cell transfers. Fluorescent intracytoplasmic inclusion bodies remained present in all the cultured cells after the decline in virus release. The cultures became resistant to superinfection with vesicular stomatitis virus (VSV) and an inhibitor with interferon-like properties

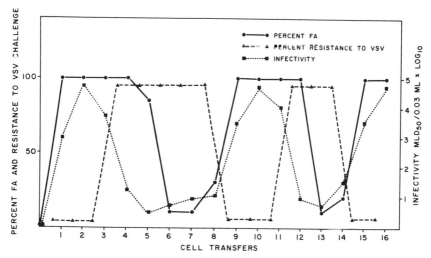

Fig. 1. Carrier-type of rabies virus infection (PM strain) in hamster cell culture (Nil-2).

was recovered from the culture medium. After this phase of infection there was a marked decrease in the number of antigen-containing cells, followed again by a gradual increase in the proportion of infected cells and in the production of infectious virus. These cycles of high and low levels of rabies infection and corresponding resistance to challenge with superinfecting virus recurred periodically.

V. Dynamics of Virus Replication *In Vitro*

An idealized single-cycle growth curve of rabies virus in cultured cells has not yet been described. Immunofluorescent examination of infected monolayer cell cultures reveals that infection proceeds asynchronously irrespective of the virus input multiplicity. The problems caused by the failure to obtain synchronous virus infection may be resolved by future studies of virus infection of synchronized cell populations.

The characteristics of virus growth under standard growth conditions have been well studied in several cell culture systems. Fluorescent antibody staining (Wiktor, 1966) revealed that both adsorption and penetration of the virus occurs relatively rapidly. Monolayers of HDCS were exposed to virus (CVS, HEP, and PM strains) at 37°C for various periods of time, after which the cells were washed to remove the unadsorbed virus and the adsorption was measured; or, they were washed and treated with antirabies serum in order to neutralize virus unproductively attached to the cells, and virus penetration could be distinguished from adsorption. The cultures were fed with fresh medium, and the incidence of cell infection was evaluated by measuring both fluorescent antigen and infectious virus production. The results suggested that adsorption and penetration of virus at early passage levels of adaptation to HDCS were not complete until 2–4 hours after exposure. With the PM virus strain at the fifty-second cell culture-passage level, however, only a few seconds of contact were needed for the virus to attach irreversibly. Penetration of the attached virus, beyond the influence of antibody, began within minutes after the initial exposure and appeared to be maximum in about 1 hour.

Electron microscopic studies of virus adsorption and penetration were performed with BHK cells infected with HEP or PM virus (Hummeler et al., 1967). Adsorbed particles were seen attached to the cell surface by fine fibers 15 min after first contact; this attachment seemed to occur at random sites on the virus particle surface. The particles passed into the cytoplasm by phagocytosis, and were enclosed, either singly or in small clusters, in pinocytotic vesicles. By 60 min after infection the virus-containing vesicles had moved deeper into the cytoplasm and disintegration of the particles was observed.

In another electron microscope study Iwasaki et al. (1973), using a high input multiplicity of virus of ERA and HEP strains to infect BHK/21 cultures, observed that numerous viral particles were attached to the cell plasma membrane or were within intracytoplasmic vesicles 5 min after exposure. At 60 min, intact virions could no longer be observed within the cell protoplasm.

The growth of Flury strain HEP virus in BHK/21 cell cultures infected at three different multiplicities (MOI) (Wiktor, 1973) is depicted in Fig. 2. Input multiplicity is shown to affect both the length of the virus eclipse and the yields of infectious virus recovered during the first 72 hours after infection. At the highest MOI [20 plaque-forming units (PFU) per cell] tested in this series of experiments, the eclipse phase lasted for 12 hours. At 12 hours postinfection, new infectious virus appeared almost simultaneously in the cells and in the supernatant fluids. The cell-associated virus titers exceeded those detected in the culture fluids for the first 30 hours after infection, but thereafter the released virus titers were higher.

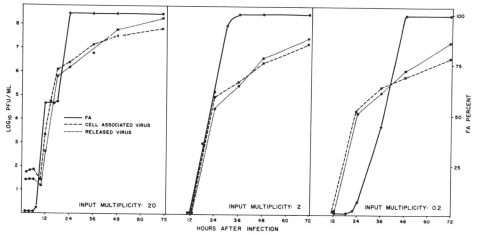

Fig. 2. Dynamics of rabies virus (HEP) replication in BHK/21 cell culture. Production of FA antigen, cell associated virus and released virus. Three input multiplicities.

Although total virus yields were directly related to the virus input for the first 72 hours, maximum virus yields were eventually obtained from cell cultures infected at a low MOI and tested after 4–7 days of incubation.

Fluorescent rabies antigen was detected a few hours prior to the appearance of infectious virus. In cells infected at an MOI of 20 PFU/cell (Fig. 2), FA staining was detected 8 hours after infection in 24% of the cells. At 10 hours after infection, 68% of the cells contained fluorescent antigen, a percentage which remained constant from hour 10 to hour 16. Subsequently, a rapid increase to 100% infected cells accompanied the second cycle of virus replication. In addition to sequential increases in the percentage of cells exhibiting antigen, the progression of virus infection is accompanied by increases in the number and size of the antigenic masses detected in each infected cell (Kaplan *et al.*, 1967).

The relationship of the production of hemagglutinin (HA) and complement-fixing (CF) rabies antigens to infectious virus production is illustrated in Fig. 3. HA was first detected in cell-culture supernatant fluids 30 hours after infection at an MOI of 20, and later in cell cultures infected at a lower MOI. The subsequent rise in HA titer paralleled the rise in infectious virus titer. CF antigens were first detected 24 hours after infection at an MOI of 20, before the appearance of HA. CF antigen titers continued to rise in parallel

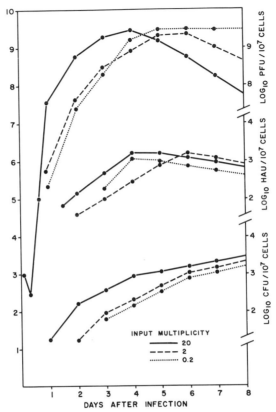

Fig. 3. Dynamics of rabies virus (HEP) replication in BHK/21 cell culture. Production of infectious virus, HA and CF antigen. Three input multiplicities.

with the increase in infectious virus. The continued increase in CF antigen titer, after titers of infectious virus and HA had reached a peak and begun to decline, indicates that CF antigens are more thermostable than virus infectivity or HA activity.

An attempt to obtain a single-cycle growth curve of the Pasteur strain of rabies virus in BHK-S13 cells has been reported by Tsiang and Atanasiu (1971). Monolayer cultures were infected with virus and after 2 hours of adsorption, the cells were washed, resuspended by trypsinization, and maintained as a suspended culture. In this system an eclipse phase of 6 hours (from the fifth to the eleventh postinfection hour) was observed followed by virus multiplication at an exponential rate between the twelfth and the thirtieth postinfection hour. However, the highest percentage of cells showing the presence of rabies FA antigen by 30 hours postinfection was only 35. A second cycle of virus multiplication started at the thirty-sixth hour and was indicated by an increase in the percentage of fluorescent cells.

VI. Virus-Specific Products of Infected Cells

In addition to infectious virus, a variety of other virus-induced products may be measured by immunologic and biochemical techniques as a further means of characterizing rabies virus-infected cells *in vitro*. Fluorescent methods developed for the detection of rabies antigens in brain tissues (Goldwasser and Kissling, 1958) were early applied to the study of rabies virus in cell culture. FA staining was extensively studied in several of the initial successful attempts to adapt rabies virus to cell culture (Kaplan *et al.*, 1960b; Fernandes *et al.*, 1963; Atanasiu *et al.*, 1963; Wiktor *et al.*, 1964) since the monitoring by FA was the most efficient method available for evaluating the progress of rabies infection in these noncytopathic systems. FA staining appears very early in the course of virus replication and eventually becomes distributed throughout the cytoplasm, but they are never seen within nuclei. Strains of rabies virus which characteristically induce pronounced Negri bodies in brain cells *in vivo* usually also induce similar large FA masses in cell culture. This observation first substantiated the actual viral antigen composition of the Negri body. Fixed non-Negrigenic strains with a long history of animal or cell culture passage usually produce multiple FA masses, ranging upward in size from the smallest resolvable dustlike particles. The typical size and distribution pattern of FA staining in a particular cell type is specific to the virus strain, but is not obviously correlated with any other virus strain characters.

Recently results similar to those obtained by fluorescein-conjugated antibody staining of rabies-infected cells have been described, using peroxidase-coupled rabies antibody conjugates (Atanasiu *et al.*, 1971).

Inclusions induced by rabies virus in cultured cells have also been studied by histochemical means. They are readily observed only in systems containing large individual antigenic masses (similar to classical Negri bodies) detectable by FA (Fig. 4). Love *et al.* (1964, 1966) determined that cytoplasmic inclusions induced by fixed rabies virus (CVS strain) in the rabbit endothelial cell line, RE, stained green by acridine orange at pH 3.5 and red at pH 7.0. This type of staining persisted after treatment of the tissue with RNase. RNA, sensitive to

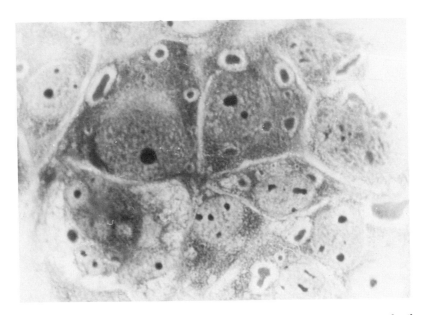

Fig. 4. Intracytoplasmic inclusions in dog kidney cell culture infected with Flury LEP strain of rabies virus. (May-Grünwald-Giemsa stain.)

RNase, was detected in the inclusions after staining by toluidine blue. It was concluded that the inclusions were composed largely of protein, with small amounts of RNA, and may represent "some form of abortive viral replication or a cellular defense mechanism." Inclusions produced by rabies virus *in vitro* were indistinguishable by histochemical methods from those characteristic of rabies infection of the central nervous system *in vivo*. In electron microscope studies mature rabies virions have been found in association with cytoplasmic inclusions formed *in vitro* or *in vivo* (Atanasiu *et al.*, 1963; Matsumoto, 1963).

HA activity in the supernatant fluids of rabies virus-infected BHK/21 cell cultures was first described by Halonen *et al.* (1968). The HA activity was detected only when the serum supplement of the cell growth medium was replaced with bovine serum albumin. The following were found to be optimal conditions for the detection of HA activity: the use of goose erythrocytes, a temperature of 4°C, and a pH of 6.2. Subsequent studies by Kuwert *et al.* (1968) revealed that rabies virus HA was produced equally well by several cell types, provided that high infectivity titers ($>10^6$ PFU/ml) were achieved.

However, in all cases, HA activity was almost exclusively limited to extracellular fluids; cell-associated virus exhibited about 15 times less HA activity than did released virus.

VII. Virion-free Rabies Antigen (Soluble Antigen) (VFRA)

In addition to infectious virus, rabies virus-infected cells produce a noninfectious material, virion-free or soluble antigen (VFRA). VFRA reacts immunologically (as measured by CF and gel-immunodiffusion techniques) with virion-specific immune serum and does not sediment under conditions which cause sedimentation of up to 95% of the virions (Wiktor *et al.*, 1969; Schlumberger *et al.*, 1970). VFRA also has the capacity to protect animals against a virulent virus challenge. This protective ability suggests the possible usefulness of VFRA in the preparation of a vaccine which would be free of rabies RNA.

VFRA can be separated from virions by the precipitation of the virions with zinc acetate, by ultrafiltration (through a membrane of 0.05 μm porosity) and by differential ultracentrifugation. Fractionation and purification of VFRA has been attempted (H. D. Schlumberger and T. J. Wiktor, unpublished data) by chromatography on Sephadex G 150. Four protein fractions were obtained. One, with a molecular weight of about 150,000, contained most of the biological activity of VFRA. This fraction reacted in the gel-diffusion technique with immune sera of different specificities in the following ways: (1) It was precipitated by immune sera prepared against virions or against coat proteins and derived from disrupted virions, giving a single sharp precipitation line; (2) it did not react with serum prepared against viral nucleocapsids; and (3) it reacted with sera prepared against either homologous- or heterologous-strain rabies intact virions.

VIII. Immune Lysis

Rabies virus-infected cells are lysed after exposure to rabies antibody and complement (Fernandes *et al.*, 1964; Wiktor *et al.*, 1968). This immune lysis can be demonstrated either by the staining of damaged cells with trypan blue (Fig. 5), or by the release from damaged cells of chromium 51 isotope. The reaction is abolished follow-

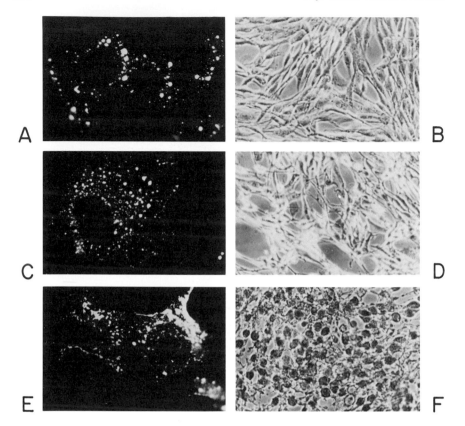

Fig. 5. Immune lysis of rabies virus (HEP) infected hamster cell culture (Nil-2). FA and trypan blue straining of cells at 12 hours (A,B), 18 hours (C,D), and 24 hours (E,F) following infection.

ing removal of bivalent cations from the serum–complement mixture by treatment with the chelating agent, ethylenediaminetetraacetate, or following inactivation of complement with heat or hydrazine.

The role of complement in immune cytolysis was investigated in rabies-infected cells treated with fluorescent antibody in the presence or absence of complement. Viable rabies-infected cells treated with antibody alone showed fluorescence only on the surface; but, in the presence of complement, intracytoplasmic staining of rabies antigen was demonstrated, indicating the penetration of the labeled antibody into the cytoplasm (Fig. 6).

The fact that the infected cells first became susceptible to immune lysis hours after the appearance of fluorescing antigen, when the newly produced virus could already be detected in the medium, in-

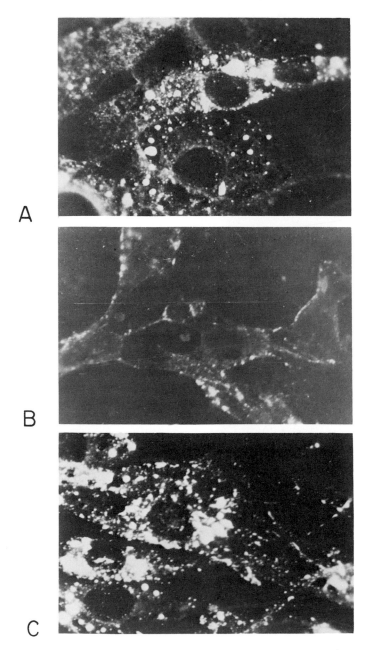

Fig. 6. Staining of PM rabies virus-infected cells with fluorescent rabies antibody. A: After fixation with acetone; B: unfixed cells in absence of complement; C: unfixed cells in presence of complement.

dicates that cell lysis is related to the process of virus release. In chronically infected cells, also, lysis can be induced only at the time when the cells are effectively producing infectious virus (Wiktor and Clark, 1972).

Both lytic and neutralizing antibody are found in the 7 S IgG fraction of human and mouse serum. In the sera of animals either immunized against rabies or in the incubation stage of the disease, however, the titers of lytic and neutralizing antibody have been found to vary independently.

IX. Production of Interferon in Rabies Virus-Infected Cells

Rabies virus-induced interferon was first isolated from tissues of infected hamsters (Stewart and Sulkin, 1966). Brain tissue, in which the virus reached its highest titer, also contained the largest amount of interferon.

Kaplan *et al.* (1960a) showed that medium from rabies virus-infected chick embryo cell monolayers was capable of inducing interference to the replication of a heterologous virus, but the inhibitor was not characterized. Wiktor *et al.* (1964) and Fernandes *et al.* (1964) were unable to demonstrate interferon in either rabies virus-infected HDCS or rabbit endothelial cells. However, Wiktor and Koprowski (1967) demonstrated that hamster (Nil-2) cells chronically infected with rabies virus were resistant to challenge with VSV and Mengo virus, and released a virus-inhibitory substance which was characterized as interferon. In this system, periodic cycles of low and high levels of virus production appeared to be related to the level of interferon production.

Recently Wiktor *et al.* (1972) were able to produce interferon in cells of human and rabbit origin treated with live or inactivated rabies virus preparations. Induction of interferon was dependent on the input MOI; only cells treated with 10 or more PFU/cell produced interferon. Virus inactivated by ultraviolet light or by β-propiolactone did not induce interferon. These results could explain the lack of success encountered by earlier workers who were using lower concentrations of virus.

Cells in tissue culture can be effectively protected from rabies virus infection by treatment with exogenous interferon. This has been demonstrated in the cells of dog (Depoux, 1965b), hamster (Wiktor and Koprowski, 1967), mouse (Barroeta and Atanasiu, 1969), and human origin (Wiktor *et al.*, 1972).

X. Cytopathic Effect of Rabies Virus in Cell Cultures

In general, no specific cytopathic effect can be observed in mono-layers of cell cultures infected with rabies virus. However, in mono-layers of chick embryo cells (Yoshino et al., 1966; Yoshino and Morishima, 1971), or in agarose-suspended cells of hamster origin (Sedwick and Wiktor, 1967), the viability of infected cells can be af-fected to the point that plaque production occurs.

Infected cells can be maintained in an actively growing state by regular trypsinization and division for prolonged periods of time. Chronically infected cells, however, may demonstrate a lower cloning efficiency as well as a slower rate of multiplication (Wiktor and Clark, 1972). Recently, a cytopathic effect was observed in fused hamster embryo cells (Díaz et al., 1973) infected with CVS strain of virus, and in pig fallopian cell line (Bouillant et al., 1974) infected with ERA strain. The use of this system was recommended for virus titration and determination of virus neutralizing antibody.

XI. Optimal Conditions for the Production of Rabies Virus in High Titer

A number of factors profoundly influence the quantity of rabies virus obtained, including the type of cell culture, the strain of virus and input multiplicity of infection, the incubation temperature, the pH of the medium, and the protein supplement in the medium.

We have found nearly every type of cultivated mammalian or avian cell, in primary culture or as an established cell line, to be suscep-tible to infection by rabies virus. Serially propagated cells are the most convenient to maintain in the laboratory, and "altered" cell lines of Syrian hamster origin, such as BHK/21 and Nil-2, seem to give the highest yields of virus. Altered cells are currently consid-ered unacceptable for human vaccine production; therefore, sub-strates used for this purpose include primary Syrian hamster kidney cells and diploid cell strains of primate origin. Maximum virus yields obtained in diploid cell strains are usually no more than 10% of those obtained in BHK/21 cells.

There has been no definitive report on a correlation between the stage of the cell cycle and susceptibility to the initiation of rabies virus infection. Total virus yields are often higher when cells are in-fected in suspension and then plated and allowed to grow to con-fluency, than when already confluent monolayers are infected *in situ*.

This suggests that rabies virus may replicate more efficiently in rapidly dividing cells. However, an enhanced susceptibility to rabies virus in monolayers of BHK/21 cells given lethal doses of UV irradiation has also been reported (Kaplan *et al.*, 1967).

Fixed virus strains with a long history of *in vitro* passage appear to give the highest yields in cell culture. ERA strain virus, with an extensive history of passage in a variety of cell culture systems (Abelseth, 1964a), appears to routinely replicate to higher titer than any other common strain; titers of $\geq 1 \times 10^9$ PFU/ml are often obtained in BHK/21 cells. Again, however, the choice of strains for human vaccine production is limited to those without a history of passage in "altered" cell lines.

The cell MOI has a profound effect on the early yield of rabies virus. Unlike several other rhabdoviruses, such as VSV (Cooper and Bellett, 1959) and Kern Canyon virus (H. G. Aaslestad and H F. Clark, unpublished data), rabies virus does not seem to exhibit autointerference when inoculated at high MOI. Thus, the level of early yield is directly proportional to the MOI, although final yields are similar at all MOI.

Incubation temperature exerts a profound effect on the yield of rabies virus. A typical example, as shown by the growth of PM strain virus in HDCS cells, is shown in Table I. Shortly after infection similar yields of virus are usually obtained over a wide temperature range, approximately 30°–38°C. However, maximal virus titers are finally obtained only in cultures incubated at a temperature of 35°C and below, with 32°–33°C being optimal (Clark and Wiktor, 1972).

The effect of pH on the yield of virus from infected HDCS is

Table I

The Effect of Temperature on Virus Yield from Rabies-Infected HDCS Cells

Temperature (°C)	Yield (PFU/ml)		
	24 hours	96 hours	14 days
34.0	4.0×10^3	4.7×10^5	1.5×10^8
35.0		2.2×10^5	1.3×10^8
35.8	5.5×10^3	4.6×10^5	9.0×10^7
36.0		3.0×10^5	1.4×10^7
37.0	6.0×10^3	2.0×10^5	2.0×10^7
38.0		3.0×10^5	1.2×10^6
38.8	1.1×10^3	3.3×10^4	1.0×10^6
39.8		4.0×10^3	1.3×10^4
42.5	$<5.0 \times 10^1$	1.0×10^1	

Table II

The Effect of Different pHs on Virus Yield from Rabies-Infected HDCS Cells

Starting pH	Final pH	Infectivity (PFU/ml × log 10)
6.7	6.4	3.0
7.1	6.5	4.0
7.5	7.0	6.2
7.9	7.2	7.2
8.3	7.7	5.8

shown in Table II. Regardless of the type of buffer employed in the medium — bicarbonate, Tris, Hepes, or others — an alkaline pH leads to enhanced virus yields. A pH of 7.6–8.0 is normally used at the initiation of virus infection.

The rate of rabies virus replication is affected by the nature of the protein supplement added to the culture medium. Replication is lowered when the culture medium is not supplemented. The addition of either human or bovine serum albumin at concentrations as low as 0.1%, or of lactalbumin hydrolysate at a concentration of ≥ 0.5%, allows virus replication to proceed at near-maximal rates for the first few days after infection of BHK/21 cells (T. J. Wiktor and H F. Clark, unpublished results). In cell types that do not support rabies virus replication as efficiently as do BHK/21 cells (such as HDCS), virus titers may be depressed in medium containing protein supplements other than whole serum.

XII. Coinfection of Cells *In Vitro* with Rabies and Other Viruses

Rabies virus has been propagated in cultured cells coinfected with canine distemper virus, with no effect on the rabies virus yield (Chang, 1965). In other instances coinfecting virus has been shown to enhance or to inhibit rabies virus replication.

As mentioned above, rabies virus replicates most efficiently in cells of the continuous cell line BHK/21, known to be infected with a native "R" type virus (Shipman *et al.*, 1969). Rabies virus is also readily grown in murine cell lines such as mouse ependymoma (Atanasiu and Lépine, 1959) and L cells which spontaneously produce budding C-type virions. In a survey of the susceptibility to rabies of several continuous cell lines of reptilian, amphibian, and fish origin (Clark, 1972), it was found that a viper cell line, VSW, which produces C-type virus in great quantity (Ziegel and Clark, 1969), yielded much higher yields of rabies virus than did any of the other cold-blooded vertebrate cell types tested. In electron microscopic examination of rabies virus-infected VSW cells, rabies virus and the indigenous C-type virus have been observed budding in very close proximity from adjacent portions of the same cell plasma membrane. It was suggested that rabies virus-infected VSW cells might provide a useful model for study of the phenotypic and genotypic interactions between these two different classes of viruses within a single cell (Lunger and Clark, 1972).

The growth of a number of strains of fixed rabies virus accidentally contaminated with lymphocytic choriomeningitis virus (LCM) was studied by Wiktor et al. (1966). The coinfection with LCM had caused a remarkable enhancement in the percentage of cells determined to develop FA staining antigen and in the final yield of infectious rabies virus obtained from cultures of HDCS or RE cells. LCM interfered with rabies growth in BHK/21 cells. The mechanism behind these phenomena has not been elucidated.

XIII. Effect of Metabolic Inhibitors on Virus Replication
In Vitro

Only a few scattered reports are available on the effects of inhibitors of macromolecular synthesis on rabies growth in cell culture. Kissling and Reese (1963) reported that replication of rabies virus was not inhibited when 5-bromo-2'-deoxyuridine (BUdR) was added to hamster kidney cell cultures in a concentration (40 μg/ml), sufficient to reduce the yields of several DNA-type viruses by more than 90%. On this basis they hypothesized that rabies contains an RNA type of nucleic acid.

Subsequently, Defendi and Wiktor (1966) reported that the induction of FA staining in infected HDCS cells was not inhibited by the DNA inhibitor 5-fluoro-2'-deoxyuridine (FUdR) and was actually enhanced in the presence of concentrations of actinomycin D (AD, an inhibitor of DNA transcription) as low as 0.01 μg/ml. Mitomycin C and guanidine were also found to be noninhibitory for rabies antigen synthesis in this system, although a profound inhibition of both antigen induction and released virus yields was observed in cultures treated with cyclohexamide, a protein synthesis inhibitor, at a concentration of 5 μg/ml.

Extended studies of the effect of several inhibitors on antigen induction and virus yields in BHK/21 cells were subsequently reported by Maes *et al.* (1967). The inhibitors of DNA replication, AD, mitomycin C, and FUdR, were found to be noninhibitory or even enhancing for rabies virus infection, whereas the protein inhibitors fluorophenylalanine and cycloheximide were both severely inhibitory. A single inhibitor of DNA replication, cytosine arabinoside (ara-C) was highly inhibitory for rabies virus at a concentration of 50 μg/ml. Studies of the inhibition of rabies synthesis by ara-C were continued by Campbell *et al.* (1968), who reported that the ara-C effect was blocked if the DNA transcription inhibitors, AD or Nogalomycin, or the RNA translation inhibitors, puromycin or cyloheximide, were added early in the course of the infection. It was concluded that ara-C acted by inducing the synthesis of a specific protein inhibitory for rabies virus.

Recently H F. Clark (unpublished data), using the sensitive plaque assay system of Sedwick and Wiktor (1967) rather than the mouse titration assays employed in the above-mentioned investigations, have encountered difficulty in reproducing some of the previously reported findings with DNA inhibitors. In this regard, both AD and ara-C present special problems, since they are so toxic in effective concentrations that specific antiviral effects, and effects resulting from nonspecific deleterious effects on cells, are often difficult to distinguish from each other, particularly in the case of rabies virus which exhibits a rather slow rate of replication at ordinary MOI.

In the case of rabies-infected cells treated with AD, we have confirmed the observation that the induction of FA staining is little affected, but we have observed substantial reductions in yields from cell cultures treated with AD. In general, we have found that the addition of 0.1 μg/ml, or more, of AD to BHK/21 cell cultures within 24 hours after infection leads to a 80–95% reduction in the total yield of released virus released at 48 hours. The inhibitory effect of AD on rabies virus has hindered efforts to characterize rabies virus specific RNA synthesis in cells infected *in vitro*.

XIV. Alteration of Rabies Virus Phenotype as a Result of Passage in Cell Culture

The effect of long-term passage *in vitro* on rabies virus characters has remained relatively untested. Indeed, many investigators have been primarily interested in demonstrating that tissue culture-propagated rabies virus possesses unaltered immunogenicity.

The adaptation of rabies virus to various cell culture substrates has often been reported to lead to the development of strains with an enhanced potential for causing "cytopathic effect" (CPE). Thus, Atanasiu and Lépine (1959) reported the appearance of CPE at the fifth passage level during adaptation of a strain of street rabies to a mouse ependymoma cell line. Kissling and Reese (1963) reported that CPE appeared during the sixteenth passage of strain CVS rabies virus in primary hamster kidney cells, and became more pronounced with further passage. Hronovský et al. (1968) reported that a street strain of rabies virus became cytopathic at the fourth passage level in primary puppy kidney cell culture. Ilyasova and Kluyeva (1969) reported the onset of CPE during the twenty-first passage of the Mochalin strain of street rabies virus in hamster kidney cell cultures. Unfortunately, none of these reported cytopathic virus strains has yet found widespread application in the laboratory. Although we have had experience at the Wistar Institute with numerous strains of fixed rabies virus serially cultivated 50–100 (or more) times in a variety of cell culture types, we have been unable to develop a virus strain of sufficient cytopathogenicity to permit the routine use of virus assay based upon CPE in cell monolayers.

Few reports of attenuation of rabies virus grown in cell culture are available. Virus of the Flury HEP strain was reported to lose its virulence for intracerebrally inoculated monkeys after 47 passages in HDCS cells, although the virus retained immunogenicity in the same species (Wiktor et al., 1964). The continued passage of the CVS strain of virus in the rabbit cell line RE caused it to exhibit a decrease in both virulence and antigenicity in mice (Fernandes et al., 1964). ERA strain fixed rabies virus, after serial passage in swine kidney cells, lost all detectable virulence for cattle while growing to high titer and retaining excellent immunogenicity (Abelseth, 1964b). During studies of the growth of strain CVS virus in reptilian cell culture (Clark, 1972), it was determined that virus passaged in a lizard cell line, GL1, decreased in virulence and immunogenicity in mice, while continued passage of the same virus in the viper cell line, VSW, led to a decrease in virulence for mice without loss in immunogenicity.

"Markers" distinguishing strains of rabies virus adapted to cell culture are essentially unknown. Clark and Wiktor (1972) demonstrate that certain rabies virus strains altered by serial passage at low temperature, or in exotic cell types, or by chemical mutagenesis, diffe from the parental virus with regard to plaque size and temperature sensitivity characters. The characters were constant for a given virus substrain, but were not regularly correlated with the presence or absence of mouse virulence.

Acknowledgment

Supported, in part, by U. S. Public Health Service Research Grant AI-09706 from the National Institute of Allergy and Infectious Diseases and by funds from the World Health Organization.

References

Abelseth, M. K. (1964a). *Can. Vet. J.* 5, 84.
Abelseth, M. K. (1964b). *Can. Vet. J.* 5, 279.
Aksenova, T. A., Selimov, M. A., Chumakov, M. P., Mironova, L. L., and Goldrin, N. E. (1966). *Acta Virol. (Prague)* 10, 276.
Allen, R., Sims, R. A., and Sulkin, S. E. (1964a). *Amer. J. Hyg.* 50, 25.
Allen, R., Sims, R. A., and Sulkin, S. E. (1964b). *Amer. J. Hyg.* 80, 11.
Atanasiu, P., and Laurent, C. (1957). *C. R. Acad. Sci.* 245, 2562–2564.
Atanasiu, P., and Lépine, P. (1959). *Ann. Inst. Pasteur, Paris* 96, 72–78.
Atanasiu, P., Favre, S., and Collombier, M. (1961). *C. R. Acad. Sci.* 252, 2029.
Atanasiu, P., Lépine, P., and Dragonas, P. (1963). *Ann. Inst. Pasteur, Paris* 105, 813.
Atanasiu, P., Dragonas, P., Tsiang, H., and Harbi, A. (1971). *Ann. Inst. Pasteur, Paris* 121, 247.
Barroeta, M., and Atanasiu, P. (1969). *C. R. Acad. Sci.* 269, 1353,
Bequignon, R., Gruest, J., Vieuchange, C., and Vieuchange, J. (1954). *C. R. Acad. Sci.* 239, 1163.
Bernkopf, H., and Kligler, I. J. (1937). *Brit. J. Exp. Pathol.* 18, 481.
Bouillant, A. M., Tabel, H., and Greig, A. S. (1974). *Can. J. Comp. Med.* 38, 118.
Cabasso, V. J., Dobkin, M. R., Roby, R. E., Hammar, A. H. (1974). *Appl. Micro.* 27, 553.
Campbell, J. B., Maes, R. F., Wiktor, T. J., and Koprowski, H. (1968). *Virology* 34, 701.
Chang, J. C.C. (1965). *Can. J. Comp. Med.* 29, 38.
Clark, H. F. (1972). *Proc. Soc. Exp. Biol. Med.* 139, 1317.
Clark, H. F., and Wiktor, T. J. (1972). *J. Infec. Dis.* 125, 637.
Cooper, P. D., and Bellett, A. J. D. (1959). *J. Gen. Microbiol.* 21, 485.
Defendi, V., and Wiktor, T. J. (1966). *Symp. Ser. Immunol. Stand.* 1, 119.
Depoux, R. (1963). *C. R. Acad. Sci.* 257, 2757.
Depoux, R. (1964). *Can. J. Microbiol.* 10, 527.
Depoux, R. (1965a). *Ann. Inst. Pasteur, Paris* 108, 566.
Depoux, R. (1965b). *C. R. Acad. Sci.* 260, 354.
Diamond, L. (1967). *Int. J. Cancer* 2, 143.
Díaz, A. M., Yager, P. A., Baer, G. M. (1973). *Arch. Gesamte. Virusforsch.* 43, 297.
Fenje, P. (1960a). *Can. J. Microbiol.* 6, 479.
Fenje, P. (1960b). *Can. J. Microbiol.* 6, 605.

178   *T. J. Wiktor and H F. Clark*

Fernandes, M. V., Wiktor, T. J., and Koprowski, H, (1963). Virology 21, 128.
Fernandes, M. V., Wiktor, T. J., and Koprowski, H. (1964). J. Exp. Med. 120, 1099.
Fox, J. P., Koprowski, H., Conwell, D. P., Black, J., and Gelfand, H. M. (1957). Bull. WHO 17, 869.
Goldwasser, R. A., and Kissling, R. E. (1958). Proc. Soc. Exp. Biol. Med. 98, 219.
Halonen, P. E., Murphy, F. A., Fields, B. N., and Reese, D. R. (1968). Proc. Soc. Exp. Biol. Med. 127, 1037.
Hayflick, L., and Moorhead, P. S. (1961). Exp. Cell Res. 25, 585.
Hronovský, V., Benda, R., and Cinatl, J. (1966). Acta Virol. (Prague) 10, 181.
Hronovsky, V., Benda, R., and Cinatl, J. (1968). Acta Virol. (Prague) 12, 233.
Hummeler, K., Koprowski, H., and Wiktor, T. J. (1967). J. Virol. 1, 152.
Ilyasova, R. Sh., and Kluyeva, D. D. (1969). Acta Virol. (Prague) 13, 156.
Iwasaki, Y., Wiktor, T. J., and Koprowski, H. (1973). Lab. Invest. 28, 142.
Kanazawa, K. (1936). Jap. J. Exp. Med. 14, 519.
Kanazawa, K. (1937). Jap. J. Exp. Med. 15, 17.
Kaplan, M. M., Wecker, E., Zlatko, R., and Koprowski, H. (1960a). Nature (London) 186, 821.
Kaplan, M. M., Forsek, Z., and Koprowski, H. (1960b). Bull. WHO 22, 434.
Kaplan, M. M., Wiktor, T. J., Maes, R. F., Campbell, J. B., and Koprowski, H. (1967). J. Virol. 1, 145.
Kissling, R. E. (1958). Proc. Soc. Exp. Biol. Med. 98, 223.
Kissling, R. E., and Reese, D. R. (1963). J. Immunol. 91, 362.
Kligler, I. J., and Bernkopf, H. (1941). Amer. J. Hyg. 33, 1.
Kondo, A. (1965). Virology 27, 199.
Koprowski, H. (1954). Bull. WHO 10, 709.
Kuwert, E., Wiktor, T. J., Sokol, F., and Koprowski, H. (1968). J. Virol. 2, 1381.
Lang, R., Petermann, H. G., Branche, R., and Soulebot, J. P. (1969). C. R. Acad. Sci. 269, 2287.
Levaditi, C. (1913). C. R. Soc. Biol. 75, 505.
Levaditi, C. (1914). C. R. Acad. Sci. 159, 284.
Levaditi, C., and Schoen, R. (1936). C. R. Acad. Sci. 202, 702.
Levaditi, C., Schoen, R., and Renie, L. (1937). Ann. Inst. Pasteur, Paris 58, 353.
Love, R., Fernandes, M. V., and Koprowski, H. (1964). Proc. Soc. Exp. Biol. Med. 116, 560.
Love, R., Fernandes, M. V., and Wiktor, T. J. (1966). Rev. Pathol. Comp. 66, 533.
Lunger, P. D., and Clark, H F. (1972). In Vitro 7, 377.
MacPherson, I., and Stoker, M. (1962). Virology 16, 147.
Maes, R. F., Kaplan, M. M., Wiktor, T. J., Campbell, J. B., and Koprowski, H. (1967). Mol. Biol. Viruses, Proc. Symp., 1966, pp. 449–462.
Martos, L., and Atanasiu, P. (1961). Ann. Inst. Pasteur, Paris 101, 448.
Matsumoto, S. (1963). J. Cell Biol. 19, 565.
Mikhailovskii, E. M. (1966). Vop. Virusol. 11, 328.
Noguchi, H. (1913). J. Exp. Med. 18, 314.
Parker, R. C., and Hollender, A. J. (1945). Proc. Soc. Exp. Biol. Med. 60, 94.
Pearson, J. E., Atanasiu, P., and Lépine, P. (1958). Ann. Inst. Pasteur, Paris 94, 1.
Plotz, J., and Reagan, R. (1942). Science 95, 102.
Schlumberger, H. D., Wiktor, T. J., and Koprowski, H. (1970). J. Immunol. 105, 291
Schoen, R. (1937). C. R. Soc. Biol. 125, 939.
Schultz, E. W., and Williams, G. F. (1937). Proc. Soc. Exp. Biol. 37, 372.
Sedwick, W. D., and Wiktor, T. J. (1967). J. Virol. 1, 1224.

Shipman, C., Vander Weide, G. C., and Ma, B. I. (1969). *Virology* **38**, 707.
Sikes, R. K., Cleary, W. F., Koprowski, H., Wiktor, T. J., and Kaplan, M. M. (1971). *Bull. WHO* **45**, 1.
Sokol, F., Kuwert, E., Wiktor, T. J., Hummeler, K., and Koprowski, H. (1968). *J. Virol.* **2**, 836.
Solis, J., and Mora, E. C. (1970). *Appl. Microbiol.* **19**, 1.
Stewart, W. E., and Sulkin, S. E. (1966). *Proc. Soc. Exp. Biol. Med.* **123**, 650.
Stoel, G. (1930). *C. R. Soc. Biol.* **104**, 851.
Tsiang, H., and Atanasiu P. (1971). *C. R. Acad. Sci.* **272**, 897.
Ver, B. A. (1965). *Indian J. Pathol. Bacteriol.* **8**, 271.
Ver, B. A., Nanavati, A. N. D., and Jhala, H. I. (1964). *Indian J. Pathol. Bacteriol.* **7**, 234.
Vieuchange, J. (1956). *C. R. Acad. Sci.* **242**, 201.
Vieuchange, J., Vialat, C., Gruest, J., and Bequignon, R. (1956a). *Ann. Inst. Pasteur, Paris* **90**, 361.
Vieuchange, J., Bequignon, R., Gruest, J., and Vialat, C. (1956b). *Bull. Acad. Nat. Med. Paris* [3] (**5/6**), 77.
Webster, L. T., and Clow, A. D. (1936). *Science* **84**, 487.
Webster, L. T., and Clow, A. D. (1937). *J. Exp. Med.* **66**, 125.
Wiktor, T. J. (1966). *Symp. Ser. Immunol. Stand.* **1**, 65.
Wiktor, T. J. (1971). *Sci. Publ., Pan-Amer. Health Org.* **226**, 66.
Wiktor, T. J. (1973). *In* "Laboratory Techniques in Rabies" (M. M. Kaplan and H. Koprowski, eds.), pp. 101–123. *Geneva. World Health Organ. Monogr. Ser.*
Wiktor, T. J., and Clark, H F. (1972). *Infection and Immunity*, **6**, 988.
Wiktor, T. J., and Koprowski, H. (1965). *Proc. Soc. Exp. Biol. Med.* **118**, 1069.
Wiktor, T. J., and Koprowski, H. (1967). *Bacteriol. Proc.* p. 166 (abstr.).
Wiktor, T. J., Fernandes, M. V., and Koprowski, H. (1964). *J. Immunol.* **93**, 353.
Wiktor, T. J., Kaplan, M. M., and Koprowski, H. (1966). *Ann. Med. Exp. Fenn.* **44**, 290.
Wiktor, T. J., Kuwert, E., and Koprowski, H. (1968). *J. Immunol.* **101**, 1271.
Wiktor, T. J., Sokol, F., Kuwert, E., and Koprowski, H. (1969). *Proc. Soc. Exp. Biol. Med.* **131**, 799.
Wiktor, T. J., Postic, B., Ho, M., and Koprowski, H. (1972). *J. Inf. Disease* **126**, 408.
Wiktor, T. J., Plotkin, S. A., Grella, D. W. (1973). *JAMA* **224**, 1170.
Yoshino, K., and Morishima, T. (1971). *Arch. Gesamte Virusforsch.* **34**, 40.
Yoshino, K., Taniguchi, S., and Arai, K. (1966). *Arch. Gesamte Virusforsch.* **18**, 370.
Ziegel, R. F., and Clark, H F. (1969). *J. Nat. Cancer Inst.* **43**, 1097.

CHAPTER 10

Pathogenesis to the Central Nervous System

George M. Baer

I. Pathogenesis after Subcutaneous or Intramuscular Introduction of Virus

In most people exposed to rabies virus the exact time and location of viral entrance are known. The treatment given thereafter must be based on a precise knowledge of the subsequent movement of virus. Rather crude methods such as tissue titration and histopathologic examination have commonly been used to study this, but recently more refined ones such as fluorescent antibody staining, radioactive labeling, and electron microscopy have been added. Yet even with these newer techniques large gaps still exist in our understanding of the chain of events that occur.

Pasteur *et al.* (1881), the first to demonstrate the role of the central nervous system (CNS) in rabies, wrote that "the central nervous system, and especially the bulb which joins the spinal cord to the brain, are particularly concerned and active in the development of the disease." Later (1882) he found virus in the spinal cord but not in the brain stem of dogs inoculated intravenously with virus and sacrificed at the first signs of paralysis.

Before the virus moves toward the CNS via the nerves, however, a complicated and little understood series of events, including entrance, absorption, and eclipse, occur at the site of introduction.

Johnson (1967) reviewed the types of infection that can occur:

a) in the most simple type of infection the virus goes into eclipse 3 hours after inoculation in the animal; the virus is logically enough in the host but cannot be recovered, but it fails to multiply; b) the virus is "fixed" in the tissue and multiplies, but cannot complete the growth-cycle; it reaches a certain stage, but does not leave the infected cell; c) the virus is "fixed," completes the growth cycle, multiplies locally, but there is no systemic invasion; d) the virus is "fixed," completes its cycle at the entrance site with subsequent systemic invasion, but without clinical signs of the disease—the animal stays healthy; e) finally there is the type of infection in which the virus enters, invades the central nervous system, and produces disease and death.

Rabies virus injected into the footpads or muscle tissue of experimental animals can be recovered from the site of inoculation for relatively short periods of time. Dean *et al.* (1963b) amputated the feet of mice inoculated with fixed virus and found that the procedure of removing the inoculated area was a lifesaving procedure for 4 hours or less after inoculation (Table I). These results are similar to (1) those found some 50 years ago by Fermi (1928), in which rats could be saved by amputation of the inoculated tail up to 5 hours after inoculation with the fixed virus, but no longer (also quoted by Kraus *et al.*, 1926), and (2) those of Bombici and Calebrese (also quoted by Kraus *et al.*, 1926) who could save rabbits that had been inoculated in the anterior chamber of the eye by ocular enucleation 24 hours

Table I

Effect of Amputation of Injected Limb on Outcome of Infection in Mice Inoculated in the Footpad with Fixed (CVS) Rabies[a]

Interval between inoculation and amputation	Results	
	Front limb	Hind limb
15 min	1/14 (HS)	0/13 (HS)
1 hour	0/10 (HS)	0/15 (HS)
2 hours	0/12 (HS)	0/14 (HS)
4 hours	2/11 (HS)	6/14 (HS)
8 hours	15/15	15/15
12 hours	14/15	15/15
24 hours	14/15	14/14
Controls	13/15	14/15

[a] Reproduced with permission of the *Bulletin of the World Health Organization*, after Dean *et al.* (1963b).

[b] Results are expressed as ratio of the number of animals dying of rabies to the number inoculated. HS indicates that the difference from the controls is highly significant

after infection, but not 36 hours. In more recent experiments fluorescent antigen was seen to be "orderly arranged" in the subcutaneous footpad tissue of mice for up to 6 hours after inoculation there with fixed virus (Schneider, 1969), but by 12 hours no fluorescence whatsoever could be noted; this corresponds very closely to the 4 hours shown by Dean *et al.* (1963b) to be the time at which fixed virus begins to leave the inoculation site. Virus could not be recovered from the inoculated left hind footpad of rats 24 hours after they had been inoculated with a low peripheral LD_{50} of a "street" virus isolate (Baer *et al.*, 1968), yet it had been recoverable immediately after inoculation (Fig. 1). Habel (1941), however, found that in some cases "street" virus isolates may persist locally for up to 96 hours after intramuscular inoculation. Sulkin *et al.* (1959) found $10^{2.5}$–10^4 mouse intracerebral LD_{50} ($MICLD_{50}$) of Mexican freetail bat strain virus in the muscular tissue of 4 of 27 hamsters inoculated intracerebrally and concluded that, terminally, virus had multiplied in muscle; this does not seem, however, to parallel the initial replication prior to multiplication of the virus in the CNS.

It appears that production of disease may depend on the area of the body exposed. Guinea pigs, for instance, died after a drop of fixed rabies virus was placed on a small hole cut in the skin of the neck, but none succumbed when the same dose was applied in the back leg (Dean *et al.*, 1963a). Similarly, 80% of red foxes died after being inoculated in the neck muscles with low egg passage Flury vaccine (developed by Koprowski and Cox, 1948) but the mortality fell to 20% when the same dose was injected in the rear leg muscles (R. L. Parker, personal communication, 1962). Statistics on human disease also indicate that wounds on the head and neck are generally more lethal than those on the hands and feet (Baltazard and Ghoddsi, 1954; Wang, 1956; Veeraraghavan, 1964).

After the short initial period of obvious viability the virus goes into eclipse, during which time it cannot be recovered from any tissue whatsoever (Remlinger and Bailly, 1928; Schindler, 1961; Kligler and Bernkopf, 1943; Johnson, 1965; Baer *et al.*, 1968; Schneider, 1969a,b), and during this eclipse period the virus may have (1) remained locally or (2) already proceeded on its pathway to or within the CNS. There is evidence (Baer *et al.*, 1965) that after footpad inoculation of virus, neural invasion may occur during eclipse, since sciatic nerve resection stopped progression of virus long before infective virus first appeared in the CNS (Table II). It appears more probable, however, that virus remains locally during most of the eclipse period. In a recent series of experiments (Baer and Cleary, 1972) mice were inoculated in the left rear footpad with approxi-

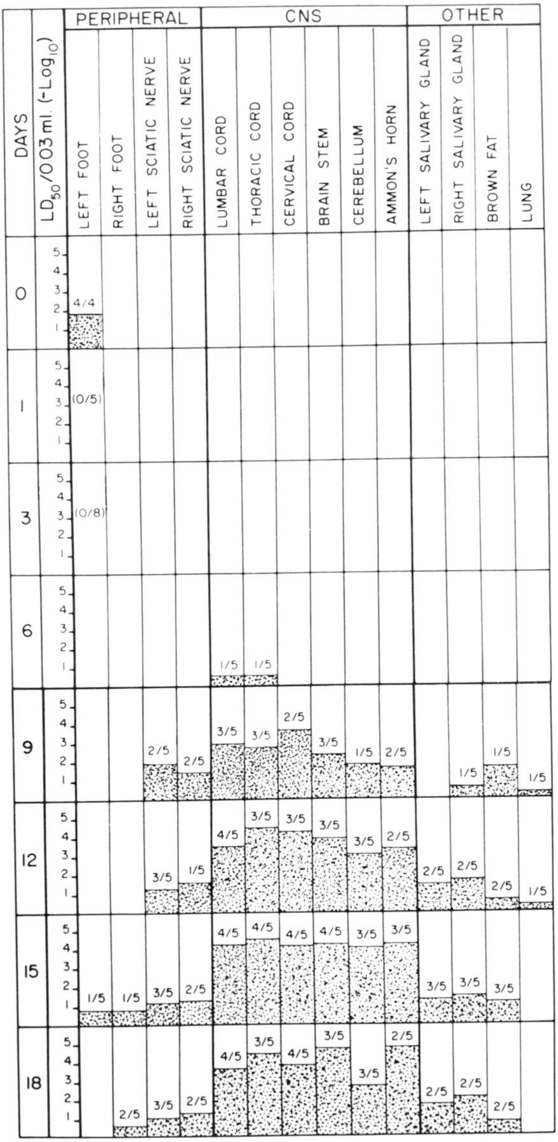

DAYS	$LD_{50}/0.03\,ml\ (-Log_{10})$	PERIPHERAL				CNS						OTHER			
		LEFT FOOT	RIGHT FOOT	LEFT SCIATIC NERVE	RIGHT SCIATIC NERVE	LUMBAR CORD	THORACIC CORD	CERVICAL CORD	BRAIN STEM	CEREBELLUM	AMMON'S HORN	LEFT SALIVARY GLAND	RIGHT SALIVARY GLAND	BROWN FAT	LUNG
0		4/4													
1		(0/5)													
3		(0/8)													
6						1/5	1/5								
9				2/5	2/5	3/5	3/5	2/5	3/5	1/5	2/5	1/5	1/5	1/5	1/5
12				3/5	1/5	4/5	3/5	3/5	3/5	3/5	2/5	2/5	2/5	2/5	1/5
15			1/5	1/5	3/5	2/5	4/5	4/5	4/5	4/5	3/5	3/5	3/5	3/5	3/5
18			2/5	3/5	2/5	4/5	3/5	4/5	3/5	3/5	2/5	2/5	2/5	2/5	

Fig. 1. Measurements of rabies virus in peripheral nervous system, central nervous system, and other organs of rats after inoculation of street virus in the left hind footpad. The numerator represents the number of animals with particular tissues infected and the denominator the number of animals killed during the period. On days 1 and 3 no tissues were infected. Reproduced with permission of *Bulletin of the World Health Organization* (1968).

Table II

*Rate of Ascent of Fixed Rabies Virus in Sciatic Nerves of Rats,
As Determined by Neurectomy or Appearance of Virus[e]*

Rabies mortality in rats challenged in the left hind footpad with fixed rabies virus, followed by neurectomy at various time intervals			Appearance of fixed rabies virus in the left sciatic nerves of rats challenged in the left hind footpad[d,e]	
Nerve removal (– hours after challenge)	Sciatic and saphenous neurectomy in 200-g[a] rats	Removal of sciatic nerve fasciculus plus saphenous neurectomy 200-g[a] rats	Mortality in mice inoculated intracerebrally with nerves	Serum-neutralizing antibodies in "immunized" rats
1	0/1[b,c]			
2	0/2			
3	0/2			
4	0/2			
5	0/2			
6	0/2	0/1		
7	0/2			
8	0/2	0/2		
9	1/2	0/2		
10	2/2	2/2		
11	2/2	1/2		
12	2/2	2/2	–	–
13	2/2	2/2		
14	2/2	1/2		
15	1/1[c]	2/2		
24			–	–
48			–	+
72			+	+
96			+	+

[a] Approximate weight.

[b] Number of rabies deaths/number of animals challenged and operated on.

[c] One rat died of causes other than rabies.

[d] As determined by mouse mortality after intracerebral inoculation or by the presence of antibody in rats "immunized" intramuscularly with pooled nerves.

[e] Reproduced with permission of the *Bulletin of the World Health Organization* (1968).

mately 10 peripheral LD_{50} of a bobcat "street" virus isolate that produced disease in 17–120 days (incubation periods similar to those often seen in man, as reviewed by Dean, 1963); 48% of those mice died less than 30 days after inoculation, 25% between the thirty-first and sixtieth days, and 12% more than 60 days after inoculation. In those groups in which the inoculated foot was amputated immediately after inoculation or 1, 3, 5, 9, or 18 days later, all animals that died did so within 30 days after inoculation (Table III), giving strong evidence that virus either stays locally for long periods (and in this case was removed by amputation even 18 days later) or advances rapidly (and those animals died with short incubation periods). Five of the 21 mice that survived the inoculation with this bobcat "street" isolate had serum neutralizing antibodies 1 year later; during this time none of the animals appeared sick, suggesting that in some cases there may be replication of the virus without production of clinical signs.

Clarification of preneural rabies pathogenesis has come with the observations recently made by Murphy *et al.* (1973), in which fixed and street virus isolates were detected in myocytes (by the fluorescent antibody technique) after intramuscular inoculation of highly susceptible young hamsters. Actual replication in myocytes was confirmed by later electron microscopy observation (see Chapter 15), and the infection was then seen to advance to the neuromuscular and neuro-tendinal spindles before its presence was noted in the peripheral and central nervous system. This remarkable finding has great importance in the study of postexposure rabies prophylaxis, since the efficacy of treatment procedures most probably depends on the accessibility of the virus before it becomes ensconced in the nervous system. As stated, this period appears to be considerably longer than 72 hours.

Another example of probable local replication of virus is the finding of antibodies to rabies in 12 of 262 (4.6%) apparently healthy foxes taken from a rabies epizootic area, suggesting that this phenomenon occurs in nature also (Tierkel, 1959), although it should be noted that these animals were not held to see whether clinical rabies would develop. Recently, however, raccoons held after capture in the wild (McLean, 1972) developed antibodies to rabies without apparent CNS involvement, once again suggesting introduction of virus without the appearance of disease, probably through contact with rabid animals of the same species in the epizootic area. The same phenomenon has been noted in bats by Burns and Farinacci (1955), who noted that up to 90% of "apparently normal healthy" colonial bats had neutralizing antibody to the virus.

The patterns of viral progression just above the inoculated footpad have been investigated by Johnson (1964, 1965), who studied herpes simplex and rabies virus pathogenesis in suckling mice, and the differences he noted were remarkable. In the mice inoculated with herpes virus the endoneural cells of small subcutaneous nerve fibers were infected (fluoresced) within 24 hours, and, in the next 4 days, infection of both endoneural and perineural cells (Schwann cells and fibroblasts) could be followed up the corresponding peripheral nerves to the dorsal root ganglions and into the appropriate segments of the spinal cord. In the animals inoculated with rabies virus, however, no fluorescence in any structure was noted prior to CNS involvement.

Once virus begins its path to the CNS it does so along nerves. DiVestea and Zagari (1887) showed that the inoculation of virus into peripheral nerves produced rabies, and that cutting or cauterizing the sciatic nerve after peripheral injection of virus in rabbits, guinea pigs, or dogs prevented "diffusion" of virus in most of the animals (DiVestea and Zagari, 1887, 1889a,b). Fermi, too (quoted by Kraus *et al.*, 1926), was able to save intramuscularly inoculated rabbits by cutting the sciatic nerve either before infection or up to 8 hours after infection. While some workers have injected virus into nerves to investigate pathogenesis (Babes, 1887; Roux, 1888; Bardach, 1888; Gantt and Ponomarew, 1929), most have investigated the distribution of virus in the body by titration of tissues at various periods after peripheral inoculation; among them were DiVestea and Zagari (1887), Cantani (quoted by Schaffer, 1889), Nicolau and Kopciowska (1934), Webster (1942), Kligler and Bernkopf (1943), Krause (1957), Huygelen and Mortelmans (1959), Huygelen (1960), and Schindler (1961), all of whom concerned themselves primarily with the central nervous system.

The role of viremia in rabies has been investigated by DiVestea and Zagari (1887), Kraus and Fukuhara (1909), and Schindler (1961), with negative findings, yet Wong and Freund (1951), Borodina (1959), Krause (1957), Frye and Enright (1964), and Kitselman and Mital (1967) found some evidence of viremia in the disease. In most of these experiments, however, the animals were given massive amounts of virus, and it is thus not surprising that "viremia" was noted.

Recent studies with six species of experimental animals, including the highly susceptible fox, have continued and extended DiVestea's and Zagari's findings of almost a century ago, and have once again shown that the spread of virus from the site of inoculation to the spinal cord is primarily by way of the nerves (Dean *et al.*, 1963b; Baer *et al.*, 1965, 1968; Johnson, 1965; Schneider, 1969). Various techniques were used in these recent studies, including the cutting of the sciatic and saphenous nerves either before or after inoculation of virus, the fluorescent antibody technique, and tissue titration.

Dean *et al.* (1963b) showed that fixed rabies virus travels along nerve pathways at a rate of approximately 3 mm/hour, a rate which is similar to that measured for poliomyelitis in monkeys by Bodian and Howe (1941). Baer *et al.* (1965) showed that in rats and hamsters inoculated with fixed virus (Table II), sciatic nerve removal 8–9 hours after footpad inoculation no longer halted viral progression (as determined by subsequent death of the animal); these data coincide

Table III

Group Mortality and Incubation Periods of Mice Inoculated with a Bobcat Rabies Isolate in Which the Left Hindfoot was Amputated at Various Periods after Virus Inoculation[a]

When amputation was done	Mortality[b]	<30 Days[c]	31–60 Days[c]	>60 Days[c]
Immediately after virus inoculation	0/15	–	–	–
1 day	2/18	13, 14	–	–
3 days	1/13	14	–	–
5 days	3/18	14, 15, 16	–	–
9 days	3/18	15, 17, 22	–	–
18 days	3/18	14, 27, 29	–	–
Controls	22/43	17, 18, 18, 20, 20, 20, 22, 23, 25, 27, 27, 29	31, 31, 35, 35, 43, 50, 60	65, 75, 120

[a] Reproduced with permission of *The Journal of Infectious Diseases* (1972).
[b] Reduction in denominator indicates that some mice died of nonspecific causes.
[c] Incubation period.

with the earlier work by Dean *et al.* (1963b). Similar results were obtained by Schneider (1969). When a street virus isolate is used, however (Baer *et al.*, 1968) the rate of progression is much slower and quite variable, and neurectomy or amputation may still be a saving procedure many days after inoculation (Tables III, IV, and V). Evidence that the virus travels passively is given by the rapidity with which fixed virus progresses along nerves, the lack of fluorescence in peripheral nerve tissues, and the fact that the first point of viral replication in the central nervous system appears to be either the spinal ganglia or the dorsal root ganglion cells corresponding to the affected peripheral nerves.

It is not known in precisely what part of the nerve virus advances. Wright (1953) suggested that movement occurs (1) in the lymphatics within the trunks; (2) in the tissue spaces in the epineurium, perineurium, or between nerve fibers; (3) along the nerve, through progressive infection of the cells in the connective tissue or Schwann sheath of the fibers; or (4) within the protoplasm of the axons.

It is apparent that the perineural pathway, although earlier incriminated as the path along which rabies virus passes flows (Gantt and Ponomarew, 1929; Krause, 1957), is not involved in the pathogenesis of the virus. To elucidate this point a series of experiments were performed (Baer *et al.*, 1965, 1968) in which the sciatic nerve peri-

Table IV

Rate of Ascent of Street Rabies Virus in Sciatic Nerves of Rats,
As Determined by Neurectomy or Appearance of Virus[a]

Rabies mortality in rats inoculated in the left hind footpad with street rabies virus followed by neurectomy at various intervals			Time of appearance of street rabies virus in left sciatic nerves[d] of rats inoculated in the left hind footpad		
	Mortality[b]				
No. of hours between challenge and surgery		Rats with sciatic nerve fasciculus removal and saphenous neurectomy	Mortality in mice inoculated intracerebrally with nerves	Fluorescent antibody staining	Presence of serum-neutralizing antibodies in "immunized" rats
0		1/13[c]			
3					
6					
9	0/10		0/5[c]	—	—
12					
24	2/10	3/18	0/5	—	—
48	2/8[c]	5/18	0/5	—	—
72	1/9[c]	3/16[c]	0/5	—	—
96	8/10	7/14[c]	1/5	—	—

[a] Reproduced with permission of *Bulletin of the World Health Organization* (1968).
[b] Ratio of number of rabies deaths to the number of animals challenged and operated on.
[c] Reduction in denominator indicates that some rats died of causes other than rabies.
[d] Nerves removed at various time periods.
[e] Number of rabies deaths/number of mice inoculated.
[f] Negative.

Table V

Effect of Amputation or Neurectomy
on Rats Challenged in the Left Hind Footpad with Street Rabies Virus[a]

No. of hours between inoculation and treatment	Mortality[b] after treatment	
	Foot amputation	Sciatic and saphenous neurectomy
0	0/8	2/8
24	0/7	1/6
48	1/7	1/6
72	1/7	0/7
96	0/7	1/7
Controls	8/12	

[a] By permission of the *Bulletin of the World Health Organization*, Baer *et al.* (1968).
[b] Ratio of number of rabies deaths to the number of animals challenged. A denominator of less than 8 indicates that some rats died of causes other than rabies.

neurium, epineurium, and perineural epithelium (Shanthaveerappa and Bourne, 1962; Fig. 2) were removed prior to inoculation; although there was some alteration of nerve physiology, as evidenced by longer incubation periods in the study animals than in the controls, mortality in both groups was virtually identical (Table VI). When the nerve fasciculus itself was removed with the perineural structures left intact and the rats were subsequently inoculated in the footpad with virus, all remained healthy, whereas all the controls died, indicating that the virus somehow progresses within the nerve fasciculus itself. When the sciatic nerve was demyelinated by nerve crush, apparently resulting in complete demyelinination and disintegration of axons, viral progression was not impeded, suggesting that perhaps the Schwann cells, the endoneurium, or associated tissue spaces play a greater role than the axis cylinder in the centripetal progression of rabies virus. Since viral progression appears almost certain to be by passive flow of the virus, it is more likely that the associated tissue spaces are used. This point remains unresolved, however, and finer techniques such as radioactive labeling will be needed to find the precise area in which rabies virus travels in nerves. Electron microscopy may be another tool, although considerable viral titer is needed before electron micrographs show presence of virus; Jenson *et al.* (1969) found developing virus particles in the perikaryon of the trigeminal ganglion cells and adjacent (un-

Table VI

*Mortality and Incubation Periods in Rats Inoculated
in the Left Hind Footpad with Street Rabies Virus after Removal
of the Sciatic Nerve Fasciculus or Perineural Structures[a]*

		Incubation period (days)	
Groups	Mortality	Median	Range
Rats with sciatic nerve fasciculus removed	0/16	–	–
Rats with sciatic perineural structures removed	9/14	19.5	16–23
Controls	7/11	16	10–25

[a] Epineurium, perineurium, and perineural epithelium. Reproduced with permission of *Bulletin of the World Health Organization*, Baer *et al.* (1968).

[b] Ratio of number of rabies deaths to the number of animals inoculated.

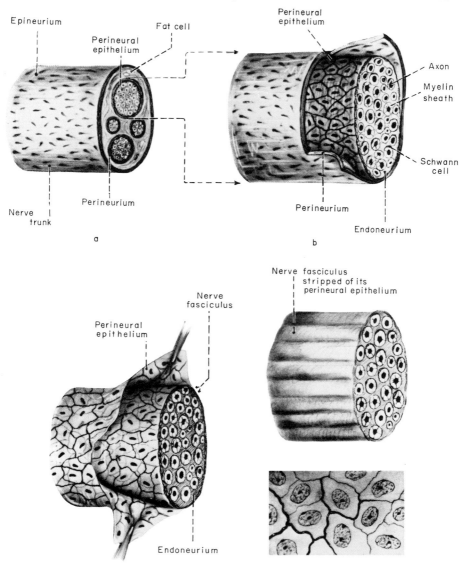

Fig. 2. Sciatic nerve showing perineurium, epineurium, and perineural epithelium. Reproduced with permission of *Journal of Anatomy* (1962). (a) Nerve trunk as a whole, showing several fasciculi along with their connective tissue components—the epineurium, perineurium, and endoneurium. (b) One nerve fasciculus removed from the trunk, along with the perineurium, perineural epithelium, and endoneurium. Part of the perineurium is removed to expose the perineural epithelium. (c) Nerve fasciculus removed from perineural connective tissue layer, leaving the multilayered perineural epithelium. (d) Nerve fasciculus stripped of its perineural epithelium, leaving the nerve fibers of the fasciculus and endoneurium intact. Isolated perineural epithelium is shown as it would appear lying flat on a glass slide.

myelinated) axons of newborn Swiss mice 6 days after intranasal instillation of a street strain of rabies virus. This does not necessarily
show that the virus travels along the channels in which it can later be
detected; the authors concluded that "the mechanism of centripetal
spread of rabies virus . . . is uncertain. . . . "

The dorsal root ganglion cells are those first noted to be involved
after the initial replication; Johnson (1965) first found fluorescence in
the cytoplasm of dorsal root ganglion cells, and in neurons of the spinal cord. Similar results were reported by Schneider (1969a, 1969b),
who noted that fluorescence first appeared in the spinal ganglia corresponding to the area of inoculation.

Once virus in the CNS has replicated to such an extent that mye-
litic or encephalitic changes are noted the pathologic changes, especially those seen early in the course of the disease, correspond to
the site of the viral introduction. Goodpasture (1925) found Negri
bodies in the Gasserian ganglia as well as in the trigeminal nerve of
rabbits that had had rabies virus injected in the masseter muscle.
The intervertebral ganglia near the site of the vampire bat bite were
severely affected in cases of human paralytic rabies (Hurst and
Pawan, 1932). The virus progresses rapidly from the ganglia to
various parts of the CNS (Schindler, 1961; Baer *et al.*, 1965, 1968;
Schneider, 1969b).

Thus, the data currently available indicate that rabies virus apparently replicates in the muscle, connective tissue, or nerves
at the site of exposure, and may remain undetectable in this initially infected tissue for weeks or months before moving up the associated nerve. It is not known what form the virus assumes during
these long periods, nor what its relation is to the adjacent tissues.

At a given time the virus appears to move passively up either the
tissue spaces between the Schwann cells and the perineural structures, or in the interstitial nerve spaces of the fasciculus, and begins
to replicate in the spinal ganglia and dorsal root ganglion cells corresponding to the involved peripheral nerves, finally multiplying in
the central nervous system.

II. Pathogenesis after Intranasal Introduction of Virus

The airborne route of infection has attracted increasing interest in
recent years, especially since Constantine (1962) demonstrated nonbite transmission of rabies to foxes, coyotes, opossums, and ringtails
in a heavily populated bat cave in Texas. Virus was subsequently

isolated from the atmosphere in that cave (Winkler, 1968), and a laboratory outbreak of similar nonbite transmission occurred when bat virus was "aerosolized" (Winkler *et al.*, 1972).

Atanasiu (1965) showed that laboratory animals could readily be infected by the intranasal route. Invasion of the nasal mucosal cells of mice was noted following infection acquired by the aerosol route (Hronovský and Benda, 1969); virus in the nasal mucosa was noted one day earlier than in the brain, following instillation of virus in the nares. Later Fischman and Schaeffer (1971) instilled CVS and dog, bat, fox, and skunk rabies isolates intranasally and noted extensive fluorescence in the deeper submucosal layer of the nasal membranes of moribund mice; no studies were made prior to the appearance of clinical signs. In both the 1969 and 1971 studies the incubation period after intranasal instillation of virus was longer than after intracerebral inoculation. As stated previously, Jenson *et al.* (1969) found developing virus particles in the trigeminal nerves (and ganglions) of intranasally inoculated suckling mice, but, again, virus was first seen long (6 days) after inoculation, and the mechanism of centripetal spread could not be clarified. No experiments have been done in which rabies virus has been intranasally instilled after olfactory bulb removal, a method successfully employed by Schultz and Gebhardt (1934) to incriminate that structure in the pathogenesis of poliomyelitis virus administered intranasally. This route of transmission may have epidemiologic importance with the extremely concentrated Mexican freetail bats (300 bats per square foot, Constantine, 1967); experimental intranasal instillation of virus from rabid Mexican freetail bats into healthy Mexican freetail bats produced both infection and antibodies (Baer and Bales, 1967), and recently Constantine and Emmons (1972) reported seeing fluorescence in the nares of rabid Mexican freetail bats.

III. Pathogenesis after Oral Administration

The pathogenesis of ingested virus has been traced in mice by Correa-Giron *et al.* (1970) and Fischman and Schaeffer (1971*), after Svet-Moldavskaya (1958), Soave (1966), and Fischman and Ward (1969) had shown that rabies virus could infect orally.

Correa-Giron *et al.* (1970) killed mice at different intervals after

---

* This article also refers to previous positive findings by Fermi and Remlinger in the first decade of this century.

Table VII

Distribution of Rabies Virus (Bovine Strain 5V132VB)
in Mice Infected by the Oral Route[a,b]

Tissue[c]	10 min	1 hr	2 hr	6 hr	12 hr	2 days	5 days	6 days	7 days	9 days	11 days
Brain	0	0	0	0	0	0	4	5	5	0	0
Buccal mucosa	4[d]	0	0	0	0	0	5	5	3	5	0
Tongue	5	3	2	0	0	0	5	5	–	0	0
Lung	1	0	0	0	0	2	3	5	4	0	0
Stomach	4	5	4	5	0	0	0	5	1	0	0
Salivary gland	0	0	0	0	0	0	4	5	4	0	0
Esophagus and trachea	0	1	0	0	0	0	4	1	1	0	0
Heart	0	0	0	0	0	0	0	3	1	0	0
Mesentery	0	0	0	0	0	0	0	3	1	0	0
Kidney	0	0	0	0	0	0	0	1	1	0	0
Intestine	0	0	0	2	0	0	0	0	0	0	0
Liver	0	0	0	0	0	0	0	0	0	0	0
Spleen	0	1	0	0	0	0	0	0	0	0	0

Time after feeding spans the date columns (10 min – 11 days).

[a] Dose = 320,000 WMICLD$_{50}$.
[b] Reproduced with permission of the American Journal of Epidemiology, after Correa-Giron *et al.* (1970).
[c] 20% suspensions of pooled tissues from 10 mice were inoculated (0.03 ml i.e.) into groups of 5 mice each.
[d] No. of mice out of 5 which died and were proved positive for rabies virus by FA test.

they had ingested infective mouse brains. The fate of one ingested virus strain (originally from a cow that died of bovine paralytic rabies in Mexico) was traced by mouse inoculation and by the fluorescent antibody technique. Virus was first noted at 10 min in the buccal mucosa, tongue, and stomach (plus a small amount in the lung), in the tongue and stomach at 1 hour (small amount in the esophagus, trachea, and spleen), again in the tongue and stomach at 2 hours, and in the stomach and intestine at 6 hours, before the eclipse period at 12 hours (Table VII). The authors state that

the demonstration of virus in tongue, stomach, esophagus, and trachea, at one hour, and in tongue and stomach at two hours after consumption of infected tissue could . . . have been due to the mechanical adsorption of virus to mucosal surfaces. . . .

but that

The results obtained in this study indicate that following oral administration rabies virus can initiate infection through the buccal and lingual mucosae, taste buds, lung, or through the intestine; however, additional studies are needed to define more clearly the exact pathway or pathways of infection exhibited by different strains of rabies virus administered orally.

Fluorescent antibody staining of frozen sections of the positive organs had shown antigen in the cytoplasm of the epithelial cells from the mucous membranes covering the internal surface of the cheeks and lips, especially in the perinuclear area of the cells of the basal layer and prickle-cell layer (the latter being the most heavily innervated, located where the intraepithelial nerves end). Specific fluorescent staining was also observed in the epidermis of the skin of the cheek and lip, and in the nerve endings in the roots of the tactile hairs.

Fischman and Schaeffer (1971), in similar experiments, and also with a variety of virus strains (fixed-CVS, dog, bat, fox, and skunk), concluded, from the fluorescence that appeared early (3 days) after feeding, that infection took place in the alimentary tract and the oral cavity. In the buccal mucosa fluorescence was noted in the cells of the stratum granulosum and stratum Malpighii, but not in the stratum corneum; nerve cells in the lamina propia frequently showed fluorescence, as did nerve bundles in the submucosal tissue and in cells associated with the large and small tactile hair follicles of the skin of the cheek. In the tongue the cells of the stratum Malpighii showed diffuse fluorescence, as did those in both filiform and fungiform papillae, and in nerve bundles traversing the tongue, similar to what Correa-Giron *et al.* (1970) had observed earlier. The authors concluded that there was no clear evidence that infection of epidermal and dermal cells preceded spread to the CNS, but rather that "since these structures . . . failed to show infection in animals dying after intracerebral or intramuscular inoculation of rabies virus . . . infection of oropharyngeal and intestinal tissues did not represent centrifugal spread, but reflected the sites of invasion following infection by the oral portal." It is interesting to note that Bell and Moore (1971) showed that skunks could be infected with a bat strain of virus by the oral route, a fact of possibly great importance epidemiologically, since Winkler and Adams (1972) have shown that this species commonly inhabits bat caves. Moreover, the precise route of infection in oral rabies vaccination of foxes (Baer *et al.*, 1971) has yet to be delineated.

IV. Pathogenesis after Intravenous Inoculation of Virus

Although viremia has been generally discounted as a common mechanism of progression of rabies virus to the CNS (see reviews by Baer *et al.*, 1965; Schneider, 1969), some recent observations have been made on pathogenesis following intravenous administration of virus. Schneider (1969) noted that intravenously injected virus reached the CNS without spinal ganglion involvement; fluorescence first appeared (and low titers of virus) within individual nerve cells of the medulla as well as the thoracic portion of the spinal cord 12 hours after inoculation of fixed virus in the tail vein; the fact that no fluorescence was noted in the capillary endothelium of these organs suggested that the virus entered the nerve structures without prior multiplication. Fischman and Schaeffer (1971) noted very long incubation periods by this route of infection, and assumed that this was because of virus dilution in the blood. Fluorescence appeared as pinpoint foci in the cells of different areas of the cerebrum and cerebellum, also at 72 hours after injection of fixed virus. One can only assume that this is an extremely rare natural route of infection in rabies, if it indeed occurs at all.

References

Atanasiu, P. (1965). *C. R. Acad. Sci.* **261**, 277–279.

Babes, V. (1887). *Virchows Arch. Pathol. Anat. Physiol.* **110**, 562–569.

Baer, G. M., and Bales, G. (1967). *J. Infec. Dis.* **117**, 82–90.

Baer, G. M., and Cleary, W. F. (1972). *J. Infec. Dis.* **125**, 520–527.

Baer, G. M., Shanthaveerappa, T. R., and Bourne, G. (1965). *Bull. WHO* **33**, 783–794.

Baer, G. M., Shantha, T. R., and Bourne, G. (1968). *Bull. WHO* **38**, 119–125.

Baer, G. M., Abelseth, M., and Debbie, J. (1971). *Amer. J. Epidemiol.* **93**, 487–490.

Baltazard, M., and Ghoddsi, M. (1954). *Bull. WHO* **10**, 797–803.

Bardach, (1888). *Ann. Inst. Pasteur, Paris* **2**, 9–14.

Bell, J. F., and Moore, G. J. (1971). *Amer. J. Epidemiol.* **93**, 176–182.

Bodian, D., and Howe, H. (1941). *Bull. Johns Hopkins Hosp.* **69**, 79–85.

Borodina, T. A. (1959). *Probl. Virol.* (*N. Y.*) **4**, 96–99.

Burns, K. F., and Farinacci, C. J. (1955). *J. Infec. Dis.* **97**, 211–215.

Constantine, D. G. (1962). *Pub. Health Rep.* **77**, 287–289.

Constantine, D. G. (1967). Univ. of New Mexico Publications in Biology, No. 7, "Activity Patterns of the Mexican Free-Tailed Bat," The University of New Mexico Press, Albuquerque. *N. Mex. Monogr.* **5**.

Constantine, D. G., and Emmons, R. (1972). *Science* **175**, 1255–1256.

Correa-Giron, E. P., Allen, R., and Sulkin, S. E. (1970). *Amer. J. Epidemiol.* **91**, 203–215.

Dean, D. J. (1963). *N. Y. State J. Med.* **63**, 3507–3513.

Dean, D. J., Baer, G. M., and Thompson, W. (1963a). *Bull. WHO* **28**, 477–486.

Dean, D. J., Evans, W., and McClure, R. (1963b). *Bull. WHO* **29**, 803–811.

DiVestea, A., and Zagari, G. (1887). *Ann. Nevrol.* **5**, 113–131.

DiVestea, A., and Zagari, G. (1889a). *G. int. Sci. Med.* **81**, 108.

DiVestea, A., and Zagari, G. (1889b). *Ann. Inst. Pasteur, Paris* **3**, 237–248.

Fermi, C. (1928). *Zentralbl. Bakteriol., Parasitenk. Infektionskr., Abt. 1: Orig.* **112**, 73.

Fischman, H. R., and Schaeffer, M. (1971). *Ann. N. Y. Acad. Sci.* **177**, 78–97.

Fischman, H. R., and Ward, F. E. (1969). *Amer. J. Epidemiol.* 88, 132–138.

Frye, F., and Enright, J. (1964). *Proc. Soc. Exp. Biol. Med.* 115, 689–691

Gantt, W., and Ponomarew, A. (1929). *Z. Gesamte Exp. Med.* 66, 582–595.

Goodpasture, E. W. (1925). *Amer. J. Pathol.* 1, 547–582.

Habel, K. (1941). *Pub. Health Rep.* 56, 692–702.

Hıonovsky, V., and Benda, R. (1969). *Acta Virol. (Prague)* 13, 193–197.

Hurst, E., and Pawan, J. (1932). *J. Pathol. Bacteriol.* 35, 301–321.

Huygelen, C. (1960). *Antonie van Leeuwenhoek; J. Microbiol. Serol.* 26, 66.

Huygelen, C., and Mortelmans, J. (1959). *Antonie van Leeuwenhoek; J. Microbiol. Serol.* 25, 265–271.

Jenson, A. B., Rabin, E., Bentinck, D., and Melnick, J. (1969). *J. Virol.* 3, 265–269.

Johnson, H. (1967). *Primer Seminario Internacional Sobre Rabia Para Las Americas,* p. 68.

Johnson, R. T. (1964). *J. Exp. Med.* 119, 343–356.

Johnson, R. T. (1965). *J. Neuropathol. Exp. Neurol.* 24, 662–674.

Kitselman, C. H., and Mital, A. K. (1967). *Can. J. Comp. Med. Vet. Sci.* 31, 122–124.

Kligler, I., and Bernkopf, H. (1943). *Brit. J. Exp. Pathol.* 24, 15–21.

Koprowski, H., and Cox, H. R. (1948). *J. Immunol.* 60, 537–554.

Kraus, R., Gerlach, F., and Schweinburg, F. (1926). "Lyssa Bei Mensch und Tier." Urban & Schwarzenberg, Berlin.

Kraus, I., and Fukuhara, Y. (1909). *Z. Immunitaetsforsch. Exp. Ther.,* 1 3, 33.

Krause, W. (1957). *Zentralbl. Bakteriol., Parasitenk. Infektionskr., Abt. 1: Orig.* 167, 481–503.

McLean, R. G. (1972). *J. Infec. Dis.* 123, 680–681.

Murphy, F. A., Bauer, S. P., Harrison, A. K., and Washington, C. W., Jr. (1973). *Lab. Invest.* 28, 361–376.

Nicolau, S., and Kopciowska, L. (1934). *C. R. Soc. Biol.* 115, 262–264.

Pasteur, L., Chamberland, S., Roux, E., and Thuillier, (1881). *C. R. Acad. Sci.* 92, 1259.

Pasteur, L., Chamberland, S., Roux, E., and Thuillier, (1882). *C. R. Acad. Sci.* 95, 1187.

Remlinger, P., and Bailly, J. (1928). *C. R. Soc. Biol.* 99, 14.

Roux, E. (1888), *Ann. Inst. Pasteur, Paris* 2, 18–26.

Schaffer, C. (1889), *Ann. Inst. Pasteur, Paris* 3, 644–649.

Schindler, R. (1961). *Bull. WHO* 25, 119–126.

Schneider, L. G. (1969a). *Zentralbl. Bakteriol., Parasitenk., Infektionskr. Hyg.* 211, 281–308.

Schneider, L. G. (1969b). *Zentralbl. Bakteriol. Parasitenk. Infektionskr. Hyg.* 212, 1–41.

Schultz, E. W., and Gebhardt, L. P. (1934). *Proc. Soc. Exp. Biol. Med.* 31, 728–730.

Shanthaveerappa, T. R., and Bourne, G. (1962). *J. Anat.* 96, 527–536.

Soave, O. A. (1966). *Amer. J. Vet. Res.* 27, 44–46.

Sulkin, S. E., Krutzsch, P. H., Allen, R., and Wallis, C. (1959). *J. Exp. Med.* 110, 369–376.

Svet-Moldavskaya, I. A. (1958). *Acta Virol. (Prague)* 2, 228–234.

Tierkel, E. S. (1959). *Adv. in Veterinary Science, Volume V,* 183–226.

Veeragahavan, N. (1963). "Annual Report of the Director." Pasteur Institute for Southern India, Coonoor, Tamilnadu, India.

Veeragahavan. N. (1964). "Scientific Report." Pasteur Institute of Southern India, Coonoor, Tamilnadu, India.

Wang, S. P. (1956). *J. Formosan Med. Ass.* 55, 548–554.

Webster, L. T. (1942). "Rabies." Macmillan, New York.

Winkler, W. G. (1968). *Bull. Wildl. Dis. Ass.* **4**, 37–40.

Winkler, W. G., and Adams, D. B. (1972). *Amer. Midl. Natur.* **87**, 191–200.

Winkler, W. G., Baker, E. F., and Hopkins, C. C. (1972). *Amer. J. Epidemiol.* **95**, 267–277.

Wong, D., and Freund, J. (1951). *Proc. Soc. Exp. Biol. Med.* **76**, 717.

Wright, G. (1953). *Proc. Roy. Soc. Med.* **46**, 319–330.

CHAPTER 11

Spread of Virus within the Central Nervous System

Lothar G. Schneider

Rabies virus spreads rapidly throughout the central nervous system (CNS) after its arrival there via the nerves, spinal ganglia, or by other routes. The particular CNS sites that support rabies virus multiplication have long been a point of considerable discussion, as have the identification of the cellular elements that contribute to virus spread.

The methods used for studying these events in the CNS are tissue titration, histopathology, immunofluorescence, and electron microscopy, but relevant data on virus spread can only be obtained as a function of time.

I. Demonstration of Infectivity

A. FIXED VIRUS IN THE CNS

Sabin *et al.* (1940) infected mice with fixed virus by nasal instillation. They detected virus in the brain 3 and 4 days after infection, with a subsequent rapid caudal spread throughout the CNS.

In mice infected with fixed virus by either intraperitoneal or subcutaneous inoculation (Kligler and Bernkopf, 1943) virus was first
demonstrated in the upper cord 72 hours after infection, and in the
entire CNS 24 hours later. After hind footpad inoculation the virus
first appeared in the lumbar and thoracic spinal cord segments at 72
hours, in the cervical cord at 96 hours, and in the brain at 120 hours.
After front footpad or intraperitoneal inoculation the earliest appearance of virus was always in the cervical cord, and only later in the
brain and lumbar cord.

Fixed virus injected into the rear footpad of mice (Johnson, 1965)
reached the lumbar cord 24–48 hours later, and was also demonstrated 1 day later in the brain. In the experiments of Baer *et al.*
(1965) fixed virus entered the CNS of rats between 48 and 72 hours
after rear footpad injection, and was shown 24 hours later in all
examined parts of the brain and spinal cord. At 50 hours after footpad
injection of mice, Schneider (1969a) demonstrated virus in the medulla and in the thoracic and lumbar spinal cord. The cervical cord
was spared until 70 hours, and the rhinencephalon, cortex, and cerebellum were found infected 96 hours after infection. Following intravenous injection of the tail vein only the medulla and thoracic
cord contained virus at 72 hours, but synchronous infection of the entire CNS was demonstrated 96 hours postinfection.

B. Infections with Street Strains

Experimental animals infected with street strains have longer incubation periods, and the events occuring at the CNS level can thus
be studied in greater detail. Figure 1 (Schneider, 1969a) illustrates
the typical caudorostral spread of street virus in the CNS, in this case
in mice inoculated in the rear footpad with fox strain virus. Virus was
first demonstrated in the lumbar cord at 112 hours, in the entire cord
and medulla between 130 and 160 hours, and in the brain 196 hours
after infection. Virus titers in the different CNS segments increased
with time, the initially infected segment having the highest titer.
Later on, higher virus titers were observed in the brain than in those
parts of the CNS initially infected. Paralysis of the hind legs was observed 196 hours after infection, only after the logarithmic phase of
virus growth had been reached in the lumbar segment of the spinal
cord. Much the same results were obtained earlier by Schindler
(1959).

When rats were inoculated with a skunk isolate that produced incubation periods of 2–3 weeks, Baer *et al.* (1968) first detected virus

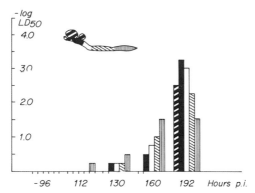

Fig. 1. Development of infectivity in brain and spinal cord segments following footpad infection of mice with street rabies virus. (After Schneider, 1969a.)

in the lumbar and thoracic cord 6 days after infection, and at 9 days in the entire CNS. In small laboratory animals it usually takes street virus 70–80 hours to spread within the CNS, compared to roughly 24 hours for fixed virus. These time periods are approximately half that necessary for the virus to reach the CNS from the site of inoculation. This is not surprising since many CNS cells are capable of supporting virus growth, and that virus within the CNS may be transported quickly via axons or the cerebrospinal fluid.

In guinea pigs inoculated in the gastrocnemius muscle with the Flury rabies strain (Huygelen and Mortelmans, 1959), virus first appeared in the lumbosacral cord 72 hours after infection, but it took another 120 hours for it to appear in the brain. After intramuscular injection of the same virus strain in the foreleg (Huygelen, 1960) the virus appeared in the cervico-thoracic cord at 96 hours, was demonstrable in the cord and medulla at 120 hours, and in the brain 144 hours after inoculation. But intravenous injection of virus resulted in synchronous infection of the entire CNS at 144 hours.

Hronovský and Benda (1969) infected suckling guinea pigs with an aerosol of a tissue culture-adapted badger strain virus, the exposure effected by means of a mechanical nebulizer. Infectious virus was first demonstrated in the nasal mucosa 6 days after infection, and 1 day later in the brain, medulla, and anterior parts of the cord, but it did not reach the lumbar cord until 9 days after infection.

Ota (1955) studied the terminal distribution of infectious virus in the CNS of rabbits, goats, and horses infected by various routes with the Nishigahara laboratory strain. In the CNS of rabbits, the virus was found equally distributed; in goats and horses, however, virus after intraspinal injection was only found in the cord, and after intracerebral inoculation in the brain and anterior parts of the cord. Combined intracerebral and intraspinal injections resulted in infection of the entire CNS. This distribution may be a reflection of strain properties, or may be due to other reasons. In general peak virus infectivity in CNS tissues is reached long before death, but terminal virus titers may be appreciably lower, especially following intracerebral inoculation (Nikolitsch, 1957; Gildemeister, 1960).

A similar finding has been noted *in vitro*. After several cycles of rabies virus multiplication infected tissue culture cells produce aberrantly formed, noninfectious virus particles which seem to interfere with fully infectious virus particles at the cell level (Hummeler *et al.*, 1967). This, and other factors, such as the production of interferon, rabies-inhibiting substance (Carski and Wilsnack, 1966), or antibody, may be involved *in vivo*, as is discussed later on in this chapter.

The results of infectivity studies give unequivocal evidence of the progressive spread of rabies virus in the CNS of experimentally infected animals. Fixed strains of rabies virus spread rapidly in mice, and stepwise CNS spread becomes obvious only if street strains that produce long incubation periods are employed, or larger animals are used.

Infectivity studies *per se* do not give evidence of the cell type or structures involved in the spread or transport of the virus in the CNS, but because of the rapidity of the process it appears as if cell-to-cell spread is unlikely, and passive transport mechanisms must be considered, either axonal, in the cerebrospinal fluid (CSF), or in the blood.

II. Histopathology

Before immunofluorescence techniques and the electron microscope became available for pathogenesis studies the location and degree of histological lesions were the only means used as indirect evidence of the sites of virus multiplication and of the path which the virus had taken. Unfortunately, pathological changes in rabies appear late during infection, and obviously cannot be correlated with the virus content of the tissues.

After experimentally infecting mice with a laboratory strain of rabies virus, Johnson (1965) observed signs of acute nerve cell disease in neurons of the hippocampus and septal nuclei, but saw little neuronophagia and glial proliferation. Most striking was the total lack of inflammatory reaction in the meninges or perivascular areas.

Mice dying after infection with street virus (Schneider and Hamann, 1969) showed vascular infiltrations at the inner and outer brain surfaces, and disseminated glial nodules and diffuse or perivascular reactions of microglial elements throughout the brain and cord. The pathologic changes in the brain were most pronounced after intracerebral injection, and in the spinal cord after footpad injection. These findings agree with those of Schaffer (1931), who found severe inflammatory reactions, glial proliferations, and nerve cell degeneration in the lumbar cord of a patient who was bitten in the leg, but only minimal glial reactions and nerve cell degeneration in the brain. From this and former experiences he concluded that the most intense lesions are found in those segments of the CNS that correspond to the site of the bite, and in which the CNS infection started. The findings of Schaffer were later confirmed by laboratory experiments of Szatmari and Salyi (1936), who found severe inflammatory and proliferative changes in the lumbar cord of rabbits following injection into the gastrocnemius muscle. Conversely, the brainstem was markedly affected after cheek injection.

Axonal spread of the virus was reported by Goodpasture (1925), who infected rabbits into the masseter muscle and demonstrated cytoplasmic inclusions resembling "lyssa bodies" in the Gasserian ganglion and within axons of the trigeminal nerve root. From our present knowledge it appears quite likely that these structures were nucleocapsid-containing rabies virus matrices, such as those recently demonstrated by electron microscopy (Jenson *et al.*, 1969) in the trigeminal nerve of suckling mice, and by Garcia-Tamayo *et al.* (1972) in human trigeminal nerve roots. Nevertheless, Seifried and Spatz (1930) assumed that the spread of virus was via the CSF, since they found a similar degree of inflammatory reactions at almost identical sites in cases of Borna disease, epidemic encephalitis, poliomyelitis, and rabies. The location of pathologic changes near the outer and inner surfaces of the brain led them to conclude that (despite the absence of meningeal reaction) the virus must have entered the brain from the meningeal surface, but especially from the inner CSF spaces.

Field (1951) injected a laboratory strain of rabies virus into the masseter muscle of rabbits, and when the animals died he found the most severe lesions in the nearby Gasserian ganglia, and then in decreasing intensity in the dorsal root ganglia of the cervical, thoracic, and lumbar segments of the spinal cord. He considered that virus passage may have occurred from the CSF of the subarachnoid space into the cord via the spinal nerve roots and dorsal root ganglia. These nerve structures had been shown to be penetrable to India ink particles (0.5–1.5 μm in diameter) injected into the CSF (Field and Brierly, 1948). It was later shown (Field, 1954a,b) that in rabbits inoculated in the cornea there were both early microglial reaction and later appearance of degenerated neurons close to the ependyma of the central spinal cord canal, suggesting the diffuse and rapid viral penetration of CNS segments via the CSF.

III. Immunofluorescence and Electron Microscopy

Johnson and Mercer (1964) studied the development of the CVS strain of rabies virus in the Purkinje cells of mouse brains, and found that rabies antigen developed only in neurons, but not in glial, meningeal, ependymal, or vascular cells. The appearance of virus antigen paralleled the infectivity, and was noted at virtually the same time in all affected neurons. At the early time periods, antigen was most commonly seen in the perikaryon, approximately 100 μm from the nuclear membrane in the dendrites. Again, it should be noted that encephalitis was not observed until after the logarithmic phase of virus growth had occurred.

In sequential pathogenesis studies done after intracerebral mouse inoculation, Johnson (1965) first found fluorescent antigen in infected neurons at 2 days. Virus development was extensive in the neurons of rhinencephalic structures but invariably more limited in the neurons of the neocortex, diencephalon, and hypothalamus. The extent of brainstem and spinal cord involvement seemed to be intermediate. Neurons in the ventral horns and dorsal root ganglia of the spinal cord were involved more consistently than neurons in the lateral or dorsal horns. Three days after footpad injection of virus, however, fluorescence in the CNS was first detected in the cytoplasm of the lumbar dorsal root ganglion cells, and in neurons of the lumbar cord, with the infection more prominent in the cells ipsilateral to the inoculated foot; 1 day later infected neurons were shown in the entire CNS, similar to that seen after intracerebral inoculation.

In suckling guinea pigs infected by aerosol (Hronovský and Benda, 1969), virus antigen was first demonstrated in epithelial cells of the nasal mucosa 6 days after infection, and in the CNS 1 day later. Early foci of virus antigen were marked in the olfactory bulbs and in the hippocampus, while irregularly dispersed foci were seen in neurons of the cortex, other parts of the brain, brainstem, cerebellum, and in the anterior portion of the spinal cord. Following the initial, extraneural multiplication of the virus, wide areas of the CNS became infected simultaneously.

Sequential immunofluorescent and virus titration studies of the CNS of mice were conducted following intracerebral and footpad injection of mice (Schneider, 1969b). The earliest demonstration of virus antigen was 40 hours after injection of 32 LD_{50} of virus into the left cerebral hemisphere, but only 24 hours after injection of 100,000 LD_{50}. Early antigen foci were demonstrated in the neocortex of both hemispheres, close to the longitudinal cerebral fissure, and some fluorescence was noted in individual neurons of the hippocampus. Within the next 24 hours the extent of involvement increased, and large fluorescent foci were seen in the superficial parts of the cortex, in the caudate nucleus of the striate body, and in the geniculate body. Diffuse foci were seen in other areas, most concentrated in brain structures close to the ventricles and to the dorsolateral and apical brain surfaces. Individual glial cells of the pia mater and the limiting membranes appeared to be involved in virus replication. Only limited involvement of the meninges and ependymal cells was seen with rabies virus, unlike the marked involvement observed after intracerebral inoculation of mice with herpesvirus (Johnson, 1964). Individual glial cells showing fluorescence therefore seemed to be infected by chance and appeared of lesser importance in the intracerebral spread of the rabies virus. Numerous medullary neurons were involved. Superficially located nerve nuclei close to the 4th ventricle seemed to be the preferential sites of early virus replication. Extensive fluorescence was seen in the dorsal and ventral horn neurons of the anterior parts of the spinal cord, with early fluorescence in the corresponding dorsal root ganglia. The posterior parts of the spinal cord were similarly involved, but at later stages of infection.

After rear footpad injection, fluorescent antigen was first demonstrated in sacral, lumbar, and thoracic ganglia ipsilateral to the infection site. The number of infected neurons in the ganglia decreased with increase in distance from the inoculation site (Table I). Antigen was also seen early in the dorsal root neurons and the dorsal and lateral horns, but rarely in neurons of the ventral horn. The infection then spread rapidly to the contralateral side and toward the brain. Fluorescent antigen was occasionally found in unidentified structures of the white matter (probably axons), and more prominently in nerve cell processes surrounding the ependyma of the central spinal

Table I

Early Sites of Virus Replication in the CNS of Mice as Demonstrated by Immunofluorescence 60 Hours after Footpad Infection of the Right Hind Leg with a Laboratory Strain of Rabies Virus[a]

	Medulla	Cervical cord	Thoracic cord	Lumbar cord Anterior	Lumbar cord Posterior	Sacral cord
Spinal ganglion						
Right	—[b]	—	++8[c,d]	+++21[c,d]	+++32[c,d]	+2[c,d]
Left	—	—	—	—	—	—
Dorsal root						
Right		—	—	+	+	—
Left		—	—	—	—	—
Dorsal horn						
Right		—	+	++	—	—
Left		—	—	—	—	—
Ventral horns, right, left		—	—	—	—	—
Lateral horn						
Right		—	+	+	—	—
Left		—	—	—	—	—
Gray commissure		—	++	+	—	—
Sympathetic trunk		—	—	—	—	—
White matter, brain	—	—	—	—	—	—
Gray matter, brain	+					

[a] Schneider, 1969a.
[b] No fluorescence noted.
[c] Number of infected neurons per spinal ganglion.
[d] + = Weak fluorescence; ++ = medium fluorescence; and +++ = strong fluorescence.

cord canal. Early involvement of the brain was demonstrated in areas of the gray matter adjacent to the ventricles, but not at the outer brain surfaces noted infected after intracerebral inoculation. The terminal distribution of virus antigen was similar to that following intracerebral inoculation, but the amount of antigen was much less.

Following intravenous (tail-vein) injection the first evidence of antigen was in irregularly disseminated foci of the spinal cord, often in close association with capillaries. It should be emphasized that, in contrast to footpad infection, involvement of spinal ganglia was observed only after CNS infection had occurred.

Electron microscopic studies of infected tissues have clearly shown the tissue structures and cells in which rabies virus multiplies. This aspect is more fully discussed in Chapters 12 and 15. The formation of virus is most common within neurons. The virus has been shown to replicate in characteristic matrices located at different sites within infected neurons: in the perikaryon (Matsumoto, 1962) and in dendrites (Johnson and Mercer, 1964) and axons of cerebrospinal and peripheral nerve fibers (Matsumoto, 1963; Jenson et al., 1969; Garcia-Tamayo et al., 1972; Murphy et al., 1973). Within the CNS, astrocytes have also been shown to support virus growth (Matsumoto, 1963).

Thus rabies virus can multiply in several types of cells and in different cell structures of the CNS, and one may assume that virus spread may be by various paths. Spread via axons and dendrites seems to be the most probable, but this would signify cell-to-cell spread, and multiplication at several sites in one cell would be required before the next neuron might be infected via connecting synapses. A passive transport mechanism within axons does not appear to be at all farfetched, since active contractions of myelin sheaths (Singer and Bryant, 1969) and ultrarapid bidirectional particle movements within axons (Burwood, 1965) have been shown to exist. It may be assumed, therefore, that the virus could travel in the CNS over long distances by either active replication or passive transport of the virus genome in axons of nerve tracts which connect distant nerve centers. Infection of astrocytes and other glial elements would theoretically allow alternative passageways but would, of course, take much longer for virus spread.

As has been shown by infectivity studies, the spread of CNS infection is most often so rapid that other dissemination mechanisms also have to be considered. Besides, cell-to-cell growth would require maturation of virus particles by budding, a phenomenon which has not been observed in rabies-infected CNS tissues. Dierks et al. (1969) could not demonstrate the budding of virus particles from marginal membranes into extracellular tissue spaces of the CNS. They, as others, also failed to show neuronal damage to a degree that would permit release of virus for the subsequent progressive infection of the brain. CNS tissue spaces allowing the spread of virus apparently do not exist. Electron microscopy has shown that neurons are tightly packed and are separated from vascular cell elements by astrocytes and oligodendroglial cells (Horstmann, 1957; de Robertis et al., 1960); the distance between neighboring cell membranes is between 120–150 Å, a dimension thought to prevent virus budding. Murphy and Fields (1967), however, gave evidence to the contrary by showing the release of Kern Canyon virus, another rhabdovirus, from infected CNS neurons into adjacent tissue spaces.

The most convincing evidence of viral spread via CSF seems to be that noted after intracerebral inoculation. Infection starts not in cells surrounding the puncture track of the needle, but at almost identical locations in both hemispheres (Mims, 1960; Johnson, 1965; Schneider, 1969b). According to Schlesinger (1949) and Cairns (1950) only 8–10% of a virus or phage inoculum remains demonstrable in the brain during the first hour of infection. The residual virus is believed to spill over into the blood, via the subarachnoid and subdural cavities. The same form of transmission seems to hold true for rabies (Wong and Freund, 1951). It should be noted here that intracerebrally inoculated India ink particles have been demonstrated in all CSF-containing cavities and spaces, in perivascular spaces of the brain, in the central canal of the spinal cord, and in the subarachnoid space extending to the intervertebral foramina (Mims, 1960), and an analogous distribution might be expected after virus injection.

Various experiments in which the CNS of rabies-infected animals was examined showed almost synchronous infection of many areas of the brain (Johnson, 1965) and of the spinal cord (Schneider, 1969a), giving indirect evidence that rabies virus spreads within the CNS via the CSF over a wide area and essentially at one time. Since rabies virus multiplies in the meningeal tissues to only a limited extent, it must be assumed that virus is carried passively through these meningeal cell layers, similar to dye particles as demonstrated by Spatz (1934) and Fleischhauer (1964).

In fact, virus antigen has been found at an early time period (Schneider, 1969b) in many parts of the gray matter close to the pia mater and ependyma (such as the hippocampus, caudate nucleus, and nerve nuclei of the medulla). The gray matter of the brain or spinal cord, covered by thick layers of white matter impenetrable to dyes, was also infected with virus, but at a later time (an example is the late involvement of the cerebellum).

The early demonstration of virus antigen and of histopathologic lesions (Seifried and Spatz, 1930; Field, 1951, 1954a,b) can only give indirect evidence for the possible participation of the CSF in the spread of virus, whereas the direct isolation of infectious virus from the CSF supports the otherwise questionable role of this fluid in the pathogenesis of the disease. Although various isolations were reported by Kerbler (1933), none were obtained in many other cases in the past (Schweinburg, 1937; Eichwald and Pitzschke, 1967). More recently, however, there has been increasing evidence of the presence of infectious rabies virus in the cerebrospinal fluid of human rabies patients at various stages of the disease (Blattner, 1961; Kent and Finegold, 1966). Isolation of Mokola virus, a member of th rabies group, was recently reported (Familusi and Moore, 1972) from the CSF of a child that had convulsions but a subsequent uneventful recovery. In many instances attempts at virus isolation from the CSF have been made only late in the disease. There are no reports of virus isolations during the incubation period. These findings are similar to that of Lipton *et al.* (1965) in poliomyelitis, in which the CSF was found noninfectious in the majority of patients. These latter authors, however, demonstrated poliovirus neutralizing antibody in the CSF of 24% of their patients. Rabies virus neutralizing antibody was found in extremely high titer in the CSF of one dog that sickened but then survived experimental infection (Arko *et al.*, 1973). The presence of neutralizing antibodies, even in low titers, would explain many of the unsuccessful isolation attempts.

IV. Clinical Signs

Recent studies of the pathogenesis of rabies in the CNS (Johnson, 1965; Schneider, 1969b) have shown that the appearance of clinical signs cannot be directly correlated with the multiplication of virus in neuronal structures; clinical signs were not observed until after several growth cycles of the virus had occurred. Similarly, nerve cell disease was not detectable until the virus had spread through the entire CNS and clinical signs were noted. Lysis of neurons was not observed and neuronophagia was rare. The noncytolytic behavior of rabies virus in cell culture seems to mirror the *in vivo* conditions, and has been called an endosymbiotic virus/host cell relationship (Fernandes *et al.*, 1964). A cytopathic action of fixed and street viruses in organized mammalian neuron cultures was only recently shown (Matsumoto and Yonezawa, 1971), and the cytopathic effect progressed from cytoplasmic granulation to complete neuronolysis.

The paucity of pathologic abnormalities in infected animal brains is in striking contrast to the severe clinical signs observed. The reason for this is unknown. Johnson (1965) assumed that disease may result from the physiologic dysfunction caused by the mass of rabies virus particles within neurons rather than from a possible (but unnoted) cytopathogenic effect of the virus. Since viruses in general do not produce toxins it is conceivable to assume that the reserves of the endoplasmatic reticulum become exhausted after only several virus growth cycles, resulting in heavy impairment of the cell function. Clinical signs make their appearance only after involvement of numerous neurons, and death appears to result from the involvement of vital nerve centers.

V. Pathogenesis of Abortive and Chronic Infection

Among groups of experimentally infected animals there are those that survive after showing characteristic signs of rabies, either with or without sequelae. This has been called abortive rabies by Koch (1930), and is more fully described in Chapter 17.

Three animal models have been reported for the study of experimentally induced abortive rabies. In the first system described by Bell (1964), Bell *et al.* (1966), and Lodmell *et al.* (1969), mice were inoculated with street rabies virus by various routes. It was shown that abortive rabies occurred consistently only after intraperitoneal inoculation of low passage level street virus. Abortive infection (in about 16% of the mice that showed signs of rabies) was characterized by absence of infectious virus and virus antigen in the brain, and by presence of neutralizing antibody in brain and serum.

In a second model, in which chickens were inoculated intracerebrally (Schneider and Burtscher, 1967), recovery from clinical rabies was demonstrated in between 11 and 53% of the cases. The course of infection in a sequential study with street virus is shown in Fig. 2. Virus multiplication in the brain stopped abruptly 15 days after infection, whereas antigen was demonstrable by the fluorescent antibody technique until 60 days after inoculation. Clinical signs appeared 20–30 days after inoculation. Illness was either acute or chronic, sometimes lasting up to 85 days, with intermittent improvements and relapses. Both forms either ended fatally or in permanent recovery. Virus-specific antibody was demonstrated in extracts of CNS tissues prior to its presence in serum, and was invariably of higher titer in brains than in the sera. Antibody appeared with the onset of clinical disease, coincident with the most marked lesions in the CNS, including massive vascular and partially perivascular infiltrates of lymphocytes, plasma cells and macrophages, of widespread perivascular proliferation of glial cells, of local edema, and of lysis of myelin sheaths. This type of reaction, similar but not quite identical to the characteristic lesions of an allergic encephalitis (Lipton and Steigman, 1961; Siller and Wight, 1965; Wight and Siller, 1965), was considered to represent the defense reaction of the organism against the virus infection, as well as the histologic evidence of an antigen–antibody reaction that led to ultimate recovery. The simultaneous demonstration of persisting virus antigen and of virus neutralizing antibody supported this view of the nature of abortive rabies.

More recently Wiktor *et al.* (1972a) presented a third model of abortive rabies, in which street virus-infected mice developed pe-

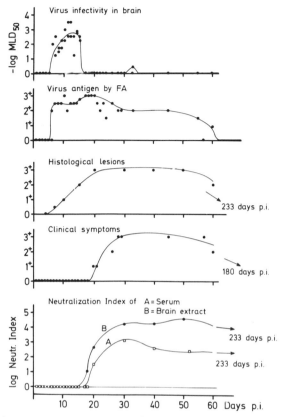

Fig. 2. Development of infectivity, viral antigen, histologic lesions, clinical signs, and virus neutralizing antibody in chickens after intracerebral injection of street rabies virus. (After Schneider and Burtscher, 1967.)

manent paralysis of the inoculated limb (survival for over 1 year) when the nonpathogenic Flury HEP strain of rabies virus was inoculated intracerebrally from 2 hours before to 24 hours after peripheral inoculation of street virus. The sparing effect was thought to be caused by interferon, which appeared at 7 and 14 hours after HEP inoculation in blood and brain, respectively, and not by the virus neutralizing antibody, which was first detected on the second day after inoculation.

There is evidence that abortive rabies also can occur after natural infection. Isolation of the virus, however, is the only unequivocal evidence of this, but, as shown in the models, is apparently possible only during the early stages of disease. Peuch (cited by Koch, 1930) described a case of a sow which developed furious rabies and paralysis for a period of 3 days followed by slow but complete recovery. Virus was isolated from the saliva, and the animal resisted a heavy challenge after recovery.

A rise of specific antibody during recovery is indirect but affirmative evidence of previous rabies infection. Baer and Olson (1972) described paralysis in four out of six pigs bitten by a rabid skunk, but all four animals recovered, and virus-neutralizing antibody was found in the sera of those pigs.

The presence of specific antibody in cerebrospinal fluid seems to be an additional indication of a previous rabies infection. Arko *et al.* (1973) found high levels of neutralizing antibody in the CSF of an experimentally infected dog that slowly recovered from severe paralysis. Therapeutic vaccination may complicate this immunologic evidence, but, as shown in a recent, well-documented, nonfatal case of rabies in a boy (Hattwick *et al.*, 1972), antibody titers rose to levels never before noted in vaccinated persons.

Virus persistence without clinical signs or antibody formation seems to be even more rare than abortive rabies; but it has been reported in experimentally infected rats (Svet-Moldavskaya, 1958; Gorshunova, 1958) and naturally infected dogs from Ethiopia (Andral and Serié, 1957). The recently described isolates from small rodents in Central Europe (Sodja *et al.*, 1971; Schneider and Schoop, 1972; 1973) form another example of rabies virus persistence in a natural host system without the production of obvious disease. Rabies virus was repeatedly isolated from CNS and salivary gland tissues of clinically healthy wild rodents by serial passage in mice. The wild rodents were shown to harbor the virus for more than 6 months without demonstrable virus excretion and without formation of antibody. The wild rodent model may yield a more precise insight into the problems governing chronic, abortive, and transient rabies in nature.

VI. Summary and Prospects

The spread of rabies infection within the CNS appears to take place by several pathways.

1. There is evidence of *active spread* of the virus by multiplication in neurons of brain, spinal cord and sympathetic trunk, and in glial cells of the CNS. Rabies virus replication has been shown to occur at different sites in affected neurons, including perikaryon, dendrites, and axons. The release of progeny virus into tissue spaces of the CNS seems to be possible, but direct evidence, also at the synapses, is still missing.

2. Many experiences provide indirect evidence for the *passive transport* of the rabies virus via either CSF or blood. Direct evidence, as obtained by the isolation of infectious virus from the CSF on several occasions, undoubtedly favors the belief that the CSF plays an important role in the pathogenesis of the disease. The presence of neutralizing antibody in the CSF seems to give further support for this idea and may well explain the reason for the failure of virus isolation attempts.

The ependymal and glial cells that line the CSF spaces have rarely been found infected, but a passive virus transport through these cell layers definitely seems possible. Virus transport by the CSF would explain the preferential sites of early virus multiplication around subarachnoidal spaces or ventricles.

There is obviously more than one path available for the virus to reach its destination — the brain — and ultimately the point of excretion for the further passage to other hosts — the salivary glands. There is no doubt today that the viral pathway to the salivary glands is through the nerves that originate near vital nerve centers. The virus passes outward through those nerves, and at the same time makes the host irritable und aggressive. The correlation of these two functions has created the precise conditions necessary for the rabies virus life cycle through the centuries.

The many CNS pathways available for rabies virus makes it difficult, if not impossible, to stop infection once the virus has reached the brain or spinal cord. Antibody, interferon, or other virus-inhibiting substances presently known do not have access to the neuraxis, and cannot stop the intracellular virus replication without stopping the vital cell function. This means that present control of the disease is possible only as long as the virus is present and multiplying outside the CNS. There is increasing evidence that rabies virus can multiply in extraneural tissues prior to its demonstration in the CNS (Schindler, 1961; Petrovic and Timm, 1969; Hronovský and Benda, 1969; Murphy *et al.*, 1973). It seems probable that early extraneural multiplication of rabies virus may be influenced by interferon as shown in the recent experiments by Wiktor *et al.* (1972b), who protected hamsters by applying rabies, Kern Canyon, or influenza virus vaccines shortly before or immediately after challenge with street rabies virus. In contrast to the preventive action of interferon, specific rabies antibody alone when applied parenterally did not protect but resulted in prolonged incubation periods (Baer and Cleary, 1972).

In abortive and chronic rabies infections the replication and spread of virus within the CNS seems amenable to attack first by the action of interferon, and only later by the specific antibody which partially prevents the further spread of the virus. Infectious virus is then no longer demonstrable, and convulsions or other clinical signs of acute nerve disease disappear. Paralysis, accompanied by severe histopathologic changes in corresponding CNS segments, may persist for longer periods of time. The exact knowledge of the sequence of events that occur in the CNS in abortive rabies infection may contribute considerably to the important questions regarding early and late measures for postexposure treatment of rabies.

References

Andral, L., and Serié, C. (1957). *Ann. Inst. Pasteur, Paris* **93**, 475.

Arko, R. J., Schneider, L. G., and Baer, G. M. (1973). *Am. J. Vet. Res.* **34**, 937.

Baer, G. M., and Cleary, W. F. (1972). *J. Infec. Dis.* **125**, 520.

Baer, G. M., and Olson, H. R. (1972). *J. Amer. Vet. Med. Ass.* **160**, 1127.

Baer, G. M., Shanthaveerappa, T. R., and Bourne, G. H. (1965). *Bull. WHO* **33**, 783.

Baer, G. M., Shantha, T. R., and Bourne, G. H. (1968). *Bull. WHO* **38**, 119.

Bell, J. F. (1964). *J. Infec. Dis.* **114**, 249.

Bell, J. F., Lodmell, D. L., Moore, G. J., and Raymond, G. H. (1966). *J. Immunol.* **97**, 747.

Blattner, R. J. (1961). *J. Pediat.* **58**, 433.

Burwood, W. O. (1965). *J. Cell Biol.* **27**, 115A.

Cairns, W. J. F. (1950). *Nature (London)* **166**, 910.

Carski, T. R., and Wilsnack, R. (1966). *Symp. Ser. Immunobiol. Stand.* **1**, 193.

de Robertis, E. D. P., Gerschenfeld, W. M., and Wald, F. (1960). *Int. Cont. Electron Microsc., Proc., 4th, 1958*, Vol. II, pp. 443–447.

Dierks, R. E., Murphy, F. A., and Harrison, A. K. (1969). *Amer. J. Pathol.* **54**, 251.

Eichwald, C., and Pitzschke, H., eds. (1967). "Die Tollwut bei Mensch und Tier." Fischer, Jena.

Familusi, J. B., and Moore, D. L. (1972). *Afr. J. Med. Sci.* **3**, 93.

Fernandes, M. V., Wiktor, T. J., and Koprowski, H. (1964). *J. Exp. Med.* **120**, 1099.

Field, E. J. (1951). *J. Comp. Pathol.* **61**, 307.

Field, E. J. (1954a). *J. Pathol. Bacteriol.* **68**, 335.

Field, E. J. (1954b). *J. Comp. Pathol.* **64**, 213.

Field, E. J., and Brierly, J. B. (1948). *Brit. Med. J.* **1**, 1167.

Fleischhauer, K. (1964). *Z. Zellforsch. Mikrosk. Anat.* **62**, 639.

Garcia-Tamayo, J., Avila-Mayor, A., and Anzola-Perez, E. (1972). *Arch. Pathol.* **94**, 11.

Gildemeister, W. (1960). *Arch. Hyg. Bakteriol.* **144**, 207.

Goodpasture, E. W. (1925). *Amer. J. Pathol.* **1**, 547.

Gorshunova, L. P. (1958). *Probl. Virol. (USSR)* **3**, 116.

Hattwick, M. A., Weis, T. T., Stechschulte, C. J., Baer, G. M., and Gregg, M. B. (1972). *Ann. Intern. Med.* **76** (6), 931.

Horstmann, E. (1957). *Naturwissenschaften* **44**, 448.

Hronovsky, V., and Benda, R. (1969). *Acta Virol. (Prague)* **13**, 198.

Hummeler, K., Koprowski, H., and Wiktor, T. J. (1967). *J. Virol.* **1**, 152.

Huygelen, C. (1960). *Antonie van Leeuwenhoek; J. Microbiol. Serol.* **26**, 66.

Huygelen, C., and Mortelmans, J. (1959). *Antonie van Leeuwenhoek; J. Microbiol. Serol.* **25**, 265.

Jenson, A. B., Rabin, E. R., Bentinck, D. C., and Melnick, J. L. (1969). *J. Virol.* **3**, 265.

Johnson, R. T. (1964). *J. Exp. Med.* **119**, 343.

Johnson, R. T. (1965). *J. Neuropathol.* **24**, 662.

Johnson, R. T., and Mercer, E. H. (1964). *Aust. J. Exp. Biol. Med. Sci.* **42**, 449.

Kent, J. R., and Finegold, S. M. (1966). *N. Engl. J. Med.* **263**, 1058.

Kerbler, F. (1933). *Z. Hyg.* **115**, 235.

Kligler, I. J., and Bernkopf, H. (1943). *Brit. J. Exp. Pathol.* **24**, 15.

Koch, J. (1930). *In* "Handbuch der pathogenen Mikroorganismen" (W. Kolle, R. Kraus, and P. Uhlenhuth, eds.), Vol. 8, Part 1, pp. 547–694. Fischer, Jena.

Lipton, M. M., and Steigman, A. J. (1961). *J. Immunol.* **86**, 445.

Lipton, M. M., Steigman, A. J., and Dizon, F. C. (1965). *J. Infec. Dis.* **115**, 356.

Lodmell, D. L., Bell, J. F., Moore, G. J., and Raymond, G. H. (1969) *J. Infec. Dis.* **119**, 569.

Matsumoto, S. (1962). *Virology* **17**, 198.

Matsumoto, S. (1963). *J. Cell Biol.* **19**, 565.

Matsumoto, S., and Yonezawa, T. (1971). *Infec. Immunity* **3**, 606.

Mims, C. A. (1960). *Brit. J. Exp. Pathol.* **41**, 52.

Murphy, F. A., and Fields, B. N. (1967). *Virology* **33**, 625.

Murphy, F. A., Bauer, S. P., Harrison, A. K., and Winn, W. C. (1973). *Lab. Invest.* **28**, 361.

Nikolitsch, M. (1957). *Arch. Hyg. Bakteriol.* **141**, 361.

Ota, Y. (1955). *Yokohama Med. Bull.* **9**, 371.

Petrovic, M., and Timm, H. (1969). *Zentralbl. Bakteriol., Parasitenk., Infektionskr., Abt. 1: Orig.* **211**, 149.

Sabin, A. B., Casals, J., and Webster, L. T. (1940). *J. Bacteriol.* **39**, 67.

Schaffer, K. (1931). *Z. Neurol.* **136**, 547.

Schindler, R. (1959). *Z. Tropenmed. Parasitol.* **10**, 450.

Schindler, R. (1961). *Bull. WHO* **25**, 119.

Schlesinger, R. W. (1949). *J. Exp. Med.* **89**, 491.

Schneider, L. G. (1969a). *Zentralbl. Bakteriol., Parasitenk., Infektionskr., Abt. 1: Orig.* **211**, 281.

Schneider, L. G. (1969b). *Zentralbl. Bakteriol., Parasitenk., Infektionskr., Abt. 1: Orig.* **212**, 1.

Schneider, L. G., and Burtscher, H. (1967). *Zentralbl. Veterinaermed., Reihe B* **14**, 598.

Schneider, L. G., and Hamann, I. (1969). *Zentralbl. Bakteriol., Parasitenk., Infektionskr., Abt. 1: Orig.* **212**, 13.

Schneider, L. G., and Schoop, U. (1972). *Ann. Inst. Pasteur, Paris* **123**, 469.

Schneider, L. G., and Schoop, U. (1973). Rabies-like viruses, *Symp. Series. Immunobiol. Stand.* (in press).

Schneider, L. G., Dietzschold, B., Dierks, R. E., Matthaeus, W., Enzmann, P. J., and Strohmaier, K. (1973). *J. Virol.* **11**, 748.

Schweinburg, F. (1937) *Ergeb. Hyg., Bakteriol., Immunitaetsforsch. Exp. Ther.* **20**, 1.

Seifried, O., and Spatz, H. (1930). *Z. Neurol.* **124**, 317.

Siller, W. G., and Wight, P. A. L. (1965). *Immunology* **8**, 223.

Singer, M., and Bryant, S. V. (1969). *Nature (London)* **221**, 1148.

Sodja, I., Lim, D., and Matouch, O. (1971). *J. Hyg., Epidemiol., Microbiol., Immunol.* **15**, 229.

Spatz, H. (1934). *Arch. Psychiat.* **101**, 267.

Svet-Moldavskaya, I. A. (1958). *Acta Virol. (Prague)* **2**, 228.

Szatmari, A., and Salyi, J. (1936). *Z. Neurol.* **156**, 424.

Wight, P. A. L., and Siller, W. G. (1965). *Res. Vet. Sci.* **6**, 324.

Wiktor, T. J., Koprowski, H., and Rorke, L. B. (1972a). *Proc. Soc. Exp. Biol. Med.* **140**, 759.

Wiktor, T. J., Postic, B., Ho, M., and Koprowski, H. (1972b). *J. Infec. Dis.* **126**, 408.

Wong, D. H., and Freund, J. (1951). *Proc. Soc. Exp. Biol. Med.* **76**, 717.

CHAPTER 12

Electron Microscopy of Central Nervous System Infection

Seiichi Matsumoto

The changes that may accompany virus infection *in vivo* do not regularly occur in all susceptible cells, and this heterogeneous character of the cell population presents difficulties in virologic research in animals compared to the increased applicability and reproducibility in tissue culture. The problem becomes more significant when virus-infected cells are observed by electron microscopy, since only a very selected area can be studied; thus, electron microscopic studies of various virus infections have been based primarily on observations in tissue culture.

The first tissue culture system highly susceptible to rabies virus was established within the last decade (Fernandes *et al.*, 1963). Accordingly, electron microscopic observations of thin sections of rabies infected tissue were first carried out on *in vivo* material, especially in the central nervous system (Matsumoto, 1962). The specimens were obtained from brains of suckling mice that had shown typical paralytic signs after intracerebral inoculation of street or fixed rabies virus. It is difficult to obtain thin sections for electron microscopy; this technical deficiency was most evident in studies of nervous tissue, and the possibility of getting satisfactory fixation of this tissue was hazardous at best. Some technical changes were therefore made in fixation procedures (Luse, 1960; Bunge *et al.*, 1960; Palay *et al.*, 1962). Since about 1960, however, the introduction of epoxy resins for embedding (Epon, Vestapol, etc.) has made it possible to obtain satisfactory results with this tissue.

The appearance of the characteristic cytoplasmic bodies (Negri, 1903) in nerve cells indicate that these cells are select targets for rabies infection. The nerve cells are located among nerve fibers and glial processes. Like the basophilic substance of glandular cells, the

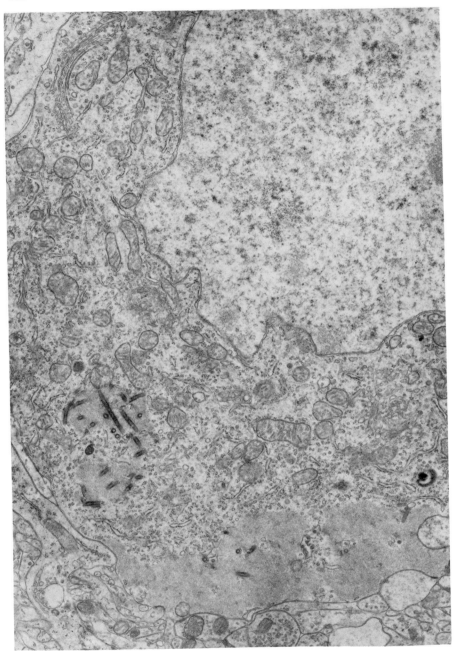

Fig. 1. A part of the nerve cell of mouse cerebellum. Near the cell membrane, two inclusion bodies containing virions cut in various planes are visible. Infection with a street virus of canine origin. ×11,000.

Nissl body is composed of endoplasmic reticulum and ribosomes measuring 10–30 nm in diameter. One component of the Nissl body appears to be part of the general endoplasmic reticulum of the nerve cells which extends throughout the entire cytoplasm, but is more condensed within the area of the Nissl body than in the rest of the cytoplasm. Another component of the Nissl body is the ribosomes, which are dispersed either in contact with the outer membranes of the endoplasmic reticulum or scattered throughout the intervening matrix (Palay and Palade, 1955). The cytoplasm around the nucleus (perikaryon) also contains many mitochondria and well-developed Golgi complexes.

The characteristic initial focus of rabies infection appears in the cytoplasm and is of variable size and irregular shape. The homogeneous ground substance of this cytoplasmic inclusion body is made up of relatively electron opaque filamentous aggregates (Fig. 1). Within or contiguous to inclusion bodies are found the rabies virions, and these in turn are found within the swollen lumens of the en-

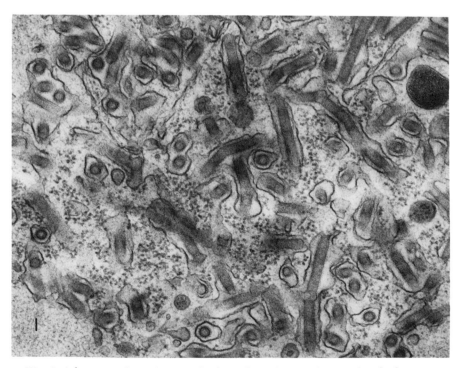

Fig. 2. A large number of virions bud out from the membrane of endoplasmic reticulum. Ribosomes, a few lysosomes, and a part of inclusion body (I) are discernible. Mouse brain infected with a street virus of canine origin. ×46,000.

doplasmic reticulum (Fig. 2). The diameter of the virion is 75–80 nm and its length is variable, but usually measures 180 nm or so. Projections or spikes 70 Å long cover the surface of the virions and can often be recognized in thin-section specimens. The core structure, with an average diameter of 40 nm, appears to be empty but some dense material is occasionally found inside (Fig. 3). The double membranes are electron dense and appear as a single layer under low magnification. The outer membrane is continuous at one end with the endoplasmic reticulum; this is seen as budding of the virion into the lumen. The size and shape of virions in nerve cells are quite similar to those of extracellular virions observed by negative staining. Additional variations in morphology may occur, depending upon the particular combination of virus strain and host cell. Three types of elongated particles are found in close relationship to the characteristic inclusion body when brain tissues infected with street rabies virus are examined (Roots and Schultze, 1963; Matsumoto,

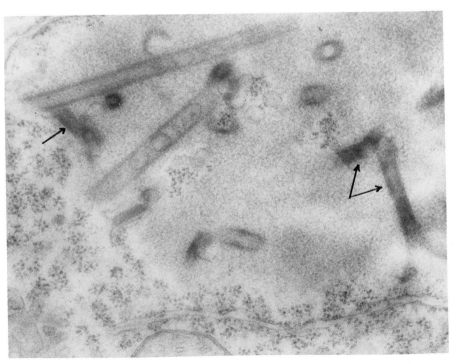

Fig. 3. A part of the inclusion body which is produced by a street virus of canine origin. Its ground substance is composed of filamentous aggregates. Two long rods covered by a single membrane contain internal structures. The second type of particles are seen within this area (arrows). ×58,300.

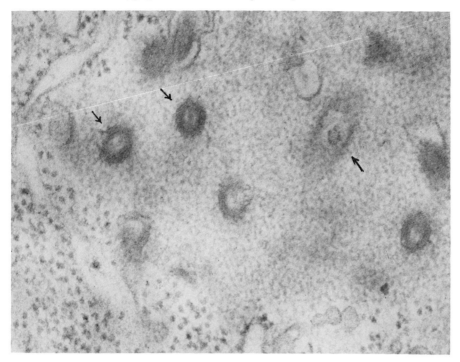

Fig. 4. A cytoplasmic part of the nerve cell is mostly replaced by inclusion body. Core-like structures are found in three particles (arrows). Infection with a street virus of canine origin. ×65,500.

1962, 1963; Johnson and Mercer, 1964; Miyamoto, 1965; Miyamoto and Matsumoto, 1967; Murphy *et al.*, 1973). The first type is 120–130 nm in diameter, has a single limiting membrane, and a light interior with a ground substance similar to that of the inclusion body (Fig. 4); the second particle is 110–120 nm in diameter and has a moderately dense peripheral space bound by a parallel double membrane (Fig. 4). It is noteworthy that neither type of particle is related to any vesicular structures, and both appear to be free within the inclusion body. The ends of the particles are open on both sides to the ground substance of the inclusion body. The last type of rod, 75–80 nm in diameter, is the smallest and appears regularly within the lumen of the endoplasmic reticulum, as described above. The first and second particles are generally less numerous than the third type. Although they are always associated with the inclusion body, no transitional relation between the first and second type of particles is demonstrable. In Fig. 5, within the Negri body we see three rods of the second type which are not associated with the endoplasmic reticulum, and

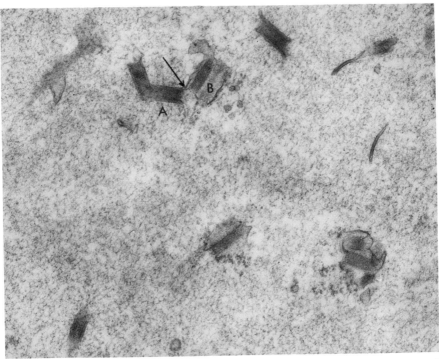

Fig. 5. A portion of an inclusion body. Four virions (type 2) are directly buried within the ground substance of this inclusion body. On the other hand, some particles (type 3) are covered by the endoplasmic reticulum. Arrows show the continuity of structure between the outer membrane of a virion (A) and the endoplasmic reticulum, and between its inner limiting membrane and the outer membrane of a virion (B). ×46,000.

one particle of the third type within the swollen endoplasmic reticulum. The outer membrane of the particle (A, second type) is continuous with the membrane of the endoplasmic reticulum, and its intermediate membrane is also connected to the outer membrane of the particle (B, third type) enclosed in a lumen. This evidence may suggest the possibility of a developmental process from the second type to the third one. It is difficult, however, to decide whether all projecting virus matures via the second type, because such figures appear infrequently compared to the large number of viruses found within the lumen of the endoplasmic reticulum. In spite of similarities between the three types of particle, their relationship can only be a matter for speculation at the present. Figure 6 shows a schematic diagram of the three types of particles found within nerve cells infected with street rabies virus isolate (Matsumoto and Miya-

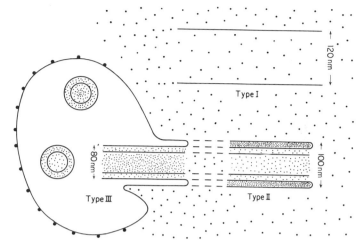

Fig. 6. Schematic diagram of three types of elongated particles found in rabies virus infected nerve cells.

moto, 1966). Branching and segmentation of the second and third type of long rods are also occasionally observed in negatively stained sections (Fig. 7; Matsumoto, 1963).

It is now concluded that the main site of rabies assembly is the cytoplasmic membrane system, and that the bullet-shaped virions are formed by a process of budding from the cytoplasmic membrane. In susceptible tissue culture systems rabies virus is assembled in variable quantities by budding at the cell surface (Hummeler *et al.*, 1967; Matsumoto and Kawai, 1969). In contrast, formation of virus is completely restricted to the inside of infected nerve cells as well as some kinds of glial cells (Fig. 8). This difference in the site of virus assembly is also observed with other combinations of virus strains and host cells; Dierks *et al.* (1969) showed that numerous virions were released from the cell surface of fox salivary gland cells infected with a street virus, but it is of particular interest that no virions were released from the surface of nerve cells in brain tissue of the same infected fox. The same predilection for virus formation inside nerve cells is noted during rabies infection of neural tissue cultivated *in vitro* (Matsumoto and Yonezawa, 1971). This morphological evidence of virus assembly at the cellular membrane must be interpreted together with biochemical analysis.

It is well known that some types of rhabdovirus such as rabies, Egtved virus (Zwillenberg *et al.*, 1965), and plaque purified stocks of the Indiana strain of vesicular stomatitis virus (Zajac and Hummeler, 1970), have been distinguished from other members of the group by

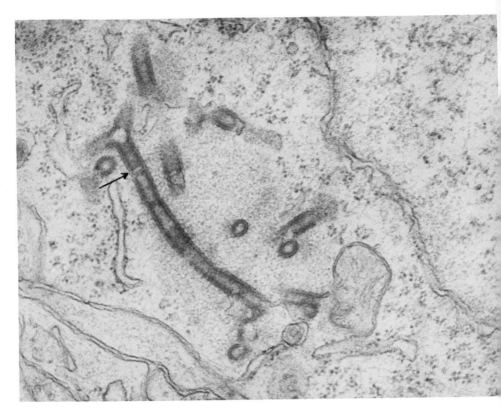

Fig. 7. Inclusion bodies containing virions with double membranes. One of the formation shows branching. A discontinuity of structure is visible (arrow). The specimen was prepared from the mouse brain infected with a street'virus of canine origin. ×49,500.

the formation of the characteristic cytoplasmic inclusion body (see Chapter 3). The presence of intracytoplasmic inclusion bodies within the nerve cell was reported by Negri (1903) as the pathognomonic finding of rabies infection. It appears that, simultaneously but independently, Bosc (1903) reported similar structures in rabid dogs. Numerous investigations have been carried out in an attempt to elucidate the nature and origin of this inclusion body. The history of these studies will be reviewed in Chapter 19. In brief, it was alleged to be: (1) a colony of viruses, (2) degenerative cellular constituents of the nerve cell, or (3) reactive products of the cell. When the characteristic inclusion body (formerly called matrix) containing rabies virions was first found in the nerve cell by electron microscopy, it

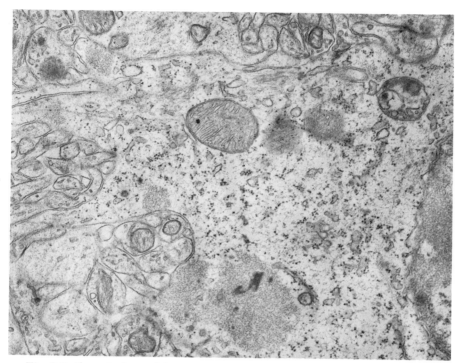

Fig. 8. In the cytoplasm of the astrocyte an inclusion body containing virions is visible. Infection with a street virus of canine origin. ×23,000.

was natural to raise the succeeding question of whether this characteristic area was identical with the Negri body (Matsumoto, 1963). Many reports confirmed that the characteristic inclusion body is quite commonly found after inoculation of either fixed or street virus strains, regardless of whether Negri bodies are identifiable by light microscopy. This appears to show that the inclusion body is not identical with the Negri body. In order to definitely show the nature of the Negri body by electron microscopy it was necessary to first exactly identify it by light microscopy. Accordingly Miyamoto and Matsumoto (1965) compared Negri bodies observed by light and electron microscopy in alternative thick (1 μm) and thin (under 100 nm) sections cut from the same nerve cell band of Ammon's horn. Comparison of light micrographs of Epon- and paraffin-embedded tissue revealed that, apart from a large number of inclusion bodies in thick sections embedded in Epon and about an equal number of Negri bodies in sections embedded in paraffin, no other pathologic formation could be found within nerve cells in the hippocampus. It was apparent, therefore, that the inclusion body seen in Epon-embedded tissue was identical with the Negri body. The electron micrographs correlated well with the light micrographs, and inclusion bodies could be readily identified as homogeneous aggregates which replaced the cytoplasmic components of nerve cells (Figs. 9 and 10). Within or contiguous to these masses of inclusion bodies we found clumps of rabies virions within swollen vesicles of the endoplasmic reticulum (Fig. 11). It was thus concluded that the Negri body corresponds to the site of virus replication. In addition, observations of consecutive thick and thin sections revealed that the so-called inner body, a characteristic constituent of the Negri body, is composed of virions associated with small amounts of cellular components. These basophilic granules which were also first described by Negri (1903, 1909), have been given much attention as regards virus classification, since they permit differentiation of the Negri body from other viral or nonviral inclusions. Goodpasture (1925) recognized Negri-like bodies containing no internal structure in the brains of rabbits infected with a street virus and termed them "lyssa bodies" for practical as well as theoretical reasons. He emphasized that "lyssa bodies" were, for the most part, small. In general, a number of small inclusion bodies were intermingled with typical Negri bodies, and small Negri bodies contained fewer inner bodies than large ones. The morphological appearance of inner bodies under the electron microscope is quite similar to that of the cytoplasmic area where virus assembly occurs, contiguous to the edges of the inclusion body. It therefore appears that Negri bodies are formed by the fusion of contiguous small inclusion bodies, and that the presence of the inner body is not essential; the term "Negri body" may thus be used in a broad sense to include "lyssa body."

Lentz (1909) first observed the extracellular structures found in nerve cells in the central nervous system of rabbits infected with the fixed virus. Lentz bodies are similar to Negri bodies in that they are eosinophilic and contain basophilic inner structures, and their exact nature is still unknown although they are thought to be the degenerative nucleus of neurons. Light microscopic observations of fixed virus infection revealed that some degenerative nerve cells were reduced in volume and had intensively eosinophilic cytoplasm. These necrotic cells, some of which had pyknotic nuclei, were found among normal or slightly damaged cells. It therefore seems likely that the Lentz bodies are severely damaged nerve cells themselves.

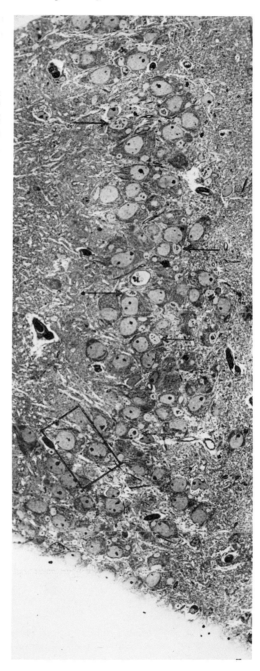

Fig. 9. A light micrograph of a section of Epon embedded hippocampus, after staining by toluidine blue. Nerve cells, most of which contain lightly stained inclusion bodies, are closely packed. Several representative inclusion bodies are indicated by arrows. The specimen was prepared from the mouse brain infected with a street virus of canine origin which readily produced Negri bodies. Electron micrograph of the rectangular area is shown in Fig. 10. ×350.

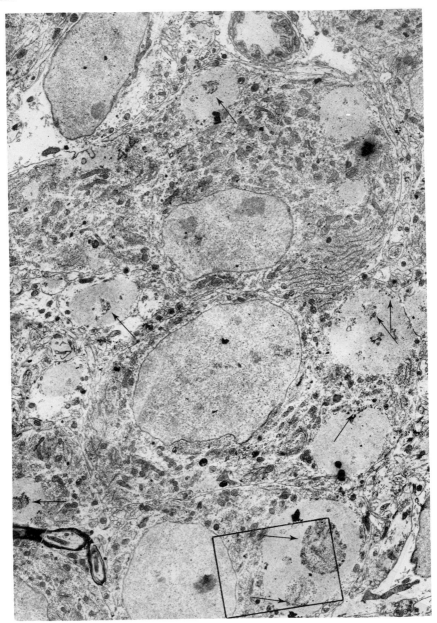

Fig. 10. A considerable number of inclusion bodies are visible in the same relation to those as in Fig. 9. Virions are found within and contiguous to the inclusion bodies (arrows). ×4500.

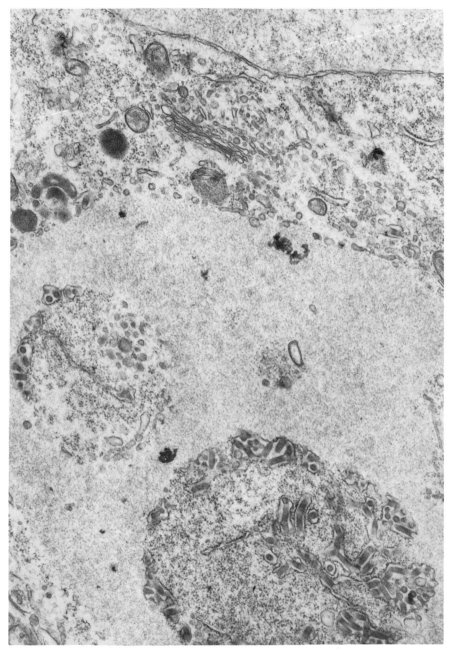

Fig. 11. A higher magnification of two inner bodies enclosed within the rectangular area shown in Fig. 10. They are composed of many virions and cytoplasmic components. ×25,000.

The fact that the Negri body corresponds to the site of virus replication immediately raises the question of why fixed rabies virus strains cannot produce Negri bodies within nerve cells, in spite of the fact that the replicating process is the same as that of the street rabies infection; fluorescent antibody staining shows the viral antigen as small Negri-like foci in nerve cells infected with fixed virus, and it seems unlikely that there is a qualitative difference between the replication of street and fixed virus (Goldwasser and Kissling, 1958). In an attempt to clarify this problem, Miyamoto and Matsumoto (1967) inoculated mice to study the comparative neuropathology of Ammon's horn infected with two strains of rabies virus; one which readily produced Negri bodies and the other (HEP Flury strain) which did not. Nerve cells containing Negri bodies appeared relatively little damaged. In striking contrast, in the case of the fixed virus infection, nerve cells showed a variety of stages of degeneration. Nerve cells with limited damage showed an increase in the number of small vesicles throughout the cytoplasm. A considerable number of lysosomes were also seen within these nerve cells. Severe necrotic alterations were found in the nucleus and the cytoplasm of the nerve cell band of Ammon's horn. Electron micrographs showed that characteristic inclusion bodies were discernible within these cells, but they were greatly reduced in volume. This suggests that the fixed virus injured nerve cells so extensively that the full development of the typical Negri body, as recognized by the light microscope, cannot occur (Figs. 12 and 13).

Other striking evidence is that fixed virus very rarely appeared within the nerve cell band of Ammon's horn (inset, Fig. 13). A higher virus titer was obtained in brains of mice infected with street virus than those inoculated with HEP Flury virus. However, various problems remain to be examined before the morphologic evidence of both virus infections can be definitely correlated with their infective titers. Different groups of neurons in the brain may be more vulnerable to virus replication. A similar phenomenon was encountered when rabies virus replication was studied in organized culture of dorsal root ganglion from rat or mouse embryos (Matsumoto and Yonezawa, 1971); only a small percentage of the inclusion bodies in nerve and glial cells were associated with virus assembly. This evidence reminds us of the existence of varying culture systems which exhibit an endosymbiotic relationship between virus and cell (Fernandes *et al.*, 1964) or a carrier-type infection of rabies virus (Wiktor, 1966, Wiktor and Clark, 1972).

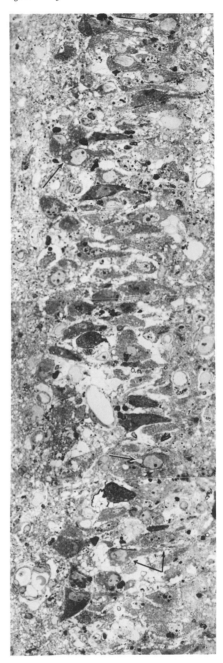

Fig. 12. A mouse cerebellum infected with a fixed virus, HEP Flury strain. A light micrograph of the nerve cell band in Ammon's horn showing marked disarrangement of neurons and the formation of vesicles in varying sizes. A considerable number of neurons are so dark that their nuclei become indistinguishable from their cytoplasms. Lightly stained inclusions in small size are found within relatively slightly damaged cells. Representative inclusions are indicated by arrows. ×350.

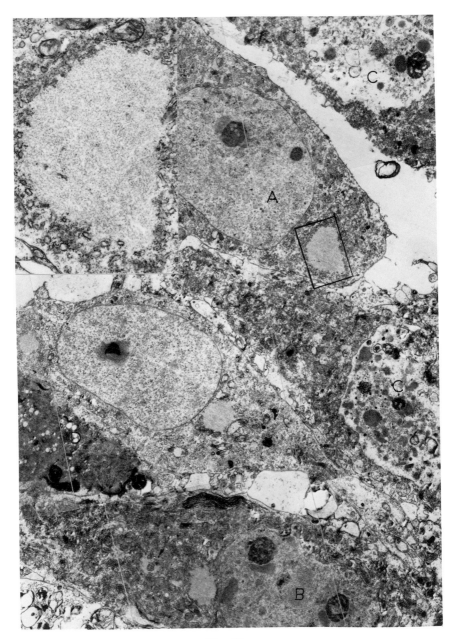

Fig. 13.

References

Bosc, F. J. (1903). *C. R. Soc. Biol.* 55, 1284–1288.
Bunge, R. P., Bunge, M. B., and Ris, H. (1960). *J. Biophys. Biochem. Cytol.* 7, 685–697.
Dierks, R. E., Murphy, F. A., and Harrison, A. K. (1969). *Amer. J. Pathol.* 54, 251–273.
Fernandes, M. V., Wiktor, T. J., and Koprowski, H. (1963). *Virology* 21, 128–130.
Fernandes, M. V., Wiktor, T. J., and Koprowski, H. (1964). *J. Exp. Med.* 120, 1099–1116.
Goldwasser, R. A., and Kissling, R. E. (1958). *Proc. Soc. Exp. Biol. Med.* 98, 219–223.
Goodpasture, E. W. (1925). *Am. J. Pathol.* 1, 547–582.
Hummeler, K., Koprowski, H., and Wiktor, T. J. (1967). *J. Virol.* 1, 152–170.
Johnson, R. T., and Mercer, E. H. (1964). *Aust. J. Exp. Biol. Med. Sci.* 42, 449–456.
Lentz, O. (1909). *Z. Hyg. Infektionskr.* 62, 63–94.
Luse, S. A. (1960). *J. Ultrastruct. Res.* 4, 108–112.
Matsumoto, S. (1962). *Virology* 17, 198–202.
Matsumoto, S. (1963). *J. Cell Biol.* 19, 565–591.
Matsumoto, S., and Miyamoto, K. (1966). *Symp. Ser. Immunobiol. Stand.* 1, 45–54.
Matsumoto, S., and Kawai, A. (1969). *Virology* 39, 449–459.
Matsumoto, S., and Yonezawa, T. (1971). *Infec. Immunity* 3, 606–616.
Miyamoto, K. (1965). *Annu. Rep. Inst. Virus Res. Kyoto Univ.* 8, 10–34.
Miyamoto, K., and Matsumoto, S. (1965). *J. Cell Biol.* 27, 677–682.
Miyamoto, K., and Matsumoto, S. (1967). *J. Exp. Med.* 125, 447–456.
Murphy, F. A., Harrison, A. K., Winn, W. C., and Bauer, S. P. (1973). *Lab. Invest.* 29, 1–16.
Negri, A. (1903). *Z. Hyg. Infektionskr.* 43, 507–528.
Negri, A. (1909). *Z. Hyg. Infektionskr.* 63, 421–443.
Palay, S. L., and Palade, G. E. (1955). *J. Biophys. Biochem. Cytol.* 1, 69–88.
Palay, S. L., McGee-Russell, S. M., Gordon, S., Jr., and Grillo, M. A. (1962). *J. Cell Biol.* 12, 385–410.
Roots, E., and Schultze, I. (1963). *Zentralbl. Bakteriol., Parasitenk., Infektionskr. Hyg., Abt. 1: Orig.* 188, 159–173.
Wiktor, T. J. (1966). *Symp. Ser. Immunobiol. Stand.* 1, 65–80.
Wiktor, T. J., and Clark, H. F. (1972). *Infec. Immunity* 6, 988–995.
Zajac, B. A., and Hummeler, K. (1970). *J. Virol.* 6, 243–252.
Zwillenberg, L. O., Jensen, M. H., and Zwillenberg, H. H. L. (1965). *Arch. Gesamte Virusforsch.* 17, 1–19.

Fig. 13. Degenerative changes of varying grades are evident. Advanced necrotic neurons (C) have nuclei showing coarse granules and watery content of low density replace the nuclear sap and nuclear membrane are disrupted in places. Cytoplasmic ground substance disappears in the vicinity of the cell membrane. A lamellate formation is visible near the cell membrane of a necrotic cell (B). The nuclear outline cannot be recognized in a necrotic cell (D) which is probably shrunken from its original size. Relatively small inclusion bodies are visible within these neurons. *Inset:* an inclusion body composed of fine filamentous ground substance. This feature resembles that of the Negri body. Note the absence of virus associated with this area. ×18,200.

CHAPTER 13

The Pathology of Rabies in the Central Nervous System

Daniel P. Perl

In spite of the striking symptoms seen in individuals or animals with rabies, there is little grossly visible alteration of the central nervous system (CNS); congestion of the meningeal vessels is usually the only externally visible abnormality of the brain. Although the congestion may be quite marked, frank subarachnoid hemorrhage is rarely seen. Clouding of the meninges has been described in a few cases of childhood rabies in which there were extensive leptomeningeal leukocytic infiltrates (Lowenberg, 1928; Tangchai *et al.*, 1970). A mild degree of cerebral edema may also be present. In a recent series of 24 autopsies of human rabies cases (Tangchai *et al.*, 1970), the brain weights were reported to be about 10–20% heavier than normal. Although a few markedly edematous brains have been reported in human cases [one weighing 1590 g (Tangchai *et al.*, 1970), one 1570 g (Berntsen and Stevenson, 1953), and another 1870 g (Erickson *et al.*, 1954)] massive cerebral swelling is rarely seen in rabies. It is difficult to determine whether respiratory insufficiency or arrest play a role in the production of this massive edema. Uncal or cerebellar herniation is rarely reported, and clinical papilledema and marked elevation of cerebrospinal fluid pressure are not noted until there are severe respiratory problems (Hattwick *et al.*, 1972; Johnson, 1972).

The parenchyma of the central nervous system also shows little gross alteration. Focal congestion may be seen in the white matter, for the most part within the brain stem, particularly in the structures comprising the floor of the fourth ventricle. Frank parenchymal hemorrhages are rarely seen. The spinal cord is also a site for focal congestion of the parenchymal and meningeal vessels.

I. Microscopic Changes

Virtually all of the significant histologic features of rabies infection in the CNS were first described in the 25-year period between the late 1870's and the first few years of the 1900's. Early in this period Benedikt (1875, 1878), Kolesnikoff (1875), Coats (1877), and Gowers (1877) all reported the accumulation of leukocytes around blood vessels of the CNS in rabid animals. These perivascular infiltrates were found primarily within the spinal cord, brain stem, and basal ganglia. Vascular congestion was also described, accompanied by diapedesis of red blood cells.

A. Inflammatory Lesions

Perivascular infiltration is undoubtedly the most frequently noted histologic change in rabies. Dupont and Earle (1965) found perivascular infiltrates in 48 of 49 cases of human rabies. Virtually all reported cases mention the presence of some perivascular infiltrates, most often found within the brain stem, particularly the pons and medulla (Fig. 1A,B). They are also frequently seen within the spinal cord, as well as the basal ganglia and cerebral cortex (Toga *et al.,* 1961; Sükrü Aksel, 1958). When the perivascular infiltrates are sparse, they are usually confined to the brain stem. As with other forms of viral encephalitis, there is nothing specific about these infiltrates; they consist primarily of round cells and occasional polymorphonuclear cells, the latter most often present in patients with a short duration of illness. Plasma cells may be present following a prolonged course of illness (Dupont and Earle, 1965; Sükrü Aksel,

---

Fig. 1A. Extensive perivascular infiltrates in the midbrain of a human case of rabies. Hematoxylin and eosin, ×50.

Fig. 1B. Perivascular infiltrate in the pons of a rabid skunk. The infiltrate is composed primarily of lymphocytes and macrophages. An occasional polymorphonuclear leukocyte is noted (arrow). H & E, ×690.

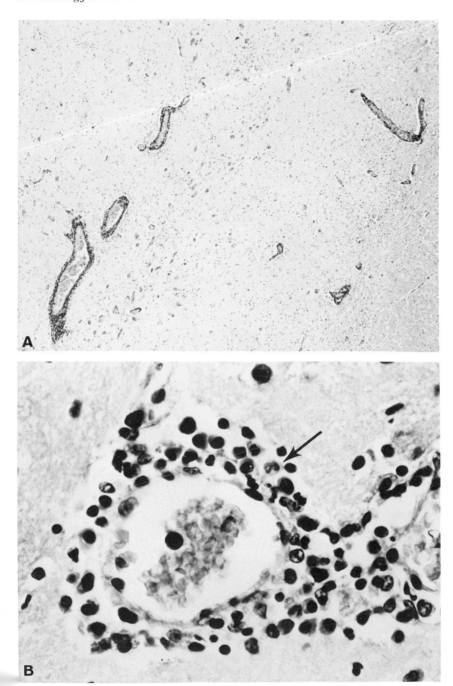

Fig. 1.

1958; Achúcarro, 1909–1910). Focal diapedesis of red blood cells is frequently seen. Frank hemorrhages are rare, but when they do occur they usually involve structures in the floor of the fourth ventricle.

Through Pasteur's dramatic report (Pasteur, 1885) in which he stated that rabies could be prevented by inoculation of fixed virus during the incubation period, a great impetus was given to the study of pathologic lesions of rabies. It now became important to rapidly establish the presence of rabies in a suspected animal. Babes (1892) stated that a specific histologic lesion of rabies was needed to replace the unreliable practice of examining the animal's stomach contents for foreign matter (its presence was considered as indicative of prior aberrant behavior). A specific histologic lesion would also supplement time-consuming rabbit inoculation, which usually provided results only after 15–18 days. Babes described perivascular infiltrates similar to those reported by the previous investigators, stating that the infiltrates were composed of "embryonal cells." In addition, he noted the presence of focal collections of "embryonal cells" away from the blood vessels, frequently surrounding a neuron or several neurons undergoing chromatolytic degeneration. He called these perineuronal cellular infiltrates "rabidic tubercules." Through the years they have come to be known as Babes' nodules (Fig. 2A,B). Babes considered the presence of parenchymal and pericellular infiltrates in the brain stem to be a specific and diagnostic histologic lesion of rabies. Although it is clear that most cases of rabies show these changes, similar findings may also be encountered in many other forms of viral encephalitis (Nieberg and Blumberg, 1972), as well as in toxic states such as uremia (Greenhouse, 1968) and chronic arsenic poisoning (Osetowska, 1971). The "embryonal cells" comprising Babes' nodules are, for the most part, the activated microglial cells characterized by del Río-Hortega (1932). The neurons near these cellular collections often show degenerative changes, appearing shrunken and containing condensed, dark-staining cytoplasm and a pyknotic nucleus. As first noted by Ramón y Cajál and García (1904) and by Achúcarro (1909–1910), coarsening of the neurofibrillar material in these cells can be seen by silver impregnation stains.

The extent of neuronal degeneration as well as inflammatory

Fig. 2A. Large Babes' nodule in the thoracic portion of the spinal cord of a monkey infected with street virus. Note the accumulation of cells around the anterior horn cells. H & E, ×160.

Fig. 2B. Neuronophagia within a Babes' nodule in the same animal. ×560.

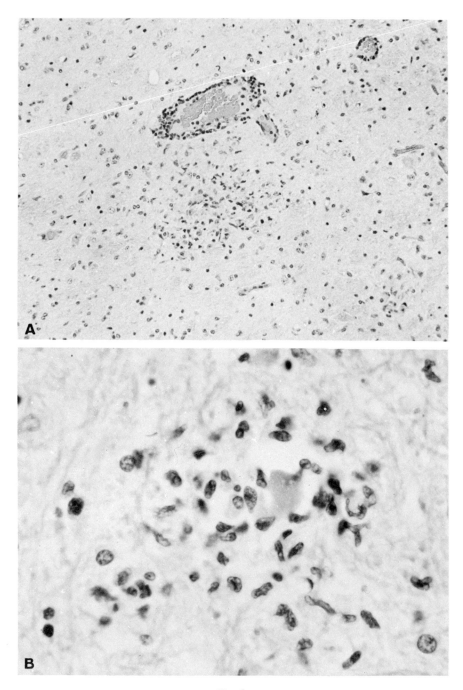

Fig. 2.

changes in cases of rabies is quite variable. A tendency for the production of severe inflammatory lesions has been noted in the dog, whereas rabies in pigs and herbivores produces little histologic evidence of neuronal degeneration or inflammation (Jubb and Kennedy, 1963). In human rabies there is a great pathologic variability, ranging from very inconspicuous inflammatory changes and virtually no evidence of neuronal degeneration to prominent, widespread perivascular inflammatory infiltrates and microglial cellular collections associated with neuronal degeneration and neuronophagia. Inflammatory changes appear to be more prominent in cases with a more fulminant course (Dupont and Earle, 1965). Some portion of this neuronal degeneration is undoubtedly secondary to coexisting processes such as anoxia and hyperpyrexia. As will be noted later, rabies is a unique form of viral encephalitis in that extensive invasion of a neuron by the virus does not, in general, give rise to significant cell disruption or lysis. Nevertheless, neuronophagia is frequently seen in rabies (Fig. 2B). Dupont and Earle (1965) identified neuronophagia in 57% of cases in their autopsy series. Lowenberg (1928) described extensive destruction of the pigmented neurons of the substantia nigra, accompanied by neuronophagia (as demonstrated by the presence of phagocytized neuromelanin) in three human rabies cases.

In virtually all cases of rabies, some minimal evidence of leptomeningeal extension of the inflammatory processes can be found (Dupont and Earle, 1965; Tangchai *et al.*, 1970). These infiltrates, particularly when they are scanty, are frequently encountered surrounding the brain stem (Fig. 3A), and are composed of the same cellular elements as the parenchymal perivascular infiltrates: lymphocytes, macrophages, and occasional plasma cells. In some cases, particularly when the inflammatory lesions are intense, polymorphonuclear cells will predominate. A general tendency has been noted for both the parenchymal and meningeal inflammatory lesions in rabies to be more intense in children than in adults (Tangchai *et al.*, 1970; Sükrü Aksel, 1958). Lowenberg (1928) described a case of

---

Fig. 3A. Leptomeningeal infiltration by chronic inflammatory cells from a case of rabies in a child. Medulla. H & E, ×180.

Fig. 3B. Van Gehuchten and Nelis lesions in a cervical spinal ganglion of a rabid raccoon. Although focal chronic inflammatory cell infiltrates are present (arrow), these are not diagnostically as significant as the capsular cell proliferation. H & E, ×450.

Fig. 3C. Several neurons showing degenerative changes. Human rabies, midbrain. H & E, ×736.

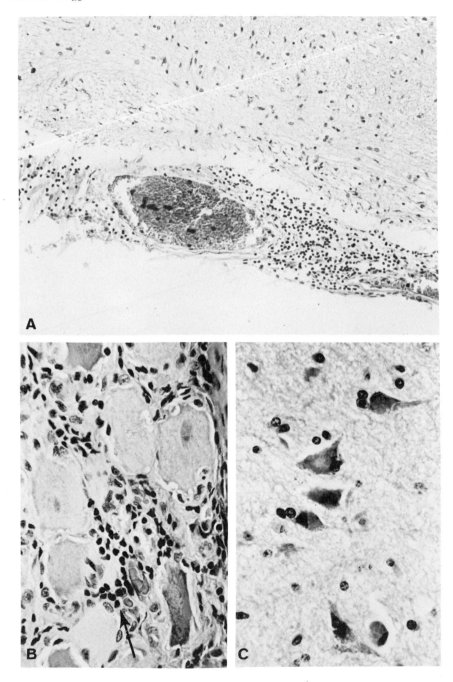

Fig. 3.

rabies in a 5-year-old girl who was bitten on the mouth by a rabid dog. Lumbar puncture 2 days after the onset of her disease revealed turbid cerebrospinal fluid containing 1032 white blood cells per cm³. The patient died on the following day, and autopsy revealed markedly congested leptomeningeal vessels. There was, however, no grossly visible clouding of the meninges. Histologic sections revealed numerous white blood cells within the leptomeninges. The parenchyma showed extensive inflammatory lesions and neuronal degeneration.

Dupont and Earle (1965) found three rabies cases with meningitis in their autopsy series, but they do not indicate the age of their patients. Tangchai *et al.*, (1970) reported four cases with meningitis, all children, and noted that there was a more intense inflammatory reaction and a shorter clinical course in these individuals.

B. GANGLIONIC LESIONS

Further attempts to discover a diagnostic histologic lesion for rabies were reported by Van Gehuchten and Nelis (1900), who criticized the lack of specificity of the lesions described by Babes in 1892. They examined the cranial nerve ganglia and spinal ganglia of a number of rabid animals and found a striking proliferation of the capsular cells surrounding the ganglionic neurons. As a result, the ganglion cells were pushed further and further apart, becoming separated by a lattice-like network of dense, proliferating capsular cells. The neuronal cells appeared compressed and were frequently undergoing varying stages of chromatolysis (Figs. 3B, and 4). The authors noticed associated gross changes within the ganglia, including an enlargement of the individual ganglia and increased firmness.

Van Gehuchten and Nelis were not the first to observe ganglionic changes in rabies, as they acknowledge in their paper. Nepveu (1872) examined the Gasserian ganglia of a man with rabies, and in passing described separation of the ganglionic neurons by proliferating cells which he interpreted to be leukocytes. Nepveu apparently did not consider the changes to be of great significance.

Although the ganglionic changes described by Van Gehuchten and Nelis have subsequently been noted by numerous investigators (Marinesco and Stroesco, 1931; Tangchai *et al.*, 1970; Innes and Saunders, 1962a; Hardenbergh and Underhill, 1916), only a few reports describe the use of these lesions in rabies diagnosis. Frothingham (1920) studied serial sections of 1100 Gasserian ganglia from

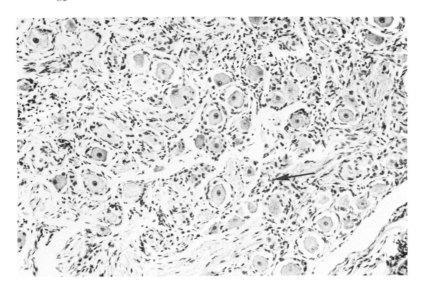

Fig. 4. Typical Van Gehuchten and Nelis lesions in a spinal ganglion in a human case of rabies. Focal round cell inflammatory infiltrates (arrow) accompany the prominent capsular cell proliferation. H & E, ×220.

suspected animals and surmised that the percentage of error was very small. Herzog (1941, 1965) compared the diagnostic efficiency of Ammon's horn examination for Negri bodies to histologic examination of the ganglion nodosum of the vagus nerve in 52 human and animal cases of rabies. All of the cases demonstrated diagnostic ganglionic changes, primarily neuronal degeneration with marked proliferation of capsular cells, but Negri bodies were noted in the hippocampus of less than 50% of the cases. Lapi *et al.*, (1952) obtained similar results in a series comparing histologic sections of Gasserian ganglion to stained smears. All of these investigators reported great variability in the presence of inflammatory cell infiltrates within ganglia, and stressed the diagnostic significance of the capsular cell proliferation and degenerative changes in ganglionic neurons (Fig. 3B).

However, the ganglionic changes described are not exclusively confined to rabies. Some other forms of viral encephalitis, such as porcine polioencephalitis (Innes and Saunders, 1962b; Jubb and Kennedy, 1963), have been shown to demonstrate similar alterations. Herzog (1941, 1965) acknowledges the nonspecific nature of the lesions, but replies that, in his experience, they are not encountered in diseases which must be considered in the differential diagnosis of rabies. Most pathologists and veterinarians are not familiar with the ganglionic lesions of Van Gehuchten and Nelis and rarely look for them. Their use in the confirmation of the diagnosis of rabies can be helpful, particularly if the brain has been destroyed. However, Negri's discovery of the diagnostic inclusions which bear his name almost completely eclipsed Van Gehuchten's and Nelis's ganglionic findings only 3 years earlier.

C. THE NEGRI BODY

It is hard to imagine the dramatic impact that the discovery of the Negri body must have had in 1903. For the next several decades, pathologic investigation of rabies centered almost exclusively around clarifying the nature, significance, and specificity of this inclusion.

Negri (1903) reported that, based on "four months of uninterrupted labor," he had detected microscopically an organism which he considered the specific etiologic agent of rabies. He described within the neuronal cytoplasm round to oval inclusion bodies which stained most consistently with the methylene blue and eosin method of Mann. They measured 1–27 μm in diameter and frequently contained a central, small dark-staining *innerkörperchen* or inner body (Figs. 5A,B; and 6A–D). Negri stated that there were privileged sites for encountering these bodies and that the large neurons of the Ammon's horn were particularly favored. The infectious nature of rabies had been described over 2000 years ago by Greek physicians (see Chapter 1), and Negri considered that he had discovered a parasitic organism which was the etiologic agent of the infection. Moreover, Negri also realized that the inclusion he described represented a specific and diagnostic lesion of rabies.

Earlier investigators had occasionally described a variety of intracytoplasmic bodies in rabies. Babes (1892) briefly noted certain rounded, ameboid bodies about 1 μm in diameter in the cytoplasm of certain neurons in rabies. Gowers (1877) described granules in the neurons in cases of rabies. It is difficult to determine, in retrospect, whether these investigators were attempting to describe Negri bodies. The important point is that they were apparently unaware of the significance of these cytoplasmic bodies and of their specificity for rabies infection. Bosc (1903a,b) independently discovered the specific inclusions of rabies infection and published his accounts almost simultaneously with Negri—history has always credited their discovery to Negri, and Bosc's name is almost unknown.

There was a rapid flurry of papers confirming Negri's observations

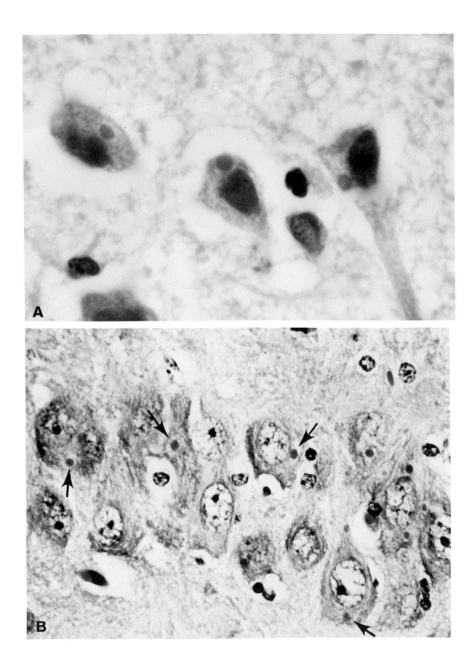

Fig. 5A. Three large neurons showing prominent Negri bodies. Ammon's horn, dog. Van Orden green stain, ×1450. (This slide provided by Miss Avis Van Orden, Pathology Section, Laboratory Division, C.D.C., Atlanta, Georgia.)

Fig. 5B. Section from the dentate gyrus of the hippocampus of the same animal, demonstrating numerous Negri bodies (arrows). H & E, ×575.

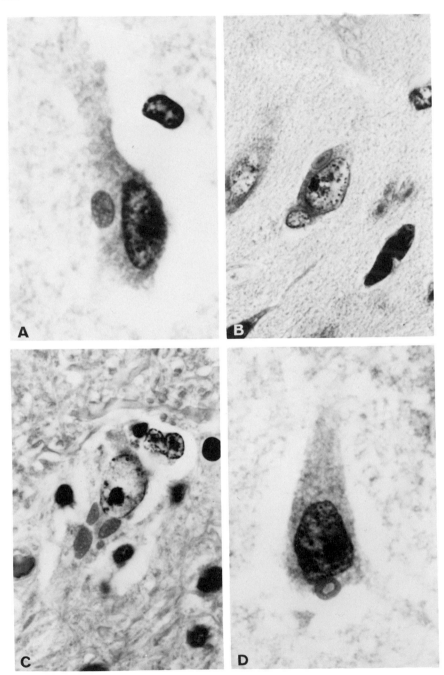

Fig. 6.

following his initial description of a distinct diagnostic, morphologic lesion of rabies (Abba and Bormans, 1905; Negri-Luzzani, 1905; Babes, 1907; Koch, 1910). It became clear that examination for Negri bodies in animals suspected of being rabid was a practical method for establishing the diagnosis. Negri-Luzzani (1913) best summarized the first 10 years of experience in the use of Negri body examination for the diagnosis of rabies. Her studies indicated that Negri bodies were present in about 90% of cases of rabies. However, confirmatory animal inoculation of the suspect material was not performed on all of those "rabid" animals. Recent studies indicate that about 75% of naturally occurring cases of rabies demonstrate Negri bodies (Dupont and Earle, 1965; World Health Organization, 1954; Tustin and Smit, 1962).

At the same time that the diagnostic efficiency of Negri body examination was being evaluated, the nature of the inclusion was also being investigated. Several theories quickly evolved. Negri (1909), of course, considered it to be a parasite which invaded the central nervous system and propagated within the neurons. In the same year as Negri's description of the "parasite," Remlinger (1903) published his classic ultrafiltration experiments. These studies indicated that the infective agent was submicroscopic. Levaditi *et al.*, (1924, 1926), aware of the ultrafiltration experiments, later still expounded the parasite theory. He suggested that the organism was a type of microsporidium, which went through a submicroscopic spore form. Upon arriving at the central nervous system from the wound site, the organism underwent proliferation into a larger "pansporoblast" form, which was seen as the Negri body. Volpino (1906) and Babes (1907) considered the basophilic kernel within the center of the Negri body (*innerkörperchen*) to be the etiologic agent of rabies. They thought that the red-staining mass around the organism was produced by the neuron in response to injury caused by the agent. Lentz (1909) and D'Amato and Faggella (1910) did not consider the Negri body to contain any etiologic agent, but instead to represent a degenerative change within the neuron, similar to the neurofibrillary tangle de-

---

Fig. 6A. Prominent Negri body in a neuron of the hippocampus of a rabid dog. H & E, ×2000.

Fig. 6B. Negri body with a prominent internal granule. Hippocampus, rabid skunk. H & E, ×1440.

Fig. 6C. Multiple large Negri bodies in a monkey experimentally infected with street virus. Pons. H & E, ×1240.

Fig. 6D. Negri body showing prominent internal structure. Hippocampus, rabid skunk. H & E, ×1800.

scribed by Alzheimer (1907). Acton and Harvey (1911) noted the morphologic similarities between the Negri body and the nucleolus, and postulated that the latter had been extruded from the nucleus into the cytoplasm. Many years later Goldwasser and Kissling (1958), through the use of fluorescent antibody techniques, demonstrated that the Negri body contained viral antigen. The viral particles within the inclusion were finally depicted ultrastructurally by Matsumoto (1962, 1963).

As one reviews the literature on the pathology of rabies, it is clear that there is a variation in the morphology of the cytoplasmic inclusions seen. Negri (1903) stressed the presence of a minute, basophilic internal granule within the inclusion, and many subsequent investigators have relied on the presence of this inner body for identification. Goodpasture (1925) made note of the difference between the classic Negri body inclusion, which contained a central, basophilic granule, and those of similar appearance displaying no internal body, which he called "lyssa bodies." Lyssa bodies have traditionally been considered unsuitable for the diagnosis of rabies. In many animal species, most notably the cat, small eosinophilic inclusions appear within the neuronal cytoplasm of normal animals (Szlachta and Habel, 1953; Tierkel, 1959; Innes and Saunders, 1962a). These nonspecific inclusions are homogeneous and do not contain an internal structure. Yet many authors on rabies do not state the criteria used for Negri body identification. Some appear to classify as Negri bodies only those inclusions which contain classic inner granules and are thus diagnostic, while others use a more general concept of the Negri body which includes any prominent intracytoplasmic inclusion. These differences in approach must be kept in mind when comparing morphologic studies on rabies.

The largest neurons involved tend to have the most prominent inclusions (Acton and Harvey, 1911; Cornwall and Kesava Pai, 1910; Tangchai *et al.*, 1970; Kraus *et al.*, 1926). The ganglion cells of the Ammon's horn configuration and the Purkinje cells of the cerebellum,

---

Fig. 7A and B. Prominent Negri body located within an axon. Hippocampus, human rabies. H & E; A: ×1440; B: ×1200.

Fig. 7C. Negri body within the neuropil in the molecular layer of the cerebellum in a monkey experimentally infected with street virus. This inclusion is most likely located within the dendritic extension of a purkinje cell. H & E, ×1040.

Fig. 7D. Several Negri bodies present within the cytoplasm of a cell appearing to be of glial origin (? oligodendroglial cell). Midbrain, monkey experimental rabies. H & E, ×960.

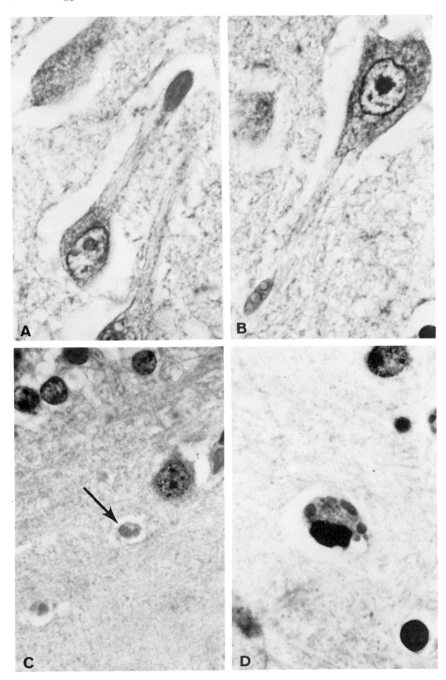

Fig. 7.

both extremely large cells, do tend to contain prominent Negri bodies, often with well-formed inner bodies (hippocampal inclusions are shown in Fig. 6B and D). Large, well-formed Negri bodies may at times be seen within axons (Fig. 7A,B). They also may be seen within dendrites, frequently appearing as a row of small, eosinophilic bodies, likened to a series of rosary beads by Marinesco and Stroesco (1931). Presumably, these axonal or dendritic inclusions have given rise to the occasional Negri body encountered within the neuropil (Fig. 7C). At times, particularly in areas of extensive Negri body formation, inclusions may be noted within glial cells (Fig. 7D). Despite the tendency for rabies virus to infect epithelial structures and thus produce cytoplasmic inclusions within the salivary glands, pancreas, etc., Negri bodies have not been noted within the choroid plexus or ependymal lining cells (Tangchai *et al.*, 1970; Sükrü Aksel, 1958; Marinesco and Stroesco, 1931).

There are also differences in Negri body morphology, depending on the species of animal infected (Acton and Harvey, 1911; van Rooyen and Rhodes, 1940). For instance, the rabbit tends to form very small, yet multiple Negri bodies (up to 2 μm) in which the inner bodies are difficult to see (Acton and Harvey, 1911; Goodpasture, 1925). The raccoon also produces small Negri bodies (Fig. 7A). On the other hand, the dog has a tendency to produce rather large Negri bodies in which there is a prominent internal granule (Iwamori and Yamagiwa, 1945) (Figs. 5A and 6A). The guinea pig (Acton and Harvey, 1911) and skunk (Moulton, 1954) also may produce very prominent inclusions (Figs. 6D and 8B). In the cow, the Negri bodies are perhaps largest of all (Acton and Harvey, 1911) and, indeed, they may at times even be seen macroscopically (G. M. Baer, personal communication, 1972). These differences appear to be related primarily to the species infected, rather than to the clinical course or the viral strain. In other words, if a dog specimen, for example, is obtained containing large Negri bodies with a prominent inner granule, rabbit inoculation with the specimen will likely produce small, multiple, "rabbitlike" inclusions with inconspicuous inner bodies (Acton and Harvey, 1911).

Crandell (1965) described the presence of intranuclear neuronal inclusions in animals inoculated with brain material from an out-

Fig. 8A. Anterior horn cell from the cervical portion of the spinal cord of a rabid raccoon demonstrating a single, small Negri body (arrow). H & E, ×1720.

Fig. 8B. Very large Negri body encountered in the basal ganglia of a rabid skunk (arrow). H & E, ×1720.

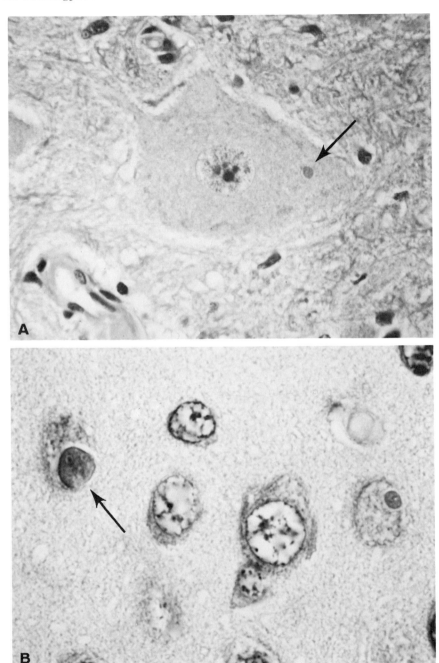

Fig. 8.

break of rabies among dogs and foxes in Greenland. The animals also showed typical intracytoplasmic Negri body inclusions. The intranuclear inclusions were eosinophilic and measured 0.5–1.5 μm. Kantorovich (1957) described the occasional appearance of similar eosinophilic inclusions in the neuronal nuclei of animals infected with "polar madness"; polar madness was considered to be a type of rabies seen in northern Russia. Sokolov and Vanag (1962), on the basis of acridine orange staining methods, have reported the presence of RNA-containing, intranuclear inclusions in the late stages of experimental rabies infection. The significance of these reports is difficult to determine. Intranuclear inclusions in both naturally occurring and experimental rabies have not been reported by others.

The question is frequently asked: What is the best site in which to find Negri bodies? Negri, of course, indicated that the hippocampus was preferentially involved. Several other investigators have indicated similar feelings, although one frequently finds that pathologic examination has been limited primarily to the hippocampus. In this location, Negri body formation is most frequently seen in the first one-third of the Ammon's horn configuration, the dentate gyrus, and in the vicinity of the fimbria (Marinesco and Stroesco, 1931) (Fig. 5a,b). The more basilar portions of the Ammon's horn are less prone to Negri body formation. Some authors have indicated that the hippocampus may not be the best site in which to look for Negri bodies. However, in these studies, the criteria for Negri body identification are not always clearly stated. One wonders whether lyssa bodies or other "intermediate" forms have been classified as Negri bodies. Tangchai *et al.*, (1970), in their recent study of the central nervous system lesions of 24 cases of human rabies, reported that Negri bodies were fairly ubiquitously distributed in the gray matter, but were more prominent in the larger nerve cells; the authors were not struck by any particular tendency for Negri body formation in the hippocampus. Dupont and Earle (1965) reviewed 49 cases of rabies from the files of the Armed Forces Institute of Pathology (AFIP). In their material, the cerebellum was the most frequent site of Negri body formation (59.5% of cases), followed by the hippocampus (42.9% of cases), and, finally, a much lower frequency in a number of other sites throughout the CNS. There may be an inherent bias in this survey, for Dupont and Earle were only able to review the material sent to the AFIP for confirmation. The studies by Tangchai *et al.* appear more representative, since a specific protocol for the wide and adequate sampling of the CNS was established and followed in all cases reported.

Thomas and Jackson (1930) were impressed by the frequency of involvement of the neurons of the oculomotor nucleus in rabies cases. They reported the results of histologic examination of the hippocampus versus the oculomotor nucleus (as seen in a cross section of the midbrain at the level of the posterior quadrigeminal bodies) on a series of 48 proven rabies cases in rabbits. They found that in 25 cases (51%), Negri bodies were more frequent in the midbrain sections than in the hippocampus. In only one case were the Negri bodies more frequent in the hippocampus than in the midbrain. Furthermore, in 11 cases (22%), Negri bodies were absent in the hippocampus but present in the midbrain, but the reverse situation was true in only one case. Horgan and McKinnon (1937) attempted to repeat this study using a series of 37 rabid animals, mostly dogs, and their findings were completely different than those of Thomas and Jackson: Of the 37 brains, 10 (27%) had Negri bodies in both hippocampus and midbrain, 18 (48.6%) in the hippocampus only, and in no case was the midbrain involved when the hippocampus was negative. More recently Tustin and Smit (1962), on the basis of histologic examination of 1074 proven cases of rabies from a wide range of animal species, concluded that, at least for diagnostic purposes, examination of the hippocampus (71% of proved cases) was more frequently positive than examination of other regions of the brain (46% of proved cases).

Although in most general reviews of rabies neuropathology the distribution of Negri bodies is described as being related to the site of the bite (Wolf, 1950), there is little detailed evidence from either naturally occurring or experimentally produced rabies infection to establish any such clear-cut correlation. The most systematic investigation into this question was made by Goodpasture (1925). He injected a small amount of street rabies virus into the right masseter muscle of rabbits, carefully followed the animals for clinical signs of rabies infection, and then sacrificed them at varying stages of the disease. The Gasserian ganglia and central nervous system, especially the trigeminal motor nuclei, were examined histologically, with particular attention paid to the asymmetry of the lesions. As noted above, he made a distinction between what he called "lyssa bodies" and typical Negri bodies; lyssa bodies were more numerous in the rabbits examined than were Negri bodies. Following inoculation of the virus in the right masseter muscle, Negri bodies were demonstrable within the right fifth nerve motor nucleus of all animals, but inclusions could also be seen in each left fifth motor nucleus and throughout the CNS. The concentration of inclusions and inflammatory lesions was most severe within the pons, medulla, and cervical spinal cord, based on the qualitative estimates that follow thorough histologic examination. But in most cases the lesions were judged to be somewhat more intense on the right side. Degenerative neuronal changes were frequently found within the Gasserian ganglia (particularly on the right side), but Negri bodies were rarely seen. The Ammon's horn in Goodpasture's animals showed few Negri bodies. Goodpasture was puzzled by this evidence, contradictory to the previously expressed view that the hippocampus is a preferred site for rabies virus involvement. It should be noted that the inoculum Goodpasture used apparently caused illness following a rather short incubation period (less than 2 weeks), and many of the animals were sacrificed early in the course of their illness.

While Goodpasture observed an asymmetry of the lesions related to the side of inoculation, it has been difficult to substantiate this in naturally occurring infection. Nevertheless, some attempts, have been made to relate the distribution of lesions to the wound site. Szatmári and Salyi (1936) as well as Schaffer (1912) concluded that the distribution of the lesions in rabies was dependent on the location of the wound, but the specific data on which these impressions were based is not stated. In contrast, Sükrü Aksel (1958) stated that the distribution of the inflammatory and neuronal changes were independent of the bite site, and as illustrations, cited cases in which the bite had been on either the extremities or the head, with a resultant identical distribution of pathologic lesions. To my knowledge, an unbiased, systematic survey of the central nervous system of rabid animals with varying wound locations has never been reported. The larger autopsy series have unfortunately failed to evaluate their material for the presence of these correlations.

Several authors have offered the impression that, in the earlier stages of the disease, Negri bodies are much smaller and less frequent than in later stages. This was the view of Marinesco and Stroesco (1931) in the review of their experience with both naturally occurring and experimentally produced rabies infection. In dogs inoculated with street virus and killed at daily intervals after onset of illness, they found an increasing percentage of cells containing Negri bodies as signs progressed. No Negri bodies were found 12 hours after the onset of illness. After 1 day of illness, 30–40% of cells examined contained Negri bodies, and after 5 days of illness, 80% were positive for Negri bodies. Unfortunately, there is no indication as to how the inoculations were standardized, nor which anatomic structures were examined.

Tierkel (1959) states, "The development of Negri bodies in the brain is directly related to the length of clinical illness in rabies." He does not clarify whether he is speaking about the size of the inclusions, their numbers, or both. However, he does comment that premature killing of suspected animals will reduce the accuracy of laboratory diagnosis.

Wolman and Behar (1952) studied by histochemical methods the production of Negri bodies in mice inoculated intracerebrally with street virus and sacrificed at daily intervals. One day after inoculation tiny basophilic granules were observed in the cytoplasm of the hippocampal neurons. Animals sacrificed 3 and 5 days after inoculation showed larger and increasing numbers of inclusions. By the sixth day following inoculation the inclusions were even more numerous and many contained typical inner bodies, which were Feulgen positive. Yet 8 days after inoculation many of the inclusions had lost their inner granules, thus having the appearance of lyssa bodies, and these inclusions were noted to be Feulgen negative. The authors concluded that there was a progressive reduction in the number of viral particles in the late stages of the disease, with a resultant loss of basophilia and Feulgen-positive material within the inclusion.

It should be emphasized that Negri bodies tend to be found in regions of the brain in which there is little inflammatory reaction (Goodpasture, 1925; Cornwall and Kesava Pai, 1910; Marinesco and Stroesco, 1931; Tangchai *et al.*, 1970; Sükrü Aksel, 1958). Conversely, Negri bodies are generally not found in areas showing a prominent inflammatory reaction. In these regions one more commonly finds evidence of neuronal degeneration in the absence of inclusion body formation. Neuronophagia is, as noted above, occasionally associated with these degenerative changes.

II. Paralytic Rabies

On occasion, rabies infection produces an illness in which flaccid paralysis is the outstanding clinical feature in the absence (particularly in the early stages of the disease) of the classic symptoms of hydrophobia and periods of excited behavior. Gamaleia (1877) reported 20 human cases of rabies in which paralysis had been the outstanding feature. All of these patients eventually developed the charteristic hydrophobic symptoms in their clinical course. Pathologic mination was not reported in any of the cases. Remlinger (1906) pointed out that rabies infection could produce a syndrome consisting predominantly of acute ascending paralysis. Marie and Chatelin (1919) described a case of paralytic rabies in an 11-year-old child. The symptoms consisted primarily of a flaccid paralysis, and the total duration of illness was 18 days. It was not until 3 days prior to death that difficulty in swallowing was noted, and hydrophobia did not become evident until just before death. Postmortem examination revealed perivascular infiltrates throughout the spinal cord, brain stem, cerebellum and, occasionally, within the cerebral cortex. The inflammatory lesions were most prominent within the spinal cord and medulla, and many Babes' nodules were also noted. Prominent Van Gehuchten and Nelis lesions were noted within the spinal ganglia. Within the spinal cord, foci of neuronal degeneration and neuronaphagia were also described. Neurons of the spinal cord contained cytoplasmic bodies which were described as resembling Negri bodies. Similar bodies were also described in the Ammon's horn, but they were noted to stain very poorly there.

Knutti (1929) described a case of ascending paralysis in a 23-year-old student nurse. The woman died 9 days following the onset of symptoms and was never noted to have developed difficulty in swallowing or hydrophobia. At autopsy, Negri bodies were discovered within the spinal cord. Love (1944) reviewed the literature on paralytic rabies and presented an additional case in a 4-year-old boy. Postmortem examination in his case revealed some congestion of the meninges and parenchyma of the central nervous system. Negri bodies were discovered within neurons of the cerebral cortex, Ammon's horn, and "internal capsule" (*sic*). Perivascular infiltrates, glial proliferation and neuronophagia were also described. There was also neuronal degeneration within the spinal cord, particularly in the posterior horns and dorsal root ganglia. Recently Lassen (1962) described a case of paralytic rabies in a 4-year-old Eskimo girl who had been bitten on the face by a dog. At autopsy, inflammatory changes were found within the entire central nervous system and spinal ganglia. Lyssa bodies are stated to have been present, but their exact localization is not given. Typical Negri bodies were formed in mice, hamsters, and dogs inoculated with material from this case.

A discussion of paralytic rabies would not be complete without reference to the outbreak of paralytic disease in Trinidad described by Hurst and Pawan (1931, 1932). These authors investigated an out break of an acute ascending myelitis which occurred in 1929 and 1930 on the island of Trinidad. Although the disease was f thought to be a form of poliomyelitis, animal inoculation sho that the causal agent was rabies virus. The patients, for the most part, demonstrated fever, headache, numbness, and paresthesias, followed by an ascending, flaccid paralysis. Dysphagia was frequently absent and, when present, appeared terminally. Clinical hydrophobia was not noted in the patients. Epidemiologic investigation revealed that at the same time there was an epizootic of cattle rabies on the island, and evidence was presented to implicate the vampire bat as a vector for the disease (see Chapter 10, Volume II). Pathologic examination of material from the Trinidad outbreak revealed that there was marked perivascular infiltration, microglial proliferation, and neuronal degeneration present within the spinal cord of these cases. The posterior and anterior horns appeared to be affected to an approximately equal extent. Negri bodies were not seen. Only mild inflammatory lesions were noted within the brain stem and cerebellum.

III. Ultrastructural Studies

There was great anticipation that with the use of electron microscopy, the nature of the Negri body would be quickly and finally established, but it was not until 1962 that Matsumoto confirmed the viral nature of the Negri body inclusion. He clearly demonstrated that the rabies virions were elongated, bullet-shaped particles. The viral particles were found to be accompanied by aggregates of a granular, electron-dense matrix, and the larger collections of matrix with contained viral particles corresponded to Negri bodies on adjacent light sections. A thorough discussion of this work can be found in Chapter 12.

It should be noted, however, that these excellent studies were limited, for the most part, to examining the hippocampus of mice infected after intracerebral inoculation (Matsumoto, 1962, 1963; Matsumoto and Miyamoto, 1966; Miyamoto and Matsumoto, 1965). Ultrastructural studies of human and animal cases of rabies are limited. Morecki and Zimmerman (1969) reported ultrastructural studies of a human case of rabies. Areas containing Negri bodies were removed from paraffin blocks, deparaffinized, and processed for electron microscopy. Viral particles similar to those described by Matsumoto were seen only in small aggregates of matrix not visible by light microscopy in adjacent thick sections. The large collections of matrix identified as Negri bodies on histologic preparations were free of identifiable viral particles.

Gonzáles-Angulo *et al.* (1968, 1970) described the ultrastructural appearance of Negri bodies in the Purkinje cells of two human cases of rabies. Their findings were similar to those of Matsumoto, but they also noted considerable cytoplasmic swelling, with disruption of rough endoplasmic reticulum. Similar changes have been described by Lemercier *et al.* (1970) in the Purkinje cells of a human case.

We have performed extensive ultrastructural studies on a rhesus monkey which died of rabies 108 days following injection of street virus into the neck muscles (Perl *et al.*, 1972; Perl and Callaway, 1974). The duration of the illness was 8 days, and there was extensive Negri body formation. Although many of our findings were similar to those previously reported, certain differences and additional observations are noteworthy. The animal showed extensive Negri body formation within the brain stem, particularly in the cranial nerve nuclei at the floor of the fourth ventricle and surrounding the aqueduct of Sylvius (Fig. 6C). Also, numerous Negri bodies were found within anterior horn cells of the cervical and thoracic spinal cord and within the thalamus and caudate nuclei. Although the neurons of the hippocampus occasionally showed large, discrete Negri bodies with a prominent inner body, this region was sparsely involved compared to the other, previously mentioned areas.

When examined ultrastructurally, the brain showed more extensive involvement by the viral infection than could be discerned from light microscopic investigation. Throughout the central nervous system there were numerous small aggregates of electron-dense, granular matrix and rabies virions which could not be seen by light microscopy in adjacent thick sections (Fig. 9). The intracytoplasmic inclusions which could be seen by light microscopy consisted of large aggregates of granular, electron-dense matrix associated with numerous virions. It was noted, on the basis of a wide sampling of the CNS, that these inclusions could be divided into three basic types.

The first type consisted of a well-circumscribed, generally round collection of matrix which contained at its periphery many of the bullet-shaped forms of the rabies virions (Figs. 9 and 10A,B). Many sections showed that there were invaginations in the external contour of these Negri bodies, giving rise to the inner body noted in histologic preparations (Fig. 10A). The virions at the periphery of the

---

Fig. 9. Neuron from caudate nucleus of monkey experimentally infected with street virus. Low power electron micrograph shows several Negri bodies. The two smaller inclusions (arrows) could not be seen by light microscopy in the adjacent thick section ×12,200.

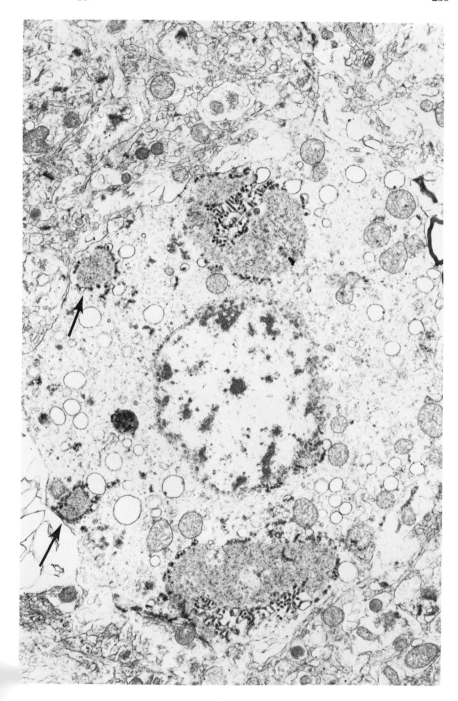

Fig. 9.

inclusion measured approximately 90 by 180 nm and were frequently attached to small, dilated portions of rough endoplasmic reticulum (Fig. 10B). The central portions of the matrix collections were generally free of viral particles. Inclusions of this type were most usually found within the neurons of the caudate nucleus and thalamus.

The second type of Negri body was found primarily within neurons of the brain stem, cerebellum, and spinal cord. In this form of inclusion, elongated tubular structures were seen, which often contained spherical internal bodies (Fig. 11). These tubular structures were seen throughout the matrix rather than at its periphery. The external contour was irregular, and at the edge of the inclusion a limiting double membrane with focal dilatations was frequently seen. The extent of membrane formation was quite variable in the inclusions studied. It was most extensive within the Purkinje cells of the cerebellum (Fig. 12A). Similar arrays of parallel membranous structures have been described in the cytoplasm of Purkinje cells by González-Angulo *et al.* (1968, 1970) and by Lemercier *et al.* (1970). These arrays appeared to be more extensive in the Purkinje cells of our animal (Fig. 12B) than in those illustrated by the cited authors. Morales and Duncan (1966) have described small parallel laminar arrays of similar configuration in the cytoplasm of Purkinje cells of the cat. These structures were thought to represent either an unusual organelle in this cell or possibly agonal or early postmortem alterations. The significance of these findings in rabies-infected Purkinje cells is unclear.

Although the two forms of inclusion could clearly be differentiated ultrastructurally in our monkey, they could not be distinguished by light microscopy. Some Negri bodies did contain bullet-shaped virions around their periphery in addition to elongated tubular forms within the center, a sort of "mixed" type. These forms were remarkably few in number.

The third type of inclusion, seen infrequently, was primarily noted within the hippocampus, and consisted of extremely large collections of matrix, often measuring 10–15 μm. These corresponded to large,

---

Fig. 10A and B. Negri bodies with bullet-shaped virions arranged at the periphery (obtained from monkey experimentally infected with street virus). A: Note attachment of viral particles to dilated segments of rough endoplasmic reticulum (arrow). ×35,000 B: Fortuitous section demonstrates an invagination of the external contour of the inclusion which gives rise to the internal structure seen by light microscopy. Cauda nucleus. ×28,000.

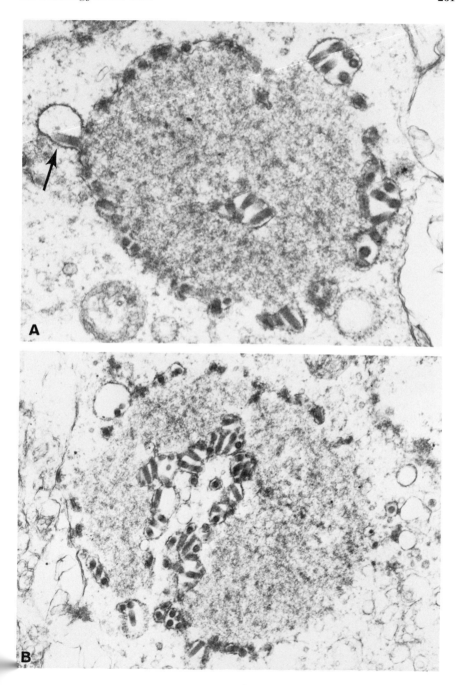

Fig. 10

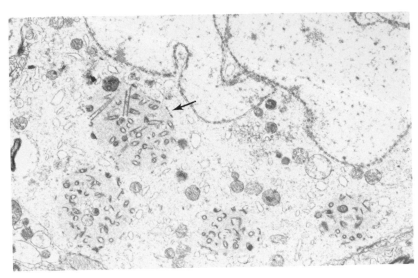

Fig. 11. Neuron from monkey infected with street rabies virus. Low power electron micrograph shows several Negri bodies containing the tubular form of the virion distributed throughout the matrix. Small fragments of a double, limiting membrane are seen (arrow). Midbrain. ×11,000.

bean-shaped Negri bodies seen in histologic preparations. Frequently no viral particles, or, at best, only one or two of the tubular forms could be identified within the large matrix aggregates (Fig. 13).

Matsumoto (1963, cf. Chapter 12) has noted small aggregates of matrix and viral particles within astrocytes, and we confirmed this observation in our animal (Fig. 14A). In addition, a few small cells were seen which appeared to be oligodendroglial cells and which contained small collections of matrix and viral particles (Fig. 14B).

A small number of bullet-shaped virions were identified within the perinuclear cistern of a few neurons in the basal ganglia. These were accompanied by small collections of matrix in the adjacent cytoplasm (Fig. 15). A similar picture has been reported by Hummeler *et al.* (1967) in DEAE-treated BKH-21 cells infected with fixed rabies virus. The significance of these findings is unclear. Some of the other

Fig. 12A. Negri body within a Purkinje cell showing extensive parallel limiting membranes (from monkey infected with street virus). Cerebellar cortex. ×22,000.

Fig. 12B. Purkinje cell cytoplasm containing two small collections of matrix in association with extensive parallel lamellar arrays (arrows). Cerebellar cortex (from monkey infected with street virus). ×21,000.

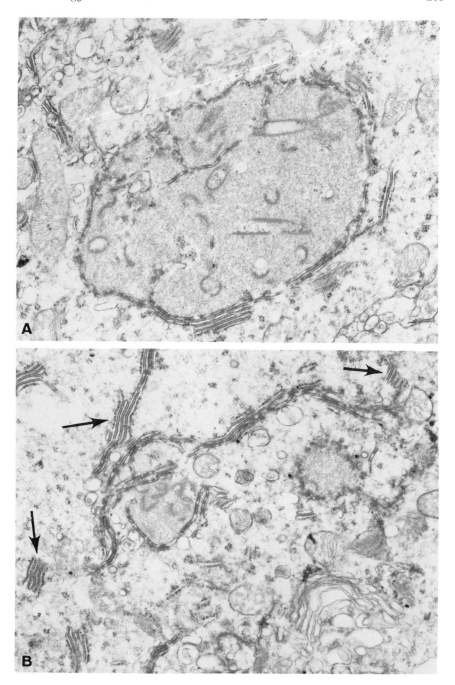

Fig. 12.

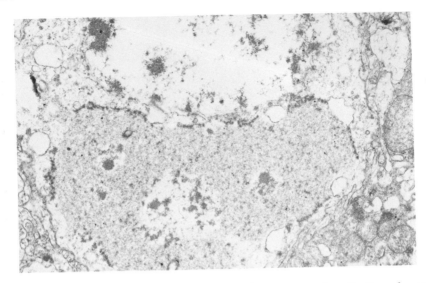

Fig. 13. Neuron with extremely large Negri body consisting of a collection of matrix material containing no recognizable viral particles. Hippocampus of monkey infected with street virus. ×19,600.

forms of rhabdovirus, particularly the plant virus varieties, have been noted to bud off the nuclear membrane (Hummeler, 1971), but rabies is not generally considered to show intranuclear involvement. We noted no viral particles within the nucleus itself, nor has this been reported by others.

Matsumoto (1963) stated that rabies virus is always accompanied by matrix. However, González-Angulo *et al.* (1968, 1970) described aggregates of viral particles without matrix within infected Purkinje cells. In our case, several small aggregates of viral particles were noted without any accompanying matrix. These collections were seen not within the perikaryon, but as isolated foci within the neuropil (Fig. 16A,B).

The route of spread of rabies infection within the CNS itself has not been clearly established (see Chapter 11). It has been suggested that the cerebrospinal fluid plays a significant role in the spread of infection. Schneider (1969), using the fluorescent antibody tech-

---

Fig. 14A. Astrocyte showing several inclusion bodies containing viral particles and matrix. Caudate nucleus from monkey infected with street virus. ×7750.

Fig. 14B. Small cell (probably oligodendroglial cell) containing a minute aggregate of matrix and viral particles (arrow). Caudate nucleus from monkey infected wit' street virus. ×8400.

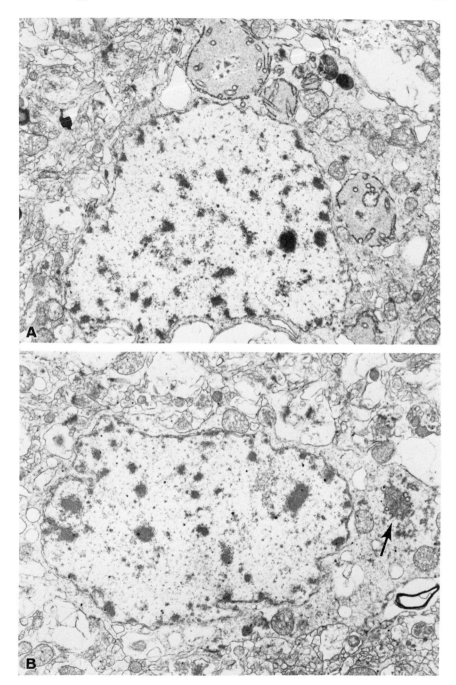

Fig. 14.

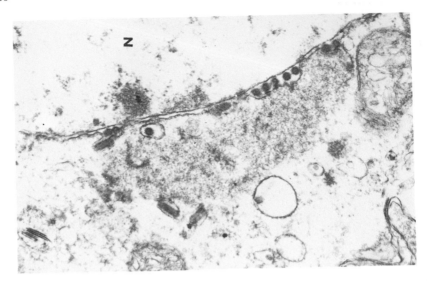

Fig. 15. Portion of a neuron containing an aggregate of perinuclear matrix with associated virions within the perinuclear cistern (N = nucleus). Caudate nucleus of monkey infected with street virus. ×46,000.

nique, demonstrated viral antigen within ependymal lining cells. The tendency for this virus to bud off secretory epithelial cells is well established (Dierks *et al.*, 1969; cf. Chapter 15), but we have been unable to find cytoplasmic inclusions within ependymal cells or the choroid plexus by light microscopy. Similarly, extensive ultrastructural study of the ependyma and choroid plexus has failed to reveal any evidence of rabies infection within these cells. Spread of the infection within the central nervous system via nerve pathways has also been considered. Viral antigen has been demonstrated within axonal processes by Yamamoto *et al.* (1965), and Jenson *et al.* (1969) have shown rabies virions within axons. We identified matrix and viral particles within axons (Fig. 17A) as well as dendrites (Fig. 17B).

In studying the neuropathology literature of rabies, it is clear that although we know a great deal about the morphologic changes pro-

Fig. 16A. Collection of matrix and viral particles encountered within the neuropil. A nearby aggregate of viral particles without matrix is noted (arrow). Caudate nucleus of monkey infected with street virus. ×40,000.

Fig. 16B. Higher magnification of the virions without matrix seen in 16A. Caudate nucleus. ×40,000.

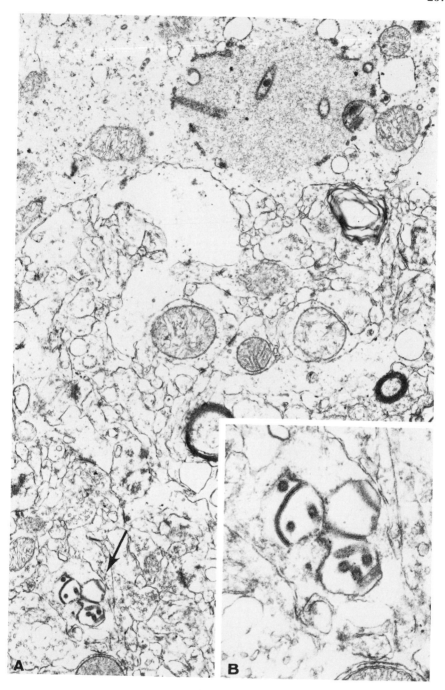

Fig. 16.

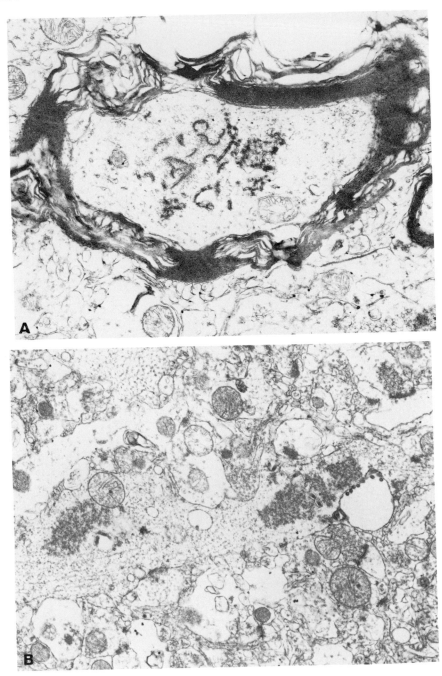

Fig. 17.

duced in the disease, many important aspects are poorly understood. In the early 1900's rabies pathology was studied extensively and much was learned from this early work. However, many questions raised by those early workers have yet to be answered despite the introduction of modern research techniques. These questions relate, for example, to the lack of cellular lysis in the face of extensive viral invasion, the mode of spread within the central nervous system, the mechanism of death in rabies, the pathologic bases for occasional paralytic forms of the disease, the causes for wide variability in the nature and distribution of histologic lesions in rabies, and the role of immune mechanisms in determining the morphologic characteristics of the disease.

With the careful application of modern techniques in virology, biochemistry, immunology, and electron microscopy, it is clear that much important data will emerge which will enable us to better understand not only rabies infection, but other forms of viral encephalitis as well.

Acknowledgments

The author wishes to acknowledge the able assistance of Miss Carey S. Callaway in the ultrastructural studies. The technical assistance of Carol Henkle and Bettyann Forbes is also gratefully acknowledged.

References

Abba, F., and Bormans, A. (1905). *Ann. Inst. Pasteur, Paris* 19, 49.
Achúcarro, N. (1909–1910). *Histol. Histopathol. Arb.* 3, 143.
Acton, H. W., and Harvey, W. F. (1911). *Parasitology* 4, 255.
Alzheimer, A. (1907). *Neurol. Zentralbl.* 18, 177.
Babes, V. (1892). *Ann. Inst. Pasteur, Paris* 6, 209.
Babes, V. (1907). *Z. Hyg. Infektionskr.* 56, 435.
Benedikt, M. (1875). *Arch. Pathol. Anat. Physiol. Klin. Med.* 64, 557.
Benedikt, M. (1878). *Arch. Pathol. Anat. Physiol. Klin. Med.* 72, 425.
Berntsen, C. A., Jr., and Stevenson, L. D. (1953). *J. Neuropathol. Exp. Neurol.* 12, 169.
Bosc, F. J. (1903a). *C. R. Soc. Biol.* 55, 1284.
Bosc, F. J. (1903b). *C. R. Soc. Biol.* 55, 1436.

Fig. 17A. Collection of viral particles and matrix within a myelinated axon. Midbrain (from monkey experimentally infected with street virus). ×20,000.

Fig. 17B. Two collections of matrix and bullet-shaped viral particles within a denrite. Hippocampus (from monkey infected with street virus). ×13,000.

Coats, J. (1877). *Lancet.* 1, 162.

Cornwall, J. W., and Kesava Pai, M. (1910). *J. Trop. Vet. Sci.* 5, 162.

Crandell, R. A. (1965). *Acta Pathol. Microbiol. Scand.* 63, 587.

D'Amato, L., and Faggella, V. (1910). *Z. Hyg. Infektionskr.* 65, 353.

del Río-Hortega, P. (1932). *In* "Cytology and Cellular Pathology of the Nervous System" (W. Penfield, ed.)., Vol. 2, p. 483. Harper (Hoeber), New York.

Dierks, R. E., Murphy, F. A., and Harrison, A. K. (1969). *Amer. J. Pathol.* 54, 251.

Dupont, J. R., and Earle, K. M. (1965). *Neurology* 15, 1023.

Erickson, E. E., Marcuse, P. M., and Halpert, B. (1954). *J. Amer. Med. Ass.* 155, 823.

Frothingham, L. (1920). *Cornell Vet.* 10, 163–175.

Gamaleia, N. (1887). *Ann. Inst. Pasteur, Paris* 1, 63–83.

Goldwasser, R. A., and Kissling, R. E. (1958). *Proc. Soc. Exp. Biol. Med.* 98, 219–223.

González-Angulo, A., Feria-Velasco, A., Márquez-Monter, H., and Zavala-Carrillo, B. J. (1968). *Bol. Estud. Med. Biol.* 25, 171–178.

González-Angulo, A., Márquez-Monter, H., Feria-Velasco, A., and Zavala-Carrillo, B. J. (1970). *Neurology* 20, 323–328.

Goodpasture, E. W. (1925). *Amer. J. Pathol.* 1, 547–582.

Gowers, W. R. (1877). *Trans. Pathol. Soc. London* 28, 10–23.

Greenhouse, A. H. (1968). *In* "Pathology of the Nervous System" (J. Minckler, ed.), Vol. 1, pp. 1029–1042. McGraw-Hill, New York.

Hardenbergh, J. B., and Underhill, B. M. (1916). *J. Amer. Vet. Med. Ass.* 49, 663–668.

Hattwick, M. A. W., Weis, T. T., Stechschulte, C. J., Baer, G. M., and Gregg, M. B. (1972). *Ann. Intern. Med.* 76, 931–942.

Herzog, E. (1941). *Bol. Soc. Biol. Concepcion* 15, 101.

Herzog, E. (1965). *Arch. Pathol.* 39, 279–280.

Horgan, E. S., and McKinnon, R. M. (1937). *J. Hyg.* 37, 340–344.

Hummeler, K. (1971). *In* "Comparative Virology" (K. Maramorosch and E. Kurstak, eds.), pp. 361–386. Academic Press, New York.

Hummeler, K., Koprowski, H., and Wiktor, T. J. (1967). *J. Virol.* 1, 152–170.

Hurst, E. W., and Pawan, J. L. (1931). *Lancet* 2, 622–628.

Hurst, E. W., and Pawan, J. L. (1932). *J. Pathol. Bacteriol.* 35, 301–321.

Innes, J. R. M., and Saunders, L. Z. (1962a). "Comparative Neuropathology," pp. 384–394. Academic Press, New York.

Innes, J. R. M., and Saunders, L. Z. (1962b). "Comparative Neuropathology," pp. 436–437. Academic Press, New York.

Iwamori, H., and Yamagiwa, S. (1945). *Jap. J. Vet. Sci.* 7, 105–115.

Jenson, A. B., Rabin, E. R., Bentinck, D. C., and Melnick, J. L. (1969). *J. Virol.* 3, 265–269.

Johnson, H. N. (1972). *In* "Viral and Rickettsial Infections of Man" (F. L. Horsfall, Jr. and I. Tamm, eds.), 4th ed., pp. 814–840. Lippincott, Philadelphia, Pennsylvania.

Jubb, K. V., and Kennedy, P. C. (1963). "Pathology of Domestic Animals," Vol. 2, pp. 352–357. Academic Press, New York.

Kantorovich, R. A. (1957). *Acta Virol. (Prague), Engl. ed.* 1, 220–228.

Knutti, R. E. (1929). *J. Amer. Med. Ass.* 93, 754–758.

Koch, J. (1910). *Z. Hyg. Infektion* 66, 443–454.

Kolesnikoff, J. (1875). *Z. Med. Wiss.* 2, 853–971.

Kraus, R., Gerlach, F., and Schweinburg, F. (1926). "Lyssa bei Mensch und Tier," pp. 172–243. Urban & Schwarzenburg, Berlin.

Lapi, A., Davis, C. L., and Anderson, W. A. (1952). *J. Amer. Vet. Med. Ass.* 120, 379–384

Lassen, H. C. A. (1962). *Lancet* 1, 247–249.

Lemercier, G., Mattei, X., Rey, M., and Collomb, H. (1970). *Pathol.-Biol.* 18, 943–949.

Lentz, O. (1909). *Z. Hyg. Infektionskr.* 62, 63–94.

Levaditi, C., Nicolau, S., and Schoen, R. (1924). *C. R. Acad. Sci.* 178, 256–258.

Levaditi, C., Nicolau, S., and Schoen, R. (1926). *Ann. Inst. Pasteur, Paris* 40, 973–1068.

Love, S. V. (1944). *J. Pediat.* 24, 312–325.

Lowenberg, K. (1928). *Arch. Neurol. Psychiat.* 19, 638–646.

Marie, P., and Chatelin, C. (1919). *Bull. Acad. Med., Paris* 81, 428–436.

Marinesco, G., and Stroesco, G. (1931). *Arch. Roum. Pathol. Exp. Microbiol.* 4, 244–288.

Matsumoto, S. (1962). *Virology* 17, 198–202.

Matsumoto, S. (1963). *J. Cell Biol.* 19, 565–591.

Matsumoto, S., and Miyamoto, K. (1966). *Symp. Ser. Immunobiol. Stand.* 1, 45–54.

Miyamoto, K., and Matsumoto, S. (1965). *J. Cell Biol.* 27, 677–682.

Morales, R., and Duncan, D. (1966). *J. Ultrastruct. Res.* 15, 480–489.

Morecki, R., and Zimmerman, H. M. (1969). *Arch. Neurol. (Chicago)* 20, 599–604.

Moulton, J. E. (1954). *Amer. J. Pathol.* 30, 533–543.

Negri, A. (1903). *Z. Hyg. Infektionskr.* 44, 519–540.

Negri, A. (1909). *Z. Hyg. Infektionskr.* 53, 421–443.

Negri-Luzzani, L. (1905). *Z. Hyg. Infektionskr.* 49, 305–324.

Negri-Luzzani, L. (1913). *Ann. Inst. Pasteur, Paris* 27, 1039–1064.

Nepveu, M. (1872). *C. R. Soc. Biol.* 4, 133–138.

Nieberg, K. C., and Blumberg, J. M. (1972). *In* "Pathology of the Nervous System" (J. Minckler, ed.), Vol. 3, pp. 2269–2323. McGraw-Hill, New York.

Osetowska, E. (1971). *Neuropatol. Pol.* 9, 1–12.

Pasteur, L. (1885). *C. R. Acad. Sci., Paris* 101, 765–772.

Perl, D. P., and Callaway, C. S. In preparation.

Perl, D. P., Callaway, C. S., and Hicklin, M. D. (1972). *J. Neuropathol. Exp. Neurol.* 31, 172–173.

Ramon y Cajál, S., and García, D. (1904). *Trab. Lab. Invest. Biol. Univ. Madrid* 3, 213.

Remlinger, P. (1903). *Ann. Inst. Pasteur, Paris* 17, 834–849.

Remlinger, P. (1906). *C. R. Soc. Biol.* 60, 818–819.

Schaffer, K. (1912). *In* "Handbuch der Neurologie" (M. von Lewandowsky, ed.), Vol. 3, pp. 980–991. Springer-Verlag, Berlin and New York.

Schneider, L. G. (1969). *Zentralbl. Bakteriol., Parasitenk., Infektionskr. Hyg., Abt. 1: Orig.* 212, 1–13.

Sokolov, N. N., and Vanag, K. A. (1962). *Acta Virol. (Prague)* 6, 452–457.

Sükrü Aksel, I. (1958). *In* "Handbuch der speziellen pathologischen Anatomie und Histologie" (O. Lubarsch, F. Henke, and R. Rössle, eds.), Vol. 13, Part 2A, pp. 418–435. Springer-Verlag, Berlin and New York.

Szatmári, A., and Sályi, J. (1936). *Z. Gesamte Neurol. Psychiat.* 156, 424–431.

Szlachta, H. L., and Habel, R. E. (1953). *Cornell Vet.* 43, 207.

Tangchai, P., and Vejjajiva, A. (1971). *Brain* 94, 299.

Tangchai, P., Yenbutr, D., and Vejjajiva, A. (1970). *J. Med. Ass. Thailand* 53, 472.

Thomas, A. D., and Jackson, C. (1930). *J. S. Afr. Vet. Med. Ass.* 1, 67.

Tierkel, E. S. (1959). *Advan. Vet. Sci.* 5, 183.

Toga, M., Payan, H., Orsini, A., and Berard-Badier, M. (1961). *Encephalitides, Proc. Symp. Neuropathol., Electroencephalogr. Biochem. Encephalitides, 1959,* pp. 67–72.

Tustin, R. C., and Smit, J. D. (1962). *J. S. Afr. Vet. Med. Ass.* 33, 295.

Van Gehuchten, A., and Nelis, C. (1900). *Bull. Acad. Roy. Med. Belg.* 14, 31–66.

van Rooyen, C. E., and Rhodes, A. J. (1940). "Virus Diseases of Man," pp. 681–690. Oxford Univ. Press, London and New York.

Volpino, G. (1906). Z. *Bakteriol.* **37**, 459.

Wolf, A. (1950). *In* "The Pathogenesis and Pathology of Viral Diseases" (J. G. Kidd, ed.), p. 194. Columbia Univ. Press, New York.

Wolman, M., and Behar, A. (1952). *J. Infec. Dis.* **91**, 69.

World Health Organization. (1954). *World Health Organ., Monogr. Ser.* **23**.

Yamamoto, T., Otani, S., and Shiraki, H. (1965). *Acta Neuropathol.* **5**, 288.

CHAPTER 14

Spread of Virus from the Central Nervous System

Lothar G. Schneider

I. Introduction

This chapter deals with the centrifugal movement of virus in nerves during the final stage of rabies infection, a phenomenon described by French authors as "neuroprobasie" or "septineuritis" to characterize the centrifugal movement of neurotropic viruses (Levaditi, 1926; Nicolau *et al.*, 1929). The term "virus generalization" is preferred by this author since it seems to more precisely characterize the events which occur in an infected organism after virus has spread within the central nervous system (CNS). Evidence for centrifugal virus spread in nerves has accumulated to such an extent that it is now widely accepted, though its precise mechanism is still a matter of discussion.

The generalization of the virus by viremia is less well documented, the missing evidence being the failure of regularly demonstrating rabies virus in the blood. Since the virus is capable of replicating a variety of non-nervous tissues, many workers consider a hematogenous virus generalization to be more reasonable than neural spread (Koch, 1930; Doerr, 1939; Wong and Freund, 1951; Krause, 1957, 1966; Becker, 1961; Katasilambros, 1962; Zunker, 1963). Most of these authors isolated virus from non-nervous organs, and occasionally from the blood, at different times after infection. From their experimental data they concluded that internal organs such as the pancreas or adrenals become infected through the blood during a viremic stage which escaped recognition due to the low sensitivity of the available isolation methods. Recent experiments in which mice were injected intravenously with virus do not support the viremic hypothesis (Schneider, 1969b; Fischman and Schaeffer, 1971); there was no evidence of infection of non-nervous organs prior to the involvement of the CNS, nor were peripheral organs terminally infected at a higher rate than after other routes of infection. The controversy concerning hematogenous virus dissemination versus the spread via nerves has not yet been definitively settled, and Russian authors recently reported a viremic phase in several animal species experimentally infected with a street virus strain (Shashenko and Kovalev, 1971). The authors detected a viremia in sheep, cattle, dogs, foxes, and cats only during the febrile phase prior to the onset of clinical signs, but not in paralyzed or dead animals. Details concerning other viremic aspects of rabies pathogenesis are further discussed in Chapter 11.

Virus isolations from peripheral nerves and non-nervous organs, and demonstration of virus specific inclusions were the methods exclusively used in the past to show the presence of the rabies virus in certain tissues. More recently the fluorescent antibody technique and electron microscopy were shown to be effective tools for the study of this aspect of rabies pathogenesis, particularly if used in sequential studies.

II. Virus Isolations from Peripheral Nerves and Non-nervous Organs

There is hardly any organ which at one time or another cannot be shown to yield rabies virus or antigen if a careful enough search is made. Virus thus obtained will usually be present in low titer only. It may originate from nerve cell structures contained in the organ, or possibly from blood spilled over terminally. Instead of discussing every individual organ from which virus has been isolated in the past, I wish to confine myself to organ systems which either serve as port of entry for the virus or through which the virus may be excreted. Tissues of epidemiologic interest are the digestive tract with the salivary glands, the respiratory system, and the urinary tract. The peripheral nerves deserve separate discussion, since they apparently represent the path for virus generalization.

The first reports on virus isolations from nerves of human rabies cases date back to the end of the last century. Nerve trunks ipsilateral and controlateral to the bite site at times contained infectious virus at the death of the patient, at other times did not (Pasteur *et al.*, 1884; Roux, 1888). Infection of other peripheral nerves was less frequent, and the virus titer was usually quite low (Lubinski and Prausnitz, 1926).

Comparative experimental data obtained by Schweinburg (1932) showed that the sciatic nerves of guinea pigs were more often infected with street virus than were nerves of animals inoculated with fixed virus. Fixed virus is apparently less frequently seen outside the CNS than is street virus (Nicolau and Serbanescu, 1928; Nicolau *et al.*, 1929; Schweinburg, 1937). This phenomenon was confirmed by more recent workers who studied rabies pathogenesis in rats (Baer *et al.*, 1965, 1968), mice (Johnson, 1965; Schneider and Hamann, 1969), and hamsters (Dean *et al.*, 1963; Petrović and Timm, 1969; Murphy *et al.*, 1973b).

The time of appearance and the progression of rabies virus in peripheral nerves, as well as in non-nervous organs, should answer the question as to how the infection of these structures is initiated, but the virus content of these tissues (as measured by infectivity) is often quite low, and virus titration is therefore not a sensitive enough method for the evaluation of the neural virus movement. This is demonstrated in the work of Nicolau (1928), in which rabbits were injected with street virus. Low titering virus was erratically demonstrated in the fore and hind leg nerves of animals sacrificed 5–7 days after infection, while virus was regularly isolated only from the eighth day until death (day 13). This indicates that during the incubation period the nerves of both fore and hind legs are almost simultaneously infected, and that the amount of virus contained in these nerves increases with time. The same conclusions may be drawn from the experiments of Baer *et al.* (1968), who injected street virus into the hind footpad of rats. Healthy appearing animals sacrificed between 9 and 18 days postinfection (p.i.) contained virus in both sciatic nerves. Similar experiments with fixed virus (Baer *et al.*, 1965) yielded neural virus inconsistently, and only shortly before death.

A. GASTROINTESTINAL TRACT

1. Salivary Glands

Among non-nervous organs, the *salivary glands* most frequently contain rabies virus. The frequency of salivary gland infection seems to vary among different animal species. We know from experimental infections that 74% of dogs, 47% of cattle (Eichwald and Pitzschke, 1967), 88% of cats (Vaughn *et al.*, 1963), 20–73% of foxes, 83% of skunks, and 63% of raccoons (Sikes, 1966; Tierkel, 1966) may harbor the virus in their glands. Naturally infected foxes, cattle, and deer showed a high rate of salivary gland involvement (90%) – independent of the animal species – when more than one gland was examined (Schaaf and Schaal, 1968). Highly susceptible animal species quite often have a higher virus titer in their salivary glands than in the brain. For example, randomly selected fox salivary glands had virus titers which exceeded those of the brain by two to three logarithms (G. M. Baer and L. G. Schneider, unpublished data). A similar situation was seen in naturally infected bats (Bell *et al.*, 1962; J. F. Bell, unpublished data), in experimentally infected foxes and skunks (Parker and Wilsnack, 1966), and in cats (Vaughn *et al.*, 1963). This is not surprising since transmission by bite is the "classic" and most common mode of rabies transmission.

More important is the question of how salivary glands become infected, and at which time during the course of infection. Experimental results by Roux and Nocard (1890) gave evidence for the centrifugal virus spread from the CNS to the salivary glands, with subsequent spillover into the saliva. At that time it was hard to believe that the strictly neurotropic rabies virus should be able to multiply in the gland tissue proper. The theory of centrifugal virus movement in nerves was further supported by the nerve-dissection experiments of Bertarelli (1904) and later by Dean *et al.* (1963), and the present working hypothesis is drawn from these studies. Another theory was that salivary gland infection occurred via the blood, believed by some people to occur soon after transmission, and independently from CNS infection (Lubinski and Prausnitz, 1926).

Virus may indeed be present in the salivary glands early during infection, either concurrent with or shortly before the onset of clinical signs. Virus was demonstrated in the saliva of dogs 3 days, of cats 1 day (Vaughn *et al.*, 1963), and of skunks 1–3 days (Sikes, 1962) prior to the appearance of clinical signs. In exceptional cases the virus may be found even earlier: Wilsnack (1966) reported on a striped skunk which shed virus in the saliva over 14 days before clinical illness. Bats may release virus over long periods without showing clinical signs. Bell *et al.* (1962), while observing naturally infected bats, demonstrated virus in the saliva of a *L. noctivagans* on several occasions over a period of 9 days. Virus has been found in the saliva of an experimentally infected *Tadarida brasiliensis mexicana* 12 days before the appearance of rabid signs (Baer and Bales, 1967). Vampire bats have been reported to carry and excrete the virus for several months (see Chapter 6, Vol. II), although this finding has not been confirmed.

In some instances virus is demonstrable in the saliva during an animal's lifetime, but cannot be detected in the salivary glands after death (Vaughn *et al.*, 1963; Parker and Wilsnack, 1966; Baer and Bales, 1967). The reason for this is not known. Possible explanations may be "autosterilization" (Levaditi *et al.*, 1928), "rabies-inhibiting substance" (Wilsnack and Parker, 1966), local antibody formation, or virus excretion during lifetime from other sources than salivary glands (oronasal mucous membranes, Malphigian cells, etc.). This phenomenon seems to occur only rarely in human cases (Emmrich *et al.*, 1970).

In experimental rabies the virus titer of salivary glands seems to be dependent on the challenge dose. In two experiments foxes given the least virus inoculum had the greatest percentage of virus shedders and their salivary glands titered highest (Sikes, 1962; Parker and Wilsnack, 1966). Similar observations have been made with dogs and mice (Schneider and Hamann, 1969); the lowest LD_{50} resulted in the most infected glands, whereas increases in the inoculum ultimately resulted in glands with no virus.

2. Gastrointestinal Mucosa

Virus isolations from the gastrointestinal tract seem to be exceedingly rare. Johnson (1966) isolated virus from the intestinal mucosa of a naturally infected striped skunk, and virus antigen was demonstrated by several investigators in the nerve elements and mucosa of stomach and intestine (see below). Virus from the mucosa, or from the pancreas or liver (Ueki and Nakamura, 1962), might theoretically be excreted together with the feces, but would more likely be inactivated by digestive enzymes. There is the remote possibility, however, that virus strains might exist which withstand gastric and other enteric fluids better than others. Correa-Giron *et al.* (1970) used a particular bovine virus strain in an oral transmission study in mice, and were able to isolate rabies virus 5 and 6 days after infection from the buccal mucosa, tongue, esophagus, stomach, mesentery, trachea, lung, heart, and kidney.

B. Respiratory System

The infectivity of lungs was stressed by Remlinger and Bailly (1931a,b, 1934, 1940) who, after using various routes of infection in different animal species, found rabies virus most frequently in the lung (37%), liver (4–40%), spleen (16–28%), and kidneys (37%). They concluded that the virus reached these organs via nerves and only multiplied in neurons or nerve fibers. Actual virus excretion through the lungs and kidneys was not confirmed. The presence of the virus in lungs and other organs has been reported following rectal instillation into hamsters (Reagan *et al.*, 1953), and after footpad injection into mice (Becker, 1961).

Two human rabies cases associated with nonbite exposure in bat caves caused Constantine (1962) to carry out transmission studies by exposing carnivores to the air of heavily populated bat caves. This successful experiment focused the attention of several research workers on the possible airborne mode of transmission.

Atanasiu (1965, 1966) recovered virus terminally from the respiratory tract after earlier exposing hamsters and mice to aerosols of street virus. On several occasions the lungs were found to contain more than $10^{3.5}$ LD_{50} of virus; virus was also recovered from fluids used to rinse the trachea. These findings indicate that the virus must have multiplied not only in nerve elements but also in other tissues, most likely in bronchial epithelium. Airborne transmission not only results in an infection of the lungs and trachea but involves the nasal mucosa, which, in the experiments of Hronovský and Benda (1969), was shown to serve as a principal port of entry for the virus. These authors exposed guinea pigs to street virus aerosols and were able to isolate rabies virus from the nasal mucosa 6 days later, one day prior to CNS involvement, and the virus could then be isolated from the nasal mucosa until death. The virus titers ($10^{4.4}$ LD_{50}) at times approximated those of the brain ($10^{4.6}$ LD_{50}). Virus in the lungs was found inconsistently. Fischman and Schaeffer (1971), in similar experiments, infected mice and hamsters by intranasal application of street and fixed virus strains. They visualized, by means of the fluorescent technique, a widespread virus generalization which included nasal mucosa, trachea and lungs, but they could not recover infectious virus from the respiratory tract. Baer and Bales (1967) infected Mexican free-tailed bats by parenteral and intranasal routes, and in five instances isolated relatively high titers of rabies virus from the lungs of moribund animals.

Naturally infected bats quite often seem to harbor the virus in the respiratory tract. Bell *et al.* (1962) showed its presence in two female *Eptesicus*. Johnson (1966) studied 24 solitary bats naturally infected with rabies, and of the 17 tested for presence of virus in lung tissue 47% were positive. Some of the lungs yielded high virus titers if they were cut open, squeezed, and the resultant fluid was then titered in mice (H. N. Johnson, personal communication). Virus was recently isolated from the nasal mucosa of 2 of 15 naturally infected Mexican free-tailed bats, and virus antigen could be demonstrated in 5 of them (Constantine *et al.*, 1972). Four of these animals had infectious virus in the lungs.

Of eight human cases studied in South America (Pizarro *et al.*, 1970), two of six had virus in the lung (liver 5/7, adrenals 4/5, heart 3/5, salivary gland 2/2, kidney 2/6, spleen 1/7) and there was one isolation each (1/1) from the diaphragm, mesentery, nerves, and intestine. Virus isolations from the lacrimal glands of human rabies cases have also been reported (Leach and Johnson, 1940).

The preceding data suggest that the respiratory system is apparently more frequently involved in a rabies infection than was generally assumed in the past. It is also evident that the respiratory system, especially the nasal mucosa, might serve as port of entry for the virus. Late findings of virus and antigen in those tissues cannot be explained by centrifugal virus spread alone (see below). The reported experiments are evidence of the dangers to be considered with rabies virus aerosols, a fact never to be underestimated; the recent human rabies case associated with aerosol exposure during rabies vaccine production should serve as a warning (Winkler *et al.*, 1973). The presumably airborne rabies outbreak in a wild carnivore colony (Winkler *et al.*, 1971) is another example; 39 animals with no known history of exposure died of rabies.

C. URINARY TRACT

Infection of the kidneys is occasionally noted in the course of natural or experimental rabies (Eichwald and Pitzschke, 1967). The infection is believed to occur via nerves late during infection, and is not considered an important route of viral excretion nor source of infection for other animals.

However, recent immunofluorescent investigations following oral, nasal, and natural infection revealed the presence of virus antigen not only in nerve elements but also in the parenchymal structures of the kidneys (Hronovský and Benda, 1969; Correa-Giron *et al.*, 1970; Debbie and Trimarchi, 1970) and in neuroepithelial tissues of the ureter, urinary bladder, and urethra (Debbie and Trimarchi, 1970). In addition, virus has been demonstrated in the urine of experimental animals (Fischman and Schaeffer, 1971) and of naturally infected foxes (Pitzschke, 1958; Kauker and Zettl, 1959; Debbie and Trimarchi, 1970) and bats (Girard *et al.*, 1965). These findings, especially the reported high incidence of urinary tract involvement among free-ranging red-foxes (Debbie and Trimarchi, 1970) raises the question of the possible epidemiologic importance of the urinary tract in rabies transmission.

The theory has been proposed by Kauker and Zettl (1959) that foxes could acquire rabies by "nosing" virus-contaminated material, trails, or urine "marks" frequently set by vixens during the mating season. Their speculation on a nonbite transmission route in sylvatic rabies does not appear too farfetched when we consider the presence of "free" virus in the urine, and the nasal mucosa or the conjunctivae as possible ports of entry in this highly susceptible animal species.

D. MAMMARY GLAND AND MILK

Little is known of the excretion of rabies virus through the milk, although the lactating mammary gland, if found infected, may represent a potential source for oral infection. Virus isolation from the milk has been reported in the past by Nocard *et al.* (1887) and by Remlinger and Bailly (1932), who found the virus in the milk on two occasions. More recently, virus was isolated from the lactating mammary glands of a spotted skunk (Johnson, 1959) and of bats (Sims *et al.*, 1963). In the light of recent successful oral transmission studies (see below) this subject seems to deserve further research.

III. Cells Involved in Virus Replication

Experimental results regarding the centrifugal virus spread are valid only if the type of cell involved in virus replication can be determined, and if the virus progression can be shown as a function of time. Until recently virus specific inclusions (Negri bodies, Babes-Koch's granules) were the pathologic indicator of terminal virus presence. Negri bodies have rarely been found in nerves. Goodpasture

(1925) demonstrated such inclusions in the Gasserian ganglion and within the intradural portion of the trigeminal nerve of rabbits inoculated into the masseter muscle. Negri bodies have further been demonstrated in the corneal epithelium of various animal species after corneal and intracerebral inoculation (Levaditi and Schoen, 1935), in the medulla of the adrenal glands (Babes, 1912; Jackson, 1921), in neurons of the salivary glands, and in neural elements of the tongue and mucosa of the mouth (Manouélian, 1935). Nicolau *et al.* (1929), using Borna and rabies virus as models, demonstrated virus specific inclusions in the neurons of lung, heart, salivary glands, pancreas, adrenals, kidney, eye, and intestine.

In 1958, Goldwasser and Kissling showed the fluorescent antibody technique of Coons *et al.* (1942) to be applicable for the diagnosis of rabies using brain and also salivary gland material (Goldwasser *et al.*, 1959). Today the fluorescent method is considered to be the best single test currently available for the rapid diagnosis of rabies (World Health Organization Expert Committee on Rabies, 1973). Soon after its development the fluorescent test was used for demonstrating virus antigen in various infected tissues, and in cell cultures also (Kaplan *et al.*, 1960).

The presence of virus antigen in peripheral nerves was first reported by Dean *et al.* (1963) and later by Yamamoto *et al.* (1965), Schneider (1966), and Baer *et al.* (1968). Virus antigen in nerves appeared as fine, dustlike granules which increased in size with time. Schneider and Hamann (1969) conducted studies of the sequential events noted during virus generalization in mice inoculated with either street or fixed virus strains. Peripheral nerves were shown to contain fluorescent antigen only after the virus had multiplied in the corresponding CNS segments. In these nerves the virus titered from trace amounts to 10^4 $LD_{50}/0.03$ ml. Following footpad injection of mice the first peripheral nerve to contain viral antigen was the sciatic nerve on the inoculated site, while nerve trunks of the other extremities became infected 1 day later, the infection there occurring almost simultaneously. With street virus the infection of peripheral nerves was noted several days before the onset of clinical signs, whereas with fixed virus peripheral infection occurred later, usually just shortly before death. The neural infection after intracerebral, footpad, or intravenous infection started at the respective CNS nerve sites, then progressed rapidly to the periphery. Viral antigen was found in either the perikaryon of Schwann cells or the periphery of axons, or both (Figs. 1–4). Early antigen was occasionally found at the Ranvier rings (Fig. 1). When antigen of different segments was

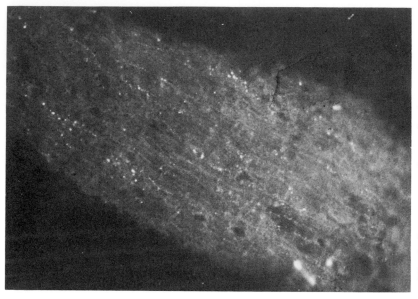

Fig. 2. Sciatic nerve, longitudinal section, discontinuous antigen foci. ×250.

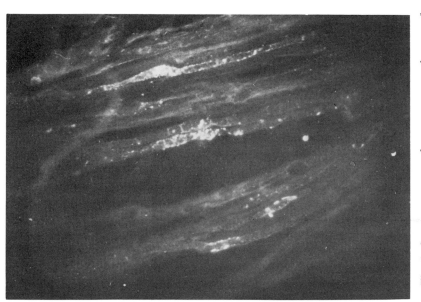

Fig. 1. Sciatic nerve, viral antigen in perikaryon of Schwann cells, at Ranvier rings, and at periphery of axons. ×400.

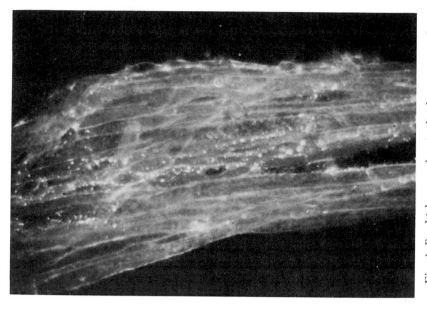

Fig. 4. Brachial nerve, longitudinal section, viral antigen forming "pearl strings." ×400.

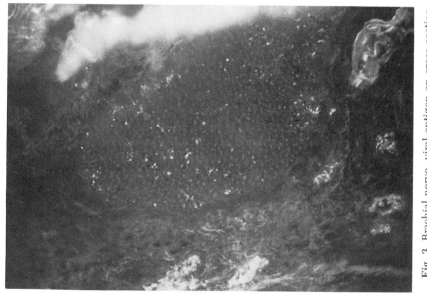

Fig. 3. Brachial nerve, viral antigen on cross section. ×250.

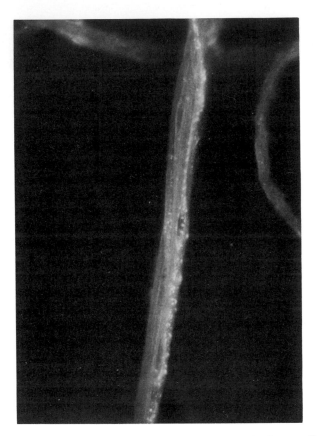

Fig. 5. Brachial nerve, "pearl string" appearance of individual nerve fiber within a fiber bundle. ×400.

confluent the nerve fibers showed a pearl stringlike appearance (Figs. 4, 5). The peripheral nerves were most involved following intracerebral inoculation (Atanasiu *et al.*, 1970b).

Recent electron microscopic studies give clear evidence of the maturation of rabies virus particles from virus specific matrices within axons (Jenson *et al.*, 1969; Garcia-Tamayo *et al.*, 1972). In the experiments of Murphy *et al.* (1973a,b) in which suckling hamsters were infected by various routes, virus particles and nucleocapsid-containing structures were demonstrated at the Ranvier rings (Fig.

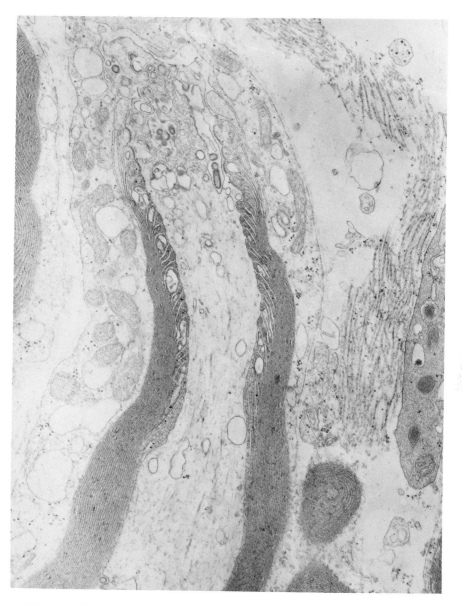

Fig. 6. Replication of rabies virus particles from virus specific matrices at the Ranvier ring of a peripheral nerve. (Kindly supplied by F. A. Murphy.)

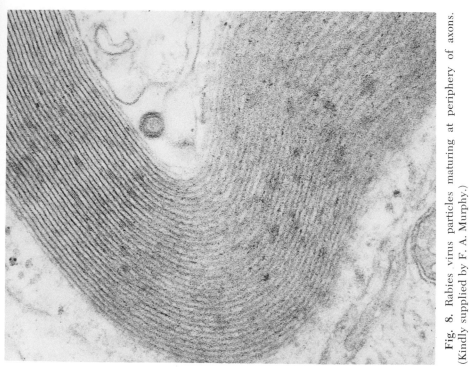

Fig. 8. Rabies virus particles maturing at periphery of axons. (Kindly supplied by F. A. Murphy.)

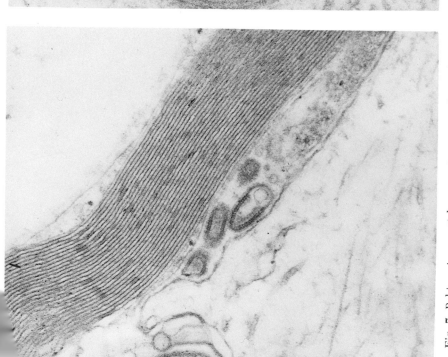

Fig. 7. Rabies virus particles maturing at periphery of axons. (Kindly supplied by F. A. Murphy.)

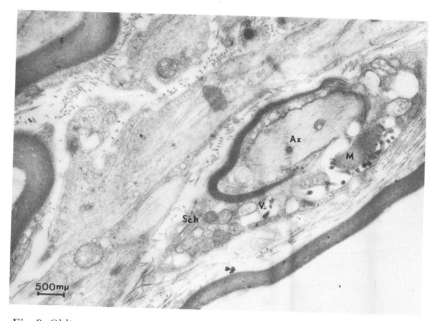

Fig. 9. Oblique section through sciatic nerve of mouse. Virus particles maturating from matrix (M) and vacuoles (V) of Schwann cell (Sch). Axon (Ax) free from virus. (Kindly supplied by P. Atanasiu.)

6), at the periphery of axons (Figs. 7 and 8), but not within Schwann cells. However, replicating virus particles in Schwann cells have been demonstrated by Atanasiu and Sisman (in preparation; Fig. 9). Rabies virus is capable of replicating in a variety of nerve structures, but it is obvious that no distinction can be made as to whether viral replication in the axoplasm of peripheral nerves is the result of centrifugal or centripetal virus movement. Antigen found late during infection might be due to centrifugal virus spread but could also be a magnification of early passage and multiplication at that site as suggested by Murphy *et al.* (1973a). In either case the presence of viral antigen is the result of continuing synthesis of excess viral structural components (mainly nucleoprotein) which remains at the site of virus replication. This has been shown to be the antigen responsible for the immunofluorescence in rabies (Schneider *et al.*, 1973).

The fluorescent and electron microscopic evidence of virus replication in nerves allows the following assumption to be made: during virus generalization the viral genome is apparently passed directly from the perikaryon of infected CNS neurons to the innervated tissues via axons, a hypothesis that would explain the rapidity of this process. Virus budding from plasma membranes (for further cell infection) would be required only at synapses. The replication observed at the Ranvier rings or elsewhere in the axoplasm may just be incidental and without pathogenetic significance, but may occasionally lead to the secondary infection of Schwann cells or other nerve-supporting structures.

A study of the distribution of fluorescent antigen in infected salivary glands was first performed by Yamamoto *et al.* (1965). They injected street virus intramuscularly into suckling mice and demonstrated virus antigen within the cytoplasm of the acinar cells of salivary glands, the fluorescence beginning with fine granules at the cell periphery and ending in massive globular structures wiuhin the acinar spaces. These findings were confirmed by Dierks *et al.* (1969) who, using the electron microscope, observed rabies virus particles budding from the plasma membranes of mucogenic acinar cells. Rabies virus was also shown to cause cellular destruction of infected salivary gland cells.

Schneider and Hamann (1969) systematically studied both the centrifugal virus spread in peripheral nerves and the virus generalization into non-nervous organs of mice infected parenterally. Virus antigen was seen in many organs (Table I, Figs. 10–20), but most frequently in richly innervated tissues. The antigen was demonstrated in nerve bundles and ganglion cells of nerves of the lung (Figs. 10 and 11), heart, pancreas, thymus, kidney (Fig. 15), ovary, uterus, and in the retina (Fig. 16), in the nerve cells and nerve fibers of the Meissner (Fig. 13) and Auerbach (Fig. 14) plexuses of the intestine, in nerve elements of smooth and skeletal muscles, in the nerve fibers of mucous membranes, and in nerve plexuses of adrenals, liver, and spleen (Fig. 12).

Virus antigen in the salivary glands first appeared in the nerves innervating the glands (Fig. 19) and only 1–3 days later in the acinar epithelial cells (Fig. 20). Corneal epithelium (Figs. 17 and 18) and multilocular fat cells of the interscapular brown fat lobes were other non-nervous tissues found to be heavily infected.

Following the intravenous injection of street and fixed virus into mice Fischman and Schaeffer (1971) did not, as expected, encounter widely spread antigen foci in parenchymatous organs. The antigen was restricted to nerve bundles near the aortic vessel and to muscle

Table I

Demonstration of Virus Antigen in Various Tissues of Moribund Mice by FA and of Infectivity of Organs after IC and Footpad Infection with Street Virus[a]

Organ	Virus antigen[b]	Infectivity[c]
CNS tissues	4/4	12/12
Spinal ganglia	4/4	n.t.
N. medianus	4/4	2/12
N. ischiadicus	4/4	3/12
Sympathetic trunk	4/4	n.t.
Lung	4/4	2/12
Heart	3/4	2/11
Popliteal lymph node	1/4	1/9
Spleen	2/4	0/12
Intestine	4/4	1/11
Liver	3/4	3/12
Pancreas	2/4	0/11
Kidney	4/4	1/12
Adrenals	4/4	2/12
Thymus gland	1/4	0/9
Uterus	3/4	0/12
Eye	4/4	5/12
Muscle tissue	3/4	3/11
Salivary glands	4/4	7/12
Brown fat	4/4	7/12

[a] Schneider and Hamann (1969).

[b] Number mice FA positive over number of mice examined.

[c] Number of individual tissues containing infectious virus over total number tested. n.t. = not tested.

spindles in the urinary bladder, adding support to the concept of centrifugal virus spread in nerves.

In their search for potential sites of the multiplication and excretion of virus other than the salivary glands Atanasiu and co-workers (1970a) demonstrated virus antigen in the Malpighian cells of the lingual epithelium, in the wall of the intestinal tract, and in nerve elements surrounding the sebaceous glands and the hair shafts in the skin of intracerebrally inoculated mice. Murphy et al. (1973b) studied rabies virus generalization in young hamsters, and stated that "the many nerve end organs of the mouth (taste buds) and nose (olfactory neuroepithelium) were much more heavily infected than salivary gland epithelium." No viral titrations were performed to determine whether the oronasal secretions yielded more infectious virus than the salivary gland tissues.

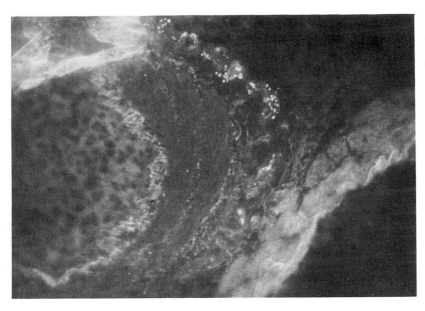

Fig. 11. Lung, viral antigen in neurons of peribronchial tissue. ×400.

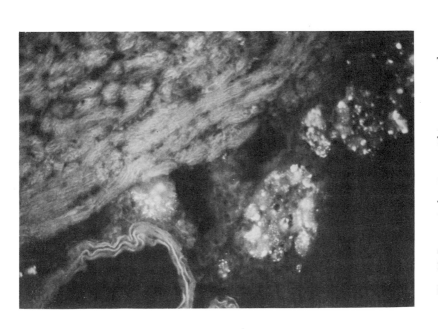

Fig. 10. Lung, viral antigen within neurons and nerve fibers alongside a bloodvessel. ×400.

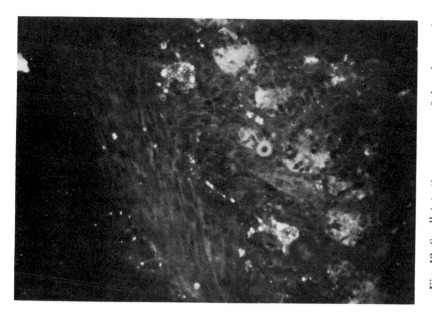

Fig. 13. Small intestine, neurons of the plexus submucosus (Meissner) containing viral antigen up to the size of Negri bodies. ×400.

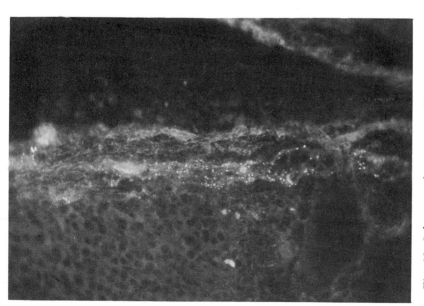

Fig. 12. Spleen, viral antigen in fibers of a nerve plexus located within trabecula. ×400.

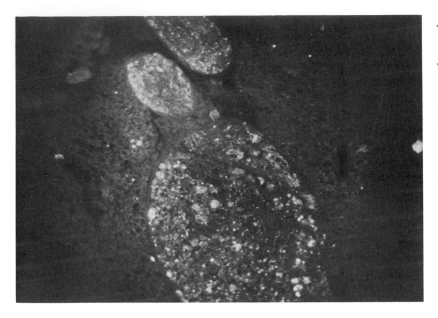

Fig. 15. Kidney, viral antigen within a ganglion and a nerve plexus of the renal pelvis. ×250.

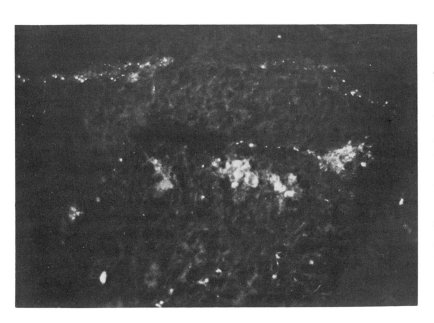

Fig. 14. Small intestine, viral antigen within nerve fibers of the plexus myentericus (Auerbach). ×400.

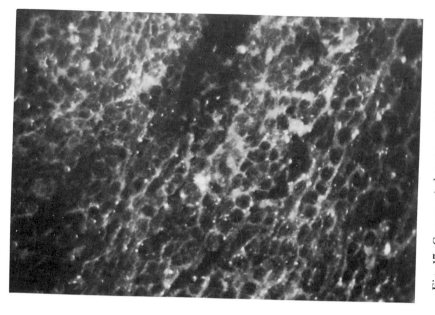

Fig. 17. Cornea, viral antigen within nervous tissue and epithelial cells. ×250.

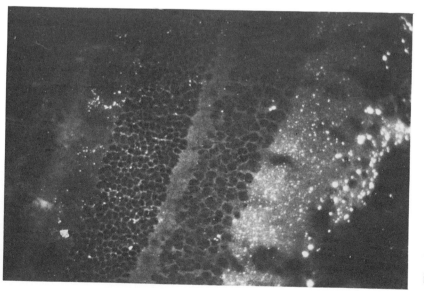

Fig. 16. Retina, viral antigen within the ganglion fasciculi optici (lower edge), within the inner reticular layer (above), and within the ganglion retinae (upper half). ×250.

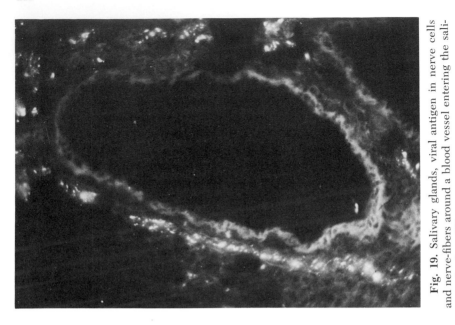

Fig. 19. Salivary glands, viral antigen in nerve cells and nerve-fibers around a blood vessel entering the salivary glands. ×400.

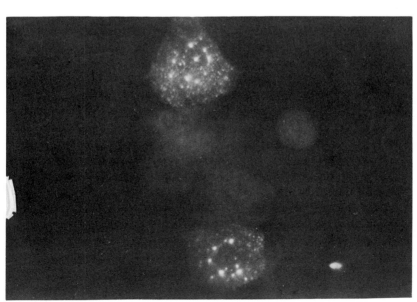

Fig. 18. Cornea, viral antigen within two corneal epithelium cells from the eye of a living mouse. ×400.

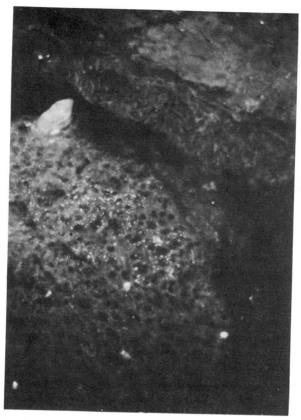

Fig. 20. Salivary glands, viral antigen in acinar epithelial cells. ×400.

Flourescent staining in the organs of naturally infected animals deserves special attention since the terminal virus dissemination reflects what is also observed in animal experiments, and allows conclusions to be drawn regarding the potential pathways for virus excretion and transmission. Schaaf and Schaal (1968) conducted a systematic study of this type of FA staining of tissue smears from 57 randomly selected rabid animals, mainly foxes, cattle, and deer. Salivary gland infection, as an indicator of virus generalization, was shown to occur at the same rate (90%) in all species tested when more than one gland was examined. Also infected were sensory organs (retina, inner ear) and the sympathetic plexuses from the mesentery. Smears from the oral and nasal mucosa were infected quite frequently, and it was assumed that not only nerve elements but also epithelial tissues contain the virus. This was convincingly shown by Debbie and Trimarchi (1970) who investigated tissues from 12 rabid, free-ranging red foxes. Numerous tissues tested from each animal were found to be infected, most frequently nerve cells and fibers of esophagus, adrenals, kidneys, urinary bladder, urethra, prostate, heart, lung, and stomach. The urinary and respiratory tracts were considered by the authors as potential sites for virus excretion since viral antigen was discernible within neuroepithelial tissues lining those tracts. Moreover, physiologic sloughing might contribute to the infectivity of oronasal secretions. It is conceivable that the nasal mucosa might also have served as a port of entry for the virus (see also below). It should be noted that the presence of virus in various organs of naturally infected bats has been reported, but the cells involved remain unidentified (Delpietro *et al.*, 1972.)

After oral infection of mice with a bovine virus strain, Correa-Giron *et al.* (1970) demonstrated virus antigen in the cytoplasm of epithelial cells from the mucous membranes of cheeks, lips, and tongue, in taste buds, in the papillae, and in nerve endings of the subepithelial nerve plexuses. Also infected were cells of the non-glandular region of the stomach, of the renal medulla, of salivary glands and nerve elements in lung, heart, and trachea. Furthermore, cells of the skin epidermis (especially those of the stratum germinativum and stratum granulosum) prickle cells, and nerve elements surrounding tactile hairs were shown to be infected. Fischman and Schaeffer (1971) repeatedly demonstrated virus antigen in the stratum granulosum of cheek mucosa and tongue of weanling mice and hamsters infected orally. The antigen found in esophagus, trachea, and intestine was limited to nerve fibers and plexuses. Both the latter groups of workers expressed the opinion that the infection of oropharyngeal tissues did not represent centrifugal virus spread but rather reflected the sites of invasion of the virus. These are apparently further examples of fluorescence observed late, hinting at early invasion paths.

In recent studies aimed at the localization of virus antigen in non-nervous structures following aerogenic infection of guinea pigs, Hronovský and Benda (1969) demonstrated virus and virus antigen in unidentified cells of the nasal mucosa, lungs, trachea, and kidneys. Virus appeared in the nasal mucosa 1 day before it was recovered from the brain. In similar studies, Fischman and Schaeffer (1971) instilled virus intranasally into mice, and the presence of virus antigen was demonstrated in cells of the nasal membrane although it was not excessive; most of the flourescence was observed in deeper submucosal layers. Virus dissemination into other organs, however, was widespread. Specific fluorescence was observed in all layers of the retina, in superficial and deep layers of the cornea, in the medulla and nerve plexuses of the adrenals, and throughout the smooth muscle layer of the urinary bladder, while acinar cells of the salivary glands, nerve cells of the trachea, and occasionally of the lungs contained scattered fluorescent foci.

These studies as well as others (Murphy et al., 1973b) seem to provide evidence for the regular involvement of the olfactory neuroepithelium in aerogenic rabies infection. Considering once more the demonstration of late antigen as a sign of early invasion at that site, these structures—more than the lungs—could serve as a likely portal of entry for the virus. Similar findings were recently reported by Constantine et al. (1972) who observed fluorescence in the nasal mucosa of naturally infected Mexican free-tail bats. This type of bat is highly colonial and might also be expected to transmit virus by the nasal route, as concluded by the authors in their discussion of the findings.

The widespread virus generalization into nonrespiratory organs following aerogenic infections (Hronovský and Benda, 1969; Fischman and Schaeffer, 1971; Murphy et al., 1973b) is obviously the result of centrifugal virus spread via nerves as judged from the terminal localization of viral antigen in nerve cells.

The mucous membranes of the oral and nasal cavities seem to play an important role in the initiation of aerogenic and oral infection. Virus multiplies in the sensory end organs of these tissues before CNS infection takes place, and may be liberated from these structures by budding or mechanical disruption of cells. This is shown by oral (Correa-Giron et al., 1970; Fischman and Schaeffer, 1971) and aerogenic transmission studies (Atanasiu, 1966; Hronovský and Benda, 1969; Fischman and Schaeffer, 1971; Murphy et al., 1973b), as well as from findings in naturally infected animals (Schaaf and Schaal, 1968; Debbie and Trimarchi, 1970; Constantine et al., 1972).

IV. Intravitam Diagnostic Tests

The findings that corneal epithelium cells may contain virus antigen even during the incubation period (Schneider and Hamann, 1969) seemed to provide a promising basis for the early diagnosis of the disease during the lifetime of the infected individual (Schneider, 1969a). A similar approach is the staining of scrapings from the oronasal mucosa (Schaaf and Schaal, 1971) and of frozen skin sections from biopsy material (Smith et al., 1972) by fluorescein-conjugated antibody. The corneal FA-test has been used by several authors and seems to be a helpful supplementary method for the diagnosis of rabies (Atanasiu *et al.*, 1970b; Emmrich *et al.*, 1970; Kovalev and Shashenko, 1970; López *et al.*, Cifuentes *et al.*, 1971; Schaaf and Schaal, 1971; Zimmermann, 1971; Larghi *et al.*, 1973). A positive result indicates rabies infection but a negative result does not rule out rabies.

V. Prevention of Virus Spread

Section of the lingual nerves of dogs prevented the infection of the mandibular glands (Bertarelli, 1904). Removal of portions of the lingual nerve and of the cranial cervical ganglion of dogs and foxes (Dean *et al.*, 1963) reduced the virus titers in the neurectomized gland about 1000-fold compared to those of the nonoperated gland, but some atrophy of the neurectomized glands occurred and the results must be considered in the light of that factor.

Antirabies vaccination is believed by French and Rumanian authors (Eichwald and Pitzschke, 1967) to prevent the infection of salivary glands to a considerable degree. Jelesić *et al.* (1963) determined the percentage of infected organs (brown fat tissue) in vaccinated and unvaccinated mice. The postinfection application of one to six doses of antirabies vaccine reduced the percentage of infected glands from 28% to zero. Passive antibody did not show this effect but, in fact, raised the percentage of infected glands to 64%. Studies on this subject certainly deserve further research. If this is confirmed, virus excretion could be prevented by postexposure treatment of previously unvaccinated animals.

References

Atanasiu, P. (1965). *C. R. Acad. Sci.* **261**, 277.
Atanasiu, P. (1966). *Symp. Ser. Immunobiol. Stand.* 1, 159-166.
Atanasiu, P., Gamet, A., Tsiang, H., Dragonas, P., and Lépine, P. (1970a). *C. R. Acad. Sci.* **271**, 2434-2436.
Atanasiu, P., Guillon, J. C., and Vallée, A. (1970b). *Ann. Inst. Pasteur, Paris* **119**, 260-269.
Babes, V. (1912). "Traité de la rage". Libraire J. B. Bailliere, Paris.
Baer, G. M., and Bales, G. L. (1967). *J. Infec. Dis.* **117**, 82-90.
Baer, G. M., Shanthaveerappa, T. R., and Bourne, G. H. (1965). *Bull. W. H. O.* **33**, 783-794.
Baer, G. M., Shantha, T. R., and Bourne, G. H. (1968). *Bull. W. H. O.* **38**, 119-125.

Becker, P. (1961). *Monatsch. Tierheilk.* 13, 90–95.

Bell, J. F., Moore, G. J., Raymond, G. H., and Tibbs, C. E. (1962). *Amer. J. Publ. Health* 52, 1293–1301.

Bertarelli, E. (1904). *Zentralbl. Bakteriol., Parasitenk. Infektionskr. Hyg., Abt. 1: Orig.* 37, 213–221.

Cifuentes, E., Calderón, E., and Bijlenga, G. (1971). *J. Trop. Med. Hyg.* 74, 23–25.

Constantine, D. G. (1962). *Pub. Health Rep.* 77, 287–289.

Constantine, D. G., Emmons, R. W., and Woodie, J. D. (1972). *Science* 175, 1255–1256.

Coons, A. H., Creech, H. J., Jones, R. N., and Berliner, E. (1942). *J. Immunol.* 45, 159–170.

Correa-Giron, E. P., Allen, R., and Sulkin, S. E. (1970). *Amer. J. Epidemiol.* 91, 203-215.

Dean, D. J., Evans, W. M., and McClure, R. C. (1963). *Bull. W. H. O.* 29, 803–811.

Debbie, J. G., and Trimarchi, C. V. (1970). *J. Wild. Dis.* 6, 500–506.

Delpietro, H., Díaz, A. M. C., Fuenzalida, E., and Bell, J. F. (1972). *Bol. Of. Sanit. Panamer.* 73, 222–230.

Dierks, R. E., Murphy, F. A., and Harrison, A. K. (1969). *Amer. J. Pathol.* 54, 251–273.

Doerr, R. (1939). In "Handbuch der Virusforschung" (R. Doerr and C. Hallauer, eds.), 1st ed., Vol. 1, Part 2, p. 761. Springer-Verlag, Berlin and New York.

Eichwald, C., and Pitzschke, H., eds. (1967). "Die Tollwut bei Mensch und Tier," Fischer, Jena.

Emmrich, P., Jüngst, B.-K., and Schneider, L. G. (1970). *Med. Klin.* (*Munich*) 65, 454–457.

Fischman, H. R., and Schaeffer, M. (1971). *Ann. N. Y. Acad. Sci.* 177, 78–97.

Garcia-Tamayo, J., Avila-Mayor, A., and Anzola-Perez, E. (1972). *Arch. Pathol.* 94, 11–15.

Girard, K. F., Hitchcock, H. B., Edsall, G., and MacCready, R. A. (1965). *N. Eng. J. Med.* 272, 75–80.

Goldwasser, R. A., and Kissling, R. E. (1958). *Proc. Soc. Exp. Biol. Med.* 98, 219–223.

Goldwasser, R. A., Kissling, R. E., Carski, T. R., and Hosty, T. S. (1959). *Bull. W. H. O.* 20, 579-588.

Goodpasture, E. W. (1925). *Amer. J. Pathol.* 1, 547–582.

Hronovský, V., and Benda, R. (1969). *Acta Virol.* (*Prague*) 13, 198-202.

Jackson, H. (1921). *J. Infec. Dis.* 29, 291.

Jelesić, Z., Vujkov, V., and Jovanovic, L. (1963). *Arch. Hyg. Bakteriol.* 146, 636–640.

Jenson, A. B., Rabin, E. R., Bentinck, D. C., and Melnick, J. L. (1969). *J. Virol.* 3, 265–269.

Johnson, H. N. (1959). *Proc. 63rd. Annu. Meet. U.S. Livestock Sanit. Ass.*, pp. 267–274.

Johnson, H. N. (1966). *Proc. Nat. Rabies Symp., 1966*, pp. 25–30.

Johnson, R. T. (1965). *J. Neuropathol. Exp. Neurol.* 24, 662–674.

Kaplan, M. M., Forsek, Z., and Koprowski, H. (1960). *Bull. W. H. O.* 22, 434–435.

Katasilambros, L. (1962). *Acta Microbiol. Hellen.* 7, 57–64.

Kauker, E., and Zettl, K. (1959). *Monatsh. Tierheilk.* 11, 129–142.

Koch, J. (1930). In "Handbuch der Pathogenen Microorganismen" (W. Kolle, R. Kraus, and P. Uhlenhuth, eds.), Vol. 8, Part 1, pp. 547–694. Fischer, Jena.

Kovalev, N. A., and Shashenko, A. S. (1970). *Veterinariya* (*Moscow*) 47, 44–46.

Krause, W. W. (1957). *Zentralbl. Bakteriol., Parasitenk., Infektionskr. Hyg., Abt. 1: Orig.* 167, 481–503.

Krause, W. W. (1966). *Symp. Ser. Immunbiol. Stand.* 1, 153–158.

Larghi, O. P., Gonzales, E., and Held, J. R. (1973). *Appl. Microbiol.* **25**, 187–189.

Leach, N., and Johnson, H. N. (1940). *Amer. J. Trop. Med.* **20**, 335–340.

Levaditi, C. (1926). "L'herpes et le zona." Masson, Paris.

Levaditi, C., Sanches-Bayarri, V., and Schoen, R. (1928). *C. R. Soc. Biol.* **98**, 911–914.

Levaditi, C., and Schoen, R. (1935). *Ann. Inst. Pasteur, Paris, Suppl. Commemorative* **55**, 69–96.

López, J. H., Alvarez-B. J., and Gil-E., J. L. (1970). *Antioquia Med.* **20**, 577–582.

Lubinski, H. and Prausnitz, C. (1926). *Ergeb. Mikrobiol., Immunitaetsforsch. Exp. Ther.* **8**, 1–164.

Manouelian, M. Y. (1935). *C. R. Soc. Biol.* **119**, 256.

Murphy, F. A., Bauer, S. P., Harrison, A. K., and Winn, W. C. (1973a). *Lab. Invest.* **28**, 361–376.

Murphy, F. A., Harrison, A. K., Winn, W. C., and Bauer, S. P. (1973b). *Lab. Invest.* **29**, 1–16.

Nicolau, S. (1928). *C. R. Soc. Biol.* **99**, 677–679.

Nicolau, S., and Serbanescu, V. (1928). *C. R. Soc. Biol.* **99**, 294–296.

Nicolau, S., Dimanesco-Nicolau, O., and Galloway, J. A. (1929). *Ann. Inst. Pasteur, Paris* **43**, 1–88.

Nocard, E., Roux, E., and Bardach (1887). *Rec. Med. Vet.* (cited by Lubinski and Prausnitz, 1926).

Parker, R. L., and Wilsnack, R. E. (1966). *Amer. J. Vet. Res.* **27**, 33-38.

Pasteur, L., Chamberland, S., and Roux, E. (1884). *C. R. Acad. Sci.* **98**, 457.

Petrović, M., and Timm, H. (1969). *Zentralbl. Bakteriol., Parasitenk., Infektionskr. Hyg., Abt. 1: Orig.* **211**, 149–161.

Pitzschke, H. (1958). *Zentralbl. Bakteriol., Parasitenk., Infektionskr. Hyg., Abt. 1: Orig.* **172**, 197–211.

Pizarro, A. L., Ruiz, O. J., de García, M. C., de Guzmán, L. E., de Carrascal, A. M., and Ramos, M. F. (1970). *Semin. Nac. Sobre Rabia, 2nd, 1970,* pp. 25–32.

Reagan, R. L., Day, W. C., Moore, S., Kehne, E. F., and Brueckner, A. L. (1953). *Amer. J. Trop. Med.* **2**, 70–73.

Remlinger, P., and Bailly, J. (1931a). *C. R. Soc. Biol.* **106**, 201–202.

Remlinger, P., and Bailly, J. (1931b). *C. R. Soc. Biol.* **106**, 1204–1205.

Remlinger, P., and Bailly, J. (1932). *C. R. Soc. Biol.* **110**, 239.

Remlinger, P., and Bailly, J. (1934). *Ann. Inst. Pasteur, Paris* **53**, 43–50.

Remlinger, P., and Bailly, J. (1940). *Ann. Inst. Pasteur, Paris* **64**, 40–46.

Roux, E. (1888). *Ann. Inst. Pasteur, Paris* **2**, 18–27.

Roux, E., and Nocard, E. (1890). *Ann. Inst. Pasteur, Paris* **4**, 163-171.

Schaaf, J., and Schaal, E. (1968). *Deut. Tieraerztl. Wochenschr.* **75**, 315–323.

Schaaf, J., and Schaal, E. (1971). *Deut. Tieraerzti. Wochenschr.* **78**, 341–346.

Schneider, L. G. (1966). *Symp. Ser. Immunobiol. Stand.* **1**, 209.

Schneider, L. G. (1969a). *Zentralbl. Veterinaermed., Reihe B* **16**, 24–31.

Schneider, L. G. (1969b). *Zentralbl. Bakteriol., Parasitenk., Infektionskr. Hyg., Abt. 1: Orig.* **211**, 281–308.

Schneider, L. G., and Hamann, I. (1969). *Zentralbl. Bakteriol., Parasitenk., Infektionskr. Hyg., Abt. 1: Orig.* **212**, 13–41. ,

Schneider, L. G., Dietzschold, B., Dierks, R. E., Matthaeus, W., Enzmann, P.-J., and Strohmaier, K. (1973). *J. Virol.* **11**, 748–755.

Schweinburg, F. (1932). *Zentralbl. Bakteriol., Parasitenk., Infektionskr. Hyg., Abt. 1: Orig.* **123**, 434–448.

Schweinburg, F. (1937). *Ergeb. Mikrobiol., 1mmunitaetsforsch. Exp. Ther.* **20**, 1–154.

Shashenko, A. S., and Kovalev, N. A. (1971). *Veterinariya (Moscow)* **5**, 42–44.

Sikes, R. K. (1962). *Amer. J. Vet. Res.* **23**, 1041–1047.

Sikes, R. K. (1966). *Proc. Nat. Rabies Symp., 1966*, pp. 31–33.

Sims, R. A., Allen, R., and Sulkin, S. E. (1963). *J. Infec. Dis.* **112**, 17–27.

Smith, W. B., Blenden, D. C., Fuh, T., and Hiler, L. L. (1972). *J. Amer. Vet. Med. Ass.* **161**, 1495–1501.

Tierkel, E. (1966). *Symp. Ser. Immunobiol. Stand.* **1**, 245–250.

Ueki, H., and Nakamura, Y. (1962). *Tokyo Lab. Med. Sci.* **165**, 29.

Vaughn, J. B., Gerhardt, P., and Paterson, J. C. S. (1963). *J. Amer. Med. Ass.* **184**, 705–708.

Wilsnack, R. E. (1966). *Symp. Series Immunobiol. Stand.* **1**, 274.

Wilsnack, R. E., and Parker, R. L. (1966). *Amer. J. Vet. Res.* **27**, 39–43.

Winkler, W. G., Baker, E. F., Jr., and Hopkins, C. C. (1971). *Amer. J. Epidemiol.* **95**, 267–277.

Winkler, W. G., Fashinell, T. R., Leffingwell, L., Howard, P., and Conomy, J. P. (1973). *J. Amer. Med. Ass.* **226**, 1219–1221.

Wong, D. H., and Freund, J. (1951). *Proc. Soc. Exp. Biol. Med.* **76**, 717–720.

World Health Organization Expert Committee on Rabies. (1973). *World Health Organ., Tech. Rep. Ser.* **523**.

Yamamoto, T., Otani, S., and Shiraki, H. (1965). *Acta Neuropathol.* **5**, 288-306.

Zimmermann, T. (1971). *Berlin. Muenchen. Tieraerztl. Wochenschr.* **84**, 172-174.

Zunker, M. (1963). *Zentralbl. Veterinaermed., Reihe B* **10**, 271–277.

CHAPTER 15

Electron Microscopy of Extraneural Rabies Infection

Richard E. Dierks

I. Extraneural Infection Prior to Invasion of the Nervous System

Morgagni (1769) first postulated that rabies virus was carried through nerves rather than veins. Since then, many studies have been conducted to elucidate the importance of neural versus hematogenous spread to and from the central nervous system (CNS). The bulk of evidence suggests that both centripetal and centrifugal spread of virus is via nervous pathways (Chapters 10, 14).

A number of studies, however, have suggested that ingress of virus appears to occur without replication at the site of inoculation (Johnson, 1971; Schindler, 1961; Ercegovac, 1969a,b; Baer *et al.*, 1965, 1968; Petrovic and Timm, 1969; Fishman, 1969; Schneider, 1969). Baer and Cleary (1972) developed an animal model for rabies with a long incubation period. Mice inoculated with virus from the salivary gland of a rabid bobcat died of rabies with incubation periods ranging from 17 to 120 days. The authors demonstrated that amputation of the inoculated foot within 18 days after inoculation was a life-saving procedure indicating that the virus was sequestered at or near the site of inoculation for most of the long incubation period. In groups of mice to which antirabies serum was administered a higher percentage of the mice died of rabies after prolonged incubation, as compared to the control group, suggesting that at least some of the virus remained at the extraneural inoculation site in a location or state inaccessable to the neutralizing action of antisera. It is possible that after the normal half-life decay of the passively administered antisera to levels below that necessary for viral neutralization the virus was then able to cross extracellular spaces, infect neural tissues and produce death. Sulkin *et al.* (1959) inoculated street virus into hamsters and observed that the virus titer in muscles at the site of inoculation occasionally approached that observed in the brain; it was concluded that viral proliferation had occurred in those tissues.

Recent studies with baby hamsters have helped in our understanding of what occurs from the time of entrance of the virus into muscle until its entrance into the nervous system. The course of infection of three rabies viruses and two rabies-like viruses, Mokola (Shope *et al.*, 1970) and Lagos bat (Boulger and Porterfield, 1958), was followed by tissue titration, histology, immunofluorescence, and electron microscopy (Murphy *et al.*, 1973a,b). As shown in previous studies, the authors found that tissue titrations were not sensitive enough to follow the early course of infection. Murphy *et al.* (1973a,b) assumed that viral antigen observed late in the infection at any site was a magnification of earlier passage and replication at that site. Early detection of antigen at a given site also indicated early invasion of the site. By immunofluorescent studies (FA), rabies antigen was first found *in* striated muscle cells near the site of inoculation followed by involvement of the peripheral nervous system and then the CNS. Electron microscopically, the authors later observed typical rhabdovirus morphogenesis occurring upon sarcoplasmic reticulum and plasma membranes of myocytes (Fig. 1). A study of the early phases of rabies pathogenesis in hamsters inoculated intramuscularly with 12 street viruses considered to be typical of strains currently being submitted to the Center for Disease Control, Atlanta, Georgia has demonstrated specific rabies immunofluorescense in a pattern similar to that observed in the earlier studies with laboratory strains and rabies-like viruses (Murphy and Bauer, 1974). Following deep intramuscular inoculation the authors demonstrated viral infection initially in striated muscle cells as plasmalemmal beaded "pinpoint" fluorescense. As the infection progressed viral antigen accumulated in muscle before involvement of any other tissues in the inoculation site or elsewhere. These studies indicate an early replication of virus in experimental infections irrespective of whether the

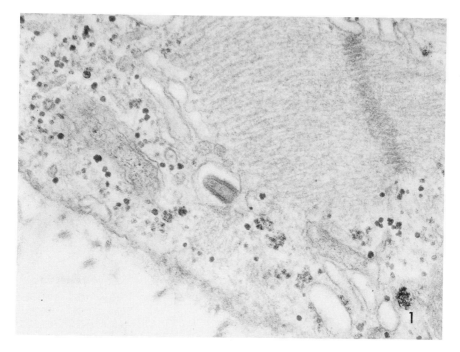

Fig. 1. Mokola virus budding into cisternea of sarcoplasmic reticulum of striated muscle cell of a hamster. ×91,000. (Photograph courtesy of F. A. Murphy.)

isolates are laboratory or street strains. These findings are discussed in detail in Chapter 2.

After inhalation exposure in suckling guinea pigs and mice, viral antigen was noted in the nasal mucosa prior to its presence in the central nervous system (Hronovský and Benda, 1969a,b; Hronovský, 1971). Viral antigen was observed 6 days after infection of suckling guinea pigs with a tissue culture adapted street rabies virus and 3 days after inoculation of suckling mice with CVS virus. In each case viral antigen was demonstrated in nasal mucosa one day before fluorescence was observed in the CNS, again suggesting that viral replication in non-neural cells may play an important role in the early pathogenesis of rabies.

The above studies provide evidence of a mechanism for the progression of infection to the nervous system if virus is not deposited in or very near nerve cells at the site of inoculation, just as viral morphogenesis on the plasma membranes of cells within the salivary glands or mucosal epithelium provides a natural mechanism for escape of the virus from its host.

II. Extraneural Infection Following Centrifugal Spread
from Nervous Tissue

Rabies virus or antigen has been demonstrated in many extraneural tissues following its multiplication in the CNS. Sequential studies give evidence favoring neuronal spread to extraneural sites (Johnson, 1971). Virus has been detected in a variety of tissues by mouse inoculation, fluorescent antibody, or electron microscopic procedures. In mice infected with street virus by the intracerebral or plantar route antigen was observed terminally in the cornea, salivary glands, brown fat, lungs, intestine, kidney, adrenal, heart, liver, uterus, and skeletal muscles (Schneider and Hamann, 1969). Extraneural multiplication occurred in epithelial tissue of the salivary glands, brown fat, and cornea, while infection was often noted in ganglion cells, nerve fibers or nerve plexuses when observed in other non-nervous organs.

Several additional studies in mice have shown similar findings. After intranasal inoculation of five rabies isolates into mice, viral antigen was found terminally in nerves or nerve plexuses of the tracheal and nasal submucosa, lung, adrenal glands, and bladder (Fishman and Schaeffer, 1971). Antigen was also found in the acinar cells of the salivary glands and other extraneural cells of the nasal mucosa, lingual papillae, and hair follicles. Following oral transmission, antigen was found in submucosal layers of the cheek and in the mucosa and papillae of the tongue. The fluorescence observed in the esophagus, trachea, and intestine was limited to nerve bundle plexuses.

Mice dying after eating mouse brains infected with vampire bat strain virus showed fluorescent antibody staining in epithelial cells of the buccal mucosa and tongue (Correa-Giron *et al.*, 1970). Antigen was also observed in kidneys and salivary glands and associated with nerves or ganglia in the lung, heart, esophagus, and trachea. In a similar study using fixed virus or fox origin street virus, positive FA findings were again observed in lingual epithelium (Atanasiu *et al.*, 1970b).

Intracytoplasmic rabies antigen has been demonstrated in the olfactory receptor cells of naturally infected Mexican free-tailed bats (*Tadarida brasiliensis mexicana*), indicating that viral replication had occurred in these tissues, and thus implicating the nasal mucosa as a possible portal of viral entry or exit (Constantine *et al.*, 1972).

After centrifugal spread of rabies and rabies-like viruses (Mokola and Lagos bat) from the CNS in hamsters, the nerve end organs in the oral and nasal cavities were heavily infected (Murphy *et al.*, 1973b). This included end organs with cells directly exposed to oral or nasal surfaces, olfactory epithelium and taste buds of the tongue, as well as a wide range of other sensory end organs normally separated from body surfaces by one or more cell layers. A wide variety of other tissues including retina, corneal epithelium, adrenal glands, pancreas, brown adipose tissue, and autonomic neuronal plexuses to visceral organs also contained viral antigen.

In another study in mice (Smith *et al.*, 1972), skin biopsies that contained large numbers of cutaneous nerves particularly near hair follicles were so consistently infected that immunofluorescent staining of frozen sections has been proposed as a routine diagnostic procedure.

Following natural rabies infection in red fox (*Vulpes fulva*), specific fluorescence was detected in submaxillary and parotid salivary glands, skeletal muscle, esophagus, stomach, intestine, pancreas, thyroid, thymus, lung, heart, adrenal glands, kidney, ureter, bladder, prostate, urethra and testicles (Debbie and Trimarchi, 1970). The liver, gall bladder, spleen, uterus, and ovaries were the only tissues studied where virus was not found. In experimentally infected foxes, fluorescent antigen was observed in salivary glands, cornea, retina, and adrenal glands, but not in pancreas or intrascapular fat (Atanasiu *et al.*, 1970a). Rabies virus has also been detected in submaxillary and parotid salivary glands, lung, pancreas, adrenal glands, nasal mucosa, oral mucosa and lingual taste buds in experimentally infected striped skunks (*Mephitis mephitis*) and spotted skunks (*Spilogale putorius*) by FA and mouse inoculation (R. E. Dierks, unpublished).

It has been shown that rabies virus titers in the salivary glands may exceed those in the brain thus indicating viral multiplication (Parker and Wilsnack, 1966; Vaughn *et al.*, 1965; Dierks *et al.*, 1969). The salivary glands have sensory nerve endings as well as sympathetic and parasympathetic efferent secretory nerves. The efferent nerves form a delicate net of epilemmal fibers around the basement membrane of acini within the gland. Small branches then penetrate through the basement lamina and form a second network of hypolemmal fibers which penetrate between the glandular cells, ramify, and end on the surfaces of the secretory cells. This nerve network provides a direct viral route to every secretory cell within the gland.

By removal of the right lingual nerve and cranial cervical ganglion in both foxes and dogs, Dean *et al.* (1963) were able to impede the spread of the virus to the denervated salivary gland. This was particularly evident in the fox and suggests that salivary glands and probably other organs customarily become infected via peripheral nerves. Sectioning of the chorda tympani in the dog, however, results in an intense degeneration and atrophy of the submaxillary and retrolingual glands (Bloom and Fawcett, 1968) similar to that indicated by the 22–52% weight loss of the neurectomized glands described by Dean *et al.* (1963). The resultant degeneration and atrophy of the mucous secreting cells may also directly reduce the virus titer by eliminating its prime site of replication, even if it reaches the gland by other routes.

Histologic changes have been shown to occur in those peripheral tissues where large amounts of antigen or virus are observed, but this has not been a consistent finding. Focal degenerative lesions have been reported in the adrenal medulla, tubular epithelium of the kidney, and acinar epithelium of the pancreas (Johnson, 1965; Debbie and Trimarchi, 1970). Severe degenerative changes of mucous acini with mononuclear infiltration have also been observed in submaxillary salivary glands (Johnson, 1965; Dierks *et al.*, 1969). The submaxillary salivary gland of the fox is a mixed gland with acini consisting primarily of pyramidal mucogenic cells and occasional serous cells (Fig. 2). In infected fox salivary glands, varying degrees of histologic change have been observed, ranging from areas of mild lymphoid infiltration to severe degenerative changes (Fig. 3). In heavily infected foci the normal acinar architecture was replaced by amorphous debri with basement membranes and stromal connective tissue remaining the only recognizable tissues left outlining the destroyed acini. By electron microscopy acinar cell cytoplasm of some abnormal cells was shown to be rarified with accumulations of intracytoplasmic viral matrices (Dierks *et al.*, 1969; Fig. 4). These cells also contained swollen mitochondria and had large spaces between secretory granules. The submaxillary salivary gland of the striped skunk is also a mixed gland but contains a higher percentage of serous secreting cells and more interstitial connective tissue (Fig. 5). Degenerative changes with accompanying lymphoid infiltration have been observed but have not been as severe as those seen in the fox (Fig. 6).

The submaxillary glands of the spotted skunk appear to contain an even higher percentage of serous secreting cells with heavy interstitial connective tissues. Occasional degenerating mucous acini have been observed, but lymphoid infiltration was the main pathologic change observed in areas where large amounts of viral antigen was detected by FA.

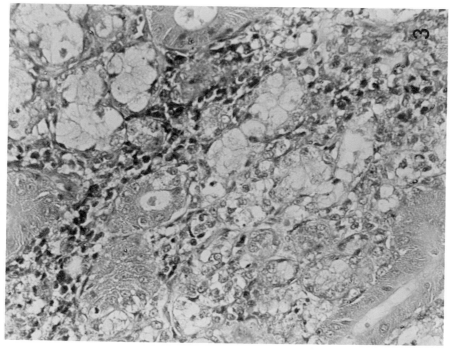

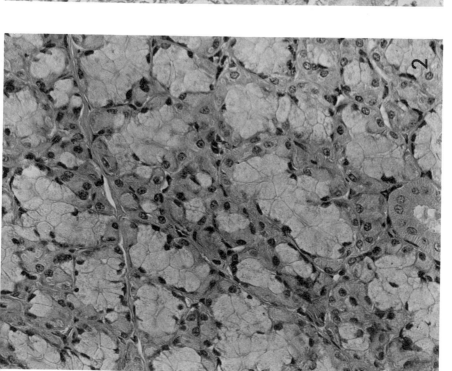

Fig. 2. Normal fox submaxillary salivary gland. Acini are predominantly mucogenic pyramidal cells. Hematoxylin and eosin stain, ×365.

Fig. 3. Infected fox submaxillary salivary gland. Mild lymphoid infiltration and severe degenerative necrosis. H & E stain, ×365.

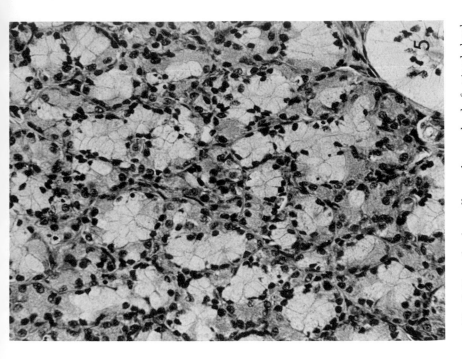

Fig. 5. Normal submaxillary salivary gland of striped skunk. Mixed gland with both mucous and serous secreting cells. H & E stain, ×365.

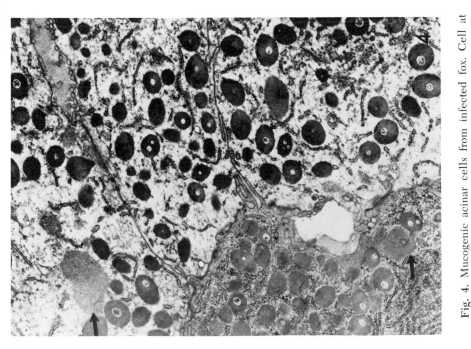

Fig. 4. Mucogenic acinar cells from infected fox. Cell at lower left has cytoplasmic density usually observed. Three cells on the right are distended and rarified. Viral inclusions in both types of cells. ×12,000. (Dierks *et al.*, 1969. Photograph by F. A.

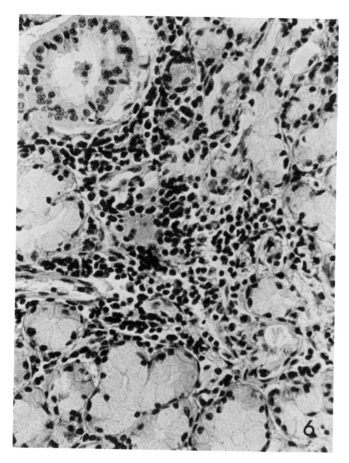

Fig. 6. Infected striped skunk submaxillary salivary gland. Lymphoid infiltration and degenerative necrosis of infected acini. H & E stain, ×365.

In all three species, fox, striped skunk, and spotted skunk, frozen sections of salivary glands showed single acini as well as whole groups of acini filled with specific fluorescent aggregates or antigen masses.

By electron microscopy, virions were observed budding from the marginal membranes of mucogenic acinar cells. This occurred on the lateral membranes of adjacent cells where dovetail interdigitations were very complex (Fig. 7) as well as upon the straighter marginal membranes and villi of intercellular canaliculi (Figs. 8 and 9). The sites of viral maturation were primarily in those areas of the cell apical to the nuclei that were rich in secretory granules but relatively

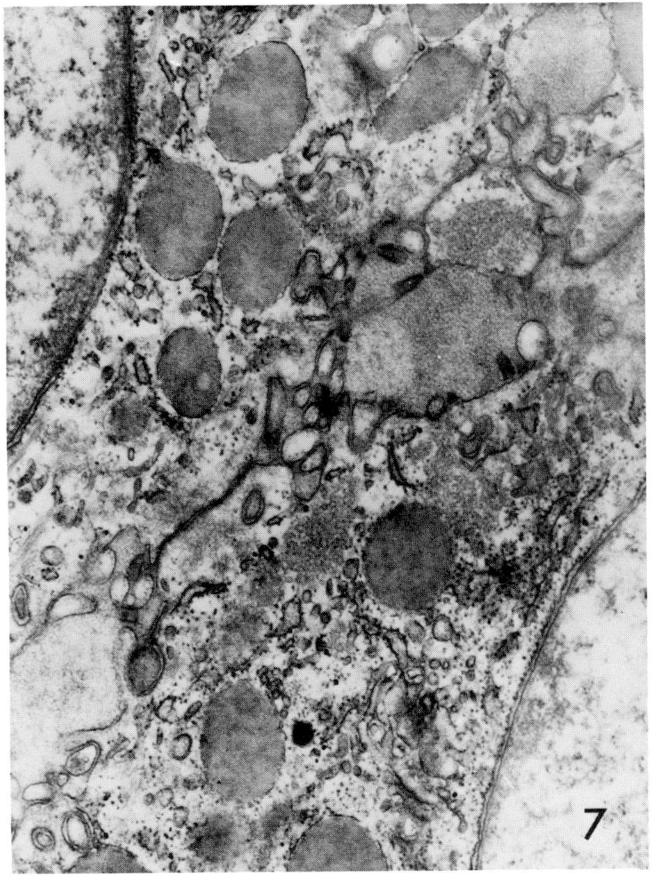

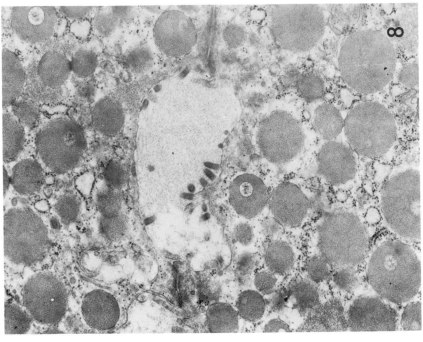

Fig. 8. Fox salivary gland. Rabies virions budding from marginal membranes of mucogenic acinar cells into intercellular canaliculus space between two adjoining cells. Large secretory granules fill cells. ×20,000. (Dierks *et al.*, 1969. Photograph by F. A. Murphy.)

Fig. 7. Fox salivary gland. Rabies virus maturing on the lateral membranes of adjacent cells where dovetail interdigitations were complex. ×21,000. (Photograph courtesy of F. A. Murphy.)

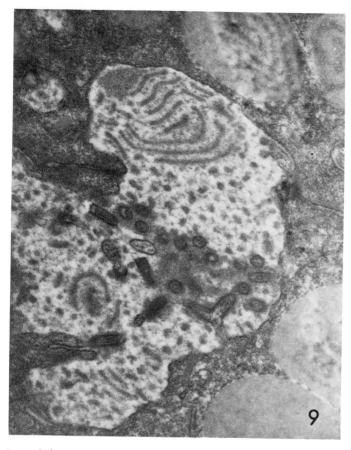

Fig. 9. Striped skunk salivary gland. Rabies virions and secretory products in an intercellular canaliculus. ×39,000.

sparse in endoplasmic reticulum or mitochondria. Intracytoplasmic viral inclusions or matrix material equivalent to that seen in neurons was often difficult to distinguish from secretory granules unless it contained virions or characteristic cylindrical structures (Fig. 10). Viral particles were occasionally found budding from the endoplasmic reticulum into cisternae and rarely found directly within the cytoplasm (Fig. 11), but maturation was most commonly observed upon apical plasma membranes of mucogenic cells resulting in direct release of virions into intercellular canaliculi and acinar lumens (Fig. 12). Virus budding was observed both upon and between microvilli protruding into the lumen of the acinus (Fig. 13).

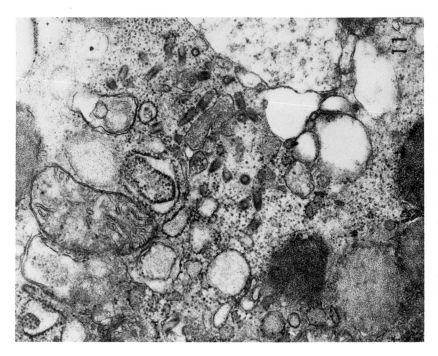

Fig. 11. Rabies particles directly in the cytoplasm of a fox mucogenic acinar cell. This distribution was rarely observed. ×33,000. (Dierks *et al.*, 1969. Photograph by F. A. Murphy.)

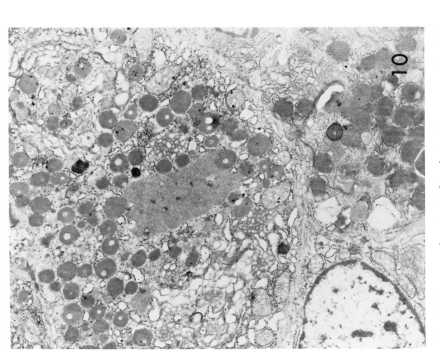

Fig. 10. Intracytoplasmic viral inclusion in mucogenic acinar cell of infected fox submaxillary salivary gland. ×8000. (Dierks *et al.*, 1969. Photograph by F. A. Murphy.)

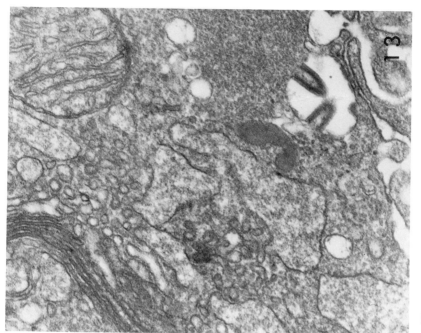

Fig. 12. Striped skunk submaxillary salivary gland. Rabies virus in the acinar lumen can be readily differentiated from microvilli. ×9000.

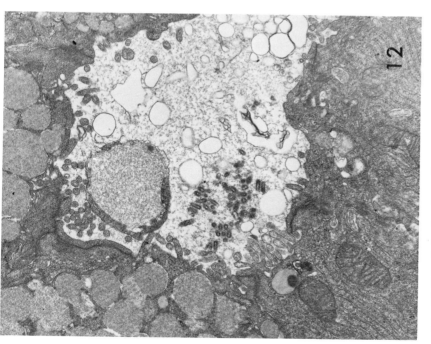

Fig. 13. Spotted skunk submaxillary salivary gland. Viral maturation on apical plasma membranes results in direct release of virions into lumen of acinus. ×56,000.

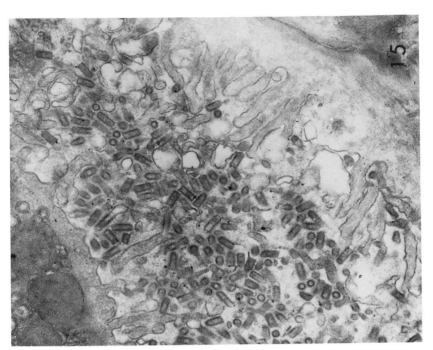

Fig. 15. Large masses of uniform bullet shaped virions in dilated lumenal space of fox salivary gland. Similar massive concentrations of virus occurred throughout infected glands. ×28,000. (Dierks *et al.*, 1969. Photograph by F. A. Murphy.)

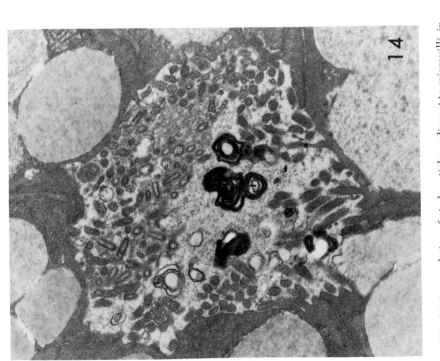

Fig. 14. Accumulation of viral particles, adjacent to microvilli, in the acinar lumen of infected striped skunk salivary gland. ×13,000.

Very large numbers of virions were intermixed with secretory granules, membranous debris, and other presumably soluble secretory products in these excretory ducts (Figs. 14 and 15). The maturation of rabies virus upon plasma membranes of extraneural cells at the site of inoculation appear to play an important role in its survival and subsequent spread to neural tissues. During its centrifugal spread within the host, rabies virus appears to have an affinity for glandular tissue and selected highly innervated epithelial tissues. Budding of infectious particles from plasma membranes into natural secretions or excretions within the salivary glands or other tissues in copious amounts provides an ideal mechanism for its maintenance in nature. The saliva of many rabies-infected carnivores has been shown to contain levels of virus as high or higher than that found in the brain. The fox and skunk, which are two of the principal wildlife reservoirs of rabies in the United States, may shed virus in their saliva for relatively long periods (7–14 days) before death, so that an important epidemiological factor in this disease is the potential for inoculating large amounts of virus into deep bite wounds. The recent observation that highly innervated nasal and oral epithelial tissues also contain large amounts of virus should be carefully studied to determine if it plays a role in the natural spread of the disease.

References

Atanasiu, P., Guillon, J. C., and Vallée, A. (1970a). *Ann. Int. Pasteur, Paris* **119**, 260.
Atanasiu, P., Gamet, A., Tsiang, H., Dragonas, P., and Lepine, P. (1970b). *C. R. Acad. Sci.* **271**, 2434.
Baer, G. M., and Cleary, W. F. (1972). *J. Inf. Dis.* **125**, 520.
Baer, G. M., Shanthaveerappa, T. R., and Bourne, G. H. (1965). *Bull. WHO* **33**, 783.
Baer, G. M., Shantha, T. R., and Bourne, G. H. (1968). *Bull. WHO* **38**, 119.
Bloom, W., and Fawcett, D. W. (1968). "Textbook of Histology," pp. 515–524. Saunders, Philadelphia, Pennsylvania.
Boulger, L. R., and Porterfield, J. S. (1958). *Trans. Roy. Soc. Trop. Med. Hyg.* **52**, 421.
Constantine, D. G., Emmons, R. W., and Woodie, J. D. (1972). *Science* **175**, 1255.
Correa-Giron, E. P., Allen, R., and Sulkin, S. E. (1970). *Amer. J. Epidemiol.* **91**, 203.
Dean, D. J., Evans, W. M., and McClure, R. C. (1963). *Bull. WHO* **29**, 803.
Debbie, J. G., and Trimarchi, C. V. (1970). *J. Wildl. Dis.* **6**, 500.
Dierks, R. E., Murphy, F. A., and Harrison, A. K. (1969). *Amer. J. Pathol.* **54**, 251.
Ercegovac, D. (1969a). *Zentralbl. Veterinaermed.* **16**, 115.
Ercegovac, D. (1969b). *Zentralbl. Veterinaermed.* **16**, 129.
Fishman, H. R. (1969). *Amer. J. Vet. Res.* **30**, 1213.
Fishman, H. R., and Schaeffer, M. (1971). *Ann. N. Y. Acad. Sci.* **177**, 78.
Hronovský, V. (1971). *Acta Virol. (Prague).* **15**, 58,

Hronovský, V., and Benda, R. (1969a). *Acta Virol. (Prague).* **13**, 193.

Hronovský, V., and Benda, R. (1969b). *Acta Virol. (Prague).* **13**, 197.

Johnson, H. N. (1965). *In* "Viral and Rickettsial Infections of Man" (F. L. Horsfall and I. Tamm, eds.), fourth edition, pp. 814–840. Lippincott, Philadelphia, Pennsylvania.

Johnson, R. T. (1971). *In* "Rabies" (Y. Nagano and F. M. Davenport, eds.), pp. 59–75. Univ. Park Press, Baltimore, Maryland.

Morgagni, J. B. (1769). Quoted from Wright (1959).

Murphy, F. A., and Bauer, S. P. (1974). *Intervirol.* **3**, 256–268.

Murphy, F. A., Bauer, S. P., Harrison, A. K., and Winn, W. C. (1973a). *Lab. Invest.* **28**, 361.

Murphy, F. A., Harrison, A. K., Winn, W. C., Jr., and Bauer, S. P. (1973b). *Lab Invest.* **29**, 1.

Parker, R. L., and Wilsnack, R. E. (1966). *Amer. J. Vet. Res.* **27**, 33.

Petrović, M., and Timm, H. (1969). *Zentralbl. Bakteriol., Parasitenk., Infektionskr. Hyg., Abt. 1: Orig.* **211**, 149.

Schindler, R. (1961). *Bull. WHO* **25**, 119.

Schindler, R. (1965). *Symp. Ser. Immunobiol. Stand.* **1**, 147–152,

Schneider, L. G. (1969). *Zentralbl. Bakteriol., Parasitenk., Infektionskr. Hyg., Abt. 1: Orig.* **211**, 281.

Schneider, L. G., and Hamann, I. (1969). *Zentralbl. Bakteriol., Parasitenk., Infektionskr. Hyg., Abt. 1: Orig.* **212**, 13.

Shope, R. E., Murphy, F. A., Harrison, A. K., Causey, O. R., Kemp, G. E., Simpson, D. I. H., and Moore, D. L. (1970). *J. Virol.* **6**, 690.

Smith, W. B., Blenden, D. C., Fuh, T., and Hiler, M. J. (1972). *J. Amer. Vet. Med. Ass.* **161**, 1495.

Sulkin, S. E., Krutzsch, P. H., Allen, R., and Wallis, C. (1959). *J. Exp. Med.* **110**, 369.

Vaughn, J. B., Gerhardt, P., and Newell, K. W. (1965). *J. Amer. Med. Ass.* **193**, 363.

Wright, G. P. (1959). *In* "Modern Trends in Pathology" (D. H. Collins, ed.). Harper (Holber), New York.

CHAPTER 16

Lipotropism in Rabies Virus Infection

S. Edward Sulkin* and Rae Allen

Viral-induced fat necrosis was first reported in early studies on the pathogenesis of certain coxsackieviruses in suckling mice; Pappenheimer and co-workers stated "the most interesting and distinctive lesions in this disease are those of the adipose tissue" (Pappenheimer et al., 1950). These lesions were found mainly in the lobules of embryonic fat (brown adipose tissue) in the cervical, axillary, and interscapular regions. Similar observations were made by other investigators that worked with the same group of viruses (Dalldorf, 1950; Godman et al., 1952). The growth of coxsackievirus in cultured mouse brown fat was accompanied by progressive cytopathic effects (Stulberg et al., 1952). Shortly thereafter, in studies concerned with the enhancing effect of cortisone administration on experimental poliovirus infection in hamsters, reproducible lesions were noted in the brown adipose tissue of animals receiving both hormone and virus (Aronson and Shwartzman, 1956). Focal necrotic lesions were also demonstrated in the brown fat of cynomolgus monkeys inoculated with poliovirus, with or without cortisone treatment (Shwartzman and Aronson, 1954). In both hamsters and monkeys the multiplication of poliovirus in brown adipose tissue preceded involvement of the central nervous system, suggesting to investigators that brown fat served as a prime extraneural site for virus replication during the preparalytic phase of the experimental disease.

The growth of rabies virus in brown adipose tissue was first demonstrated in experimentally infected Mexican free-tailed bats (*Tadarida brasiliensis mexicana*) in the initial phases of studies concerning the possible role of insectivorous bats as reservoir hosts for this agent (Sulkin et al., 1957). At the time of these studies the true

---

* Deceased.

function of brown fat had not been defined, although this tissue had attracted the attention of anatomists, physiologists and biochemists for hundreds of years, and much information had accumulated concerning its gross and microscopic anatomy and biochemical constituents. Brown adipose tissue had been described in many mammalian species and in certain species of bats and other hibernating animals. The interscapular brown fat, being a well-developed organized structure, was called "the hibernating gland" (Rasmussen, 1923). For many years a point of controversy existed as to whether the tissue was simply a reserve of energy necessary to sustain the inactive animal, or whether it functioned in controlling periods of dormancy. This structure, histogenetically distinct from white fat and physiologically more active, had been shown to store glycogen in concentrations comparable with that of the liver (Tuerkischer and Wertheimer, 1942; Wertheimer and Shapiro, 1948; Fawcett, 1952). In addition to being a rich source of certain lipids, brown adipose cells of various animal species were known to contain ascorbic acid, α-amino acids, mucoproteins, water-soluble polysaccharides, glycogen, amine oxidase, cytochrome oxidase, alkaline phosphatase, succinic dehydrogenase, and esterase (Fawcett, 1952; Menschik, 1953; Aronson and Shwartzman, 1956; Remillard, 1958). The tissue was also known to be highly vascularized and to have an abundant nerve supply (Rasmussen, 1923; Fawcett, 1952; Sidman and Fawcett, 1954; Remillard, 1958). Brown fat remains a metabolically active tissue even during hibernation, as indicated by the studies of Hook and Barron (1941), which demonstrated that slices of brown fat incubated at 8°C exhibited greater respiratory activity than did kidney tissue. In a 1959 review of reports concerned with the physiologic function of brown fat, it was concluded that this tissue appeared to be involved in the regulation of body temperature (Johansson, 1959). Evidence that brown fat is, indeed, a thermogenic tissue first appeared in 1961 (Smith, 1961). Since that time many studies have been carried out on the role of brown adipose tissue as a site of nonshivering thermogenesis and a thermogenic effector of arousal in hibernating animals (cf. Smith and Horwitz, 1969; Lindberg, 1970).

Investigators were prompted to look for rabies virus in brown fat because of the high metabolic activity of this tissue and its proposed vital function in connection with periods of dormancy in hibernating animals such as bats. Also, the earlier studies demonstrating the lipotropism of certain coxsackieviruses and polioviruses (Dalldorf, 1950; Pappenheimer *et al.*, 1950; Godman *et al.*, 1952; Stulberg *et al.*, 1952; Shwartzman and Aronson, 1954; Aronson and Shwartzman,

1956) indicated that brown adipose tissue would provide a suitable substrate for virus growth, and might prove to be an important focus of rabies virus infection, (apart from the central nervous system) in the inapparently infected bat.

In the initial studies demonstrating the growth of rabies virus in the interscapular brown fat of Mexican free-tailed bats, little brown bats (*Myotis lucifugus*), and hamsters, a highly neurotropic strain of canine origin was used (Sulkin *et al.*, 1957, 1959). Virus was inoculated intramuscularly and bats were tested for evidence of rabies infection from 2 to 12 weeks postinoculation by the assay of brain, salivary gland, and interscapular brown fat tissue. Although virus was present in brain tissue more frequently than in the other tissues tested, the demonstration of rabies virus in the brown fat of 22% of the infected Mexican free-tailed bats indicated that even this highly neurotropic strain of virus exhibited some affinity for brown adipose tissue. The course of experimental infection was essentially the same in *Myotis* inoculated with this same strain of rabies virus; the frequency of isolation of rabies virus from the brain, brown fat, and salivary glands of infected bats was 92%, 30%, and 17%, respectively. Hamsters proved to be highly susceptible to intramuscular inoculation of this strain of rabies virus, and there was marked lipotropism in this host. In contrast to the lesions induced by multiplication of coxsackievirus in suckling mouse brown fat, no histopathologic alterations were observed in the brown fat of bats or hamsters infected with rabies virus, even though high titers of virus were present in the tissue.

Following the suggestion that interscapular brown adipose tissue could be an important site of rabies virus multiplication in the bat and the demonstration of lipotropic characteristics of a canine strain in experimentally infected bats (Sulkin *et al.*, 1957, 1959), investigators began to look for this virus in the brown fat of bats being examined for evidence of natural rabies infection. The first isolation of rabies virus from the brown fat of a naturally infected bat was reported by Bell and Moore (1960), who recovered the agent from the pooled interscapular tissue from two *Myotis lucifugus* which were obtained in a routine collection, and which exhibited no apparent signs of rabies at the time of sacrifice. Additional early isolations of rabies virus from the brown fat of naturally infected bats have been summarized elsewhere (Sulkin, 1962). Since that time rabies virus has been demonstrated in the brown fat of experimentally infected bats by several investigators (Sulkin and Allen, Chapter 6, Volume II, this treatise) and has been isolated from the brown adipose tissue of naturally infected insectivorous bats in various parts of the United States (Bell et al., 1962, 1966; Girard et al., 1965), in Mexico (Villa-R. and Alvarez-L., 1963), and in Canada (Beauregard, 1969), providing support for the hypothesis that the growth of rabies virus in brown fat may contribute to the ability of these animals to serve as reservoir hosts for this agent.

Information relating to the lipotropism of rabies virus was also obtained during studies done to determine the effect of pregnancy on the susceptibility of Mexican free-tailed bats to inoculation with a canine strain of rabies virus (Sims et al., 1963). Although the susceptibility of the gravid and nongravid bats to experimental infection did not differ significantly, the frequency of isolation of virus from interscapular brown adipose tissue varied among the groups. In groups of bats which received virus during the mid-gestation period and in the early postpartum period, virus was subsequently demonstrated in the brown fat of infected animals with about equal frequency (22% and 17%, respectively). In contrast, rabies virus was isolated from the brown fat tissue of only 2.3% of the infected bats which had received virus late in the gestation period. Moreover, the frequency of isolation of virus from the brown fat of animals in all three gravid groups was less than in the nongravid bats. During the course of these studies differences were noted in the gross appearance of the interscapular brown fat lobes of bats in various stages of the gestation period; the amount of tissue was notably depleted in animals at the time of delivery and in the early postpartum period. Histologic examination of the brown fat of Mexican free-tailed bats throughout the gestation period revealed marked variations in the lipid content of this tissue (Sims et al., 1962). The amount of lipid in the brown fat cells was found to increase as pregnancy progressed, reaching a peak late in the period and decreasing precipitously during and shortly after parturition. The brown fat lobes of bats netted 2–3 weeks after the delivery period had already begun to increase in size, indicating that the observed depletion during parturition is of short duration. Cortisone was found to exert a similar effect on the brown fat of male bats, suggesting that adrenal activity plays an important role in directing alterations in the lipid content of the brown fat of gravid bats.

The results obtained in these studies indicated that fluctuations in the lipid content of brown fat influenced the growth of rabies virus in this tissue, and prompted additional experiments designed to quantitate the effect of lipid deposition on the multiplication of rabies virus in brown fat cells (Sims et al., 1967). Since the canine strain of rabies

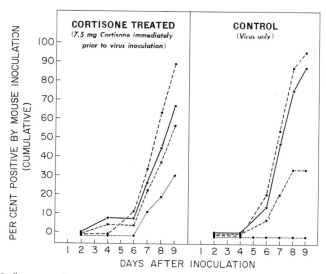

Fig. 1. Influence of cortisone on frequency of demonstration of rabies virus in brown fat (—), brain (--), salivary glands (---) and blood (·····) of hamsters shown to be infected following intramuscular inoculation. (Modified from Sims *et al.*, 1967.)

virus used in previous studies in this series was highly infectious for Syrian hamsters and exhibited marked lipotropic characteristics in this host (Sulkin *et al.*, 1959) and since Aronson and co-workers (1954) had shown that cortisone induced lipid hypertrophy in the interscapular brown fat of hamsters, this model was used in these experiments. It was found that in hamsters experimentally infected with rabies virus, cortisone-induced lipid hypertrophy of the brown fat exerted a suppressive effect on the invasion and multiplication of virus in this tissue (Fig. 1). Although rabies virus was recovered from the brown fat of 67% of the infected cortisone-treated hamsters, the agent was demonstrable in 87% of the animals that received virus alone, and levels of virus were higher in the brown fat of the latter group. In contrast, cortisone treatment appeared to enhance viral invasion of salivary gland tissue. Also, rabies virus was demonstrated in the blood of 30% of the infected cortisone-treated hamsters, whereas viremia was not evident in infected animals which had received virus alone.

The brown fat of normal hamsters is rather compact, composed of cells with dense, granular cytoplasm containing small lipid droplets; white adipose tissue, which often overlies the subscapular region of the brown fat lobes, appears along the periphery (Fig. 2). In-

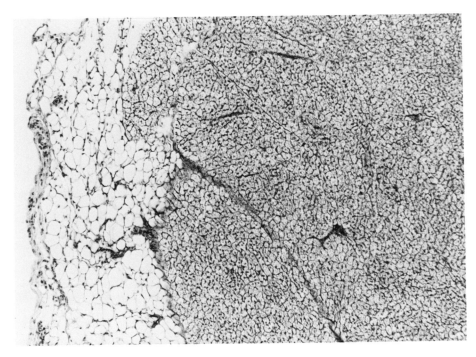

Fig. 2. Microscopic section of the interscapular brown fat of a normal hamster. A portion of the white fat tissue which overlies the brown fat lobes is seen on the left margin of this section. Hematoxylin and eosin, ×85.

tramuscular administration of cortisone results in rapid hypertrophy of brown fat, characterized by increased cell diameter with coalesced lipid vacuoles which tend to displace the nucleus to a peripheral location. Hypertrophied blood vessels were also apparent in the brown fat of cortisone-treated hamsters. In this regard, increased blood flow through the brown fat of cortisone treated rats has been reported (Kuroshima *et al.*, 1968). Sections of infected brown fat from hamsters which received rabies virus alone revealed no evidence of necrosis, hemorrhage, or other signs of histopathology. The tissue remained relatively compact and the amount of lipid in the lobules paralleled that of the normal controls. On the other hand, sections of brown fat from infected animals which had received cortisone in addition to rabies virus revealed marked histologic changes, characterized by progressive lesion formation resulting in large, focal areas of necrosis within the brown fat lobes (Fig. 3). Hypertrophied blood vessels were evident, coursing through lesions, and intimate association between red blood cells and brown fat cells was observed in these areas. The extensive histopathology observed in the brown fat of cortisone-treated hamsters infected with rabies virus would indicate an enhancement of rabies virus growth in this tissue, similar to that reported by Aronson and Shwartzman (1956) for poliovirus in brown fat of cortisone-treated hamsters; instead there was an apparent suppression of viral growth compared to the levels demonstrated in the brown fat of animals receiving virus alone. It was not established whether virus growth was actually suppressed by increased amounts of lipid in brown fat of cortisone-treated hamsters, or whether tissue degeneration may have destroyed some virus.

Each instance of isolation of rabies virus from the blood of cortisone-treated hamsters was correlated with the presence of areas of necrosis and hemorrhage in infected brown fat tissue of the animal. Viremia was not seen in infected hamsters that had not received the hormone and in which infected brown fat appeared histologically normal. The hypertrophied blood vessels and areas of hemorrhage observed in association with lesions in infected brown fat of cor-

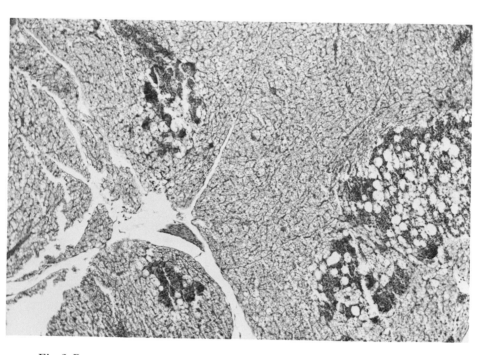

Fig. 3. Representative microscopic section of the brown fat of a hamster 8 days after receiving rabies virus and a single dose of cortisone. Note foci of lesion formation. H & E, ×85.

tisone-treated hamsters suggested that virus from the blood of these animals could have entered the bloodstream as a result of the pathologic condition of the brown adipose tissue. If one assumes that there is a similar histologic picture in the brown fat of gravid Mexican free-tailed bats naturally infected with rabies virus, the possible spillover of virus from brown fat into the blood would increase the chances of transplacental transmission which has been demonstrated in experimentally infected *Tadarida* (Sims *et al.*, 1963).

It has been demonstrated in experimental rabies infection of little brown bats that strains of rabies virus may differ in their lipotropic characteristics (Sulkin *et al.*, 1959); one of the virus isolates inoculated came from the pooled brown fat of naturally infected *Myotis* (Bell and Moore, 1960). This strain exhibited a marked affinity for the interscapular brown fat of bats which became infected following intramuscular inoculation. Virus was demonstrated in the brown fat of 92% of the infected bats, only 50% of which had virus present in brain tissue. Thus the lipotropism of this strain was significantly greater than that of the canine strain used in the same series of experiments. Also, only one bat infected with the lipotropic bat strain developed signs of rabies whereas the neurotropic canine strain induced overt disease in many infected animals (Sulkin *et al.*, 1959, 1960). These strains could also be differentiated on the basis of incubation period and symptomatology in weanling mice, infectivity for intramuscularly inoculated suckling hamsters, infectivity for weanling mice via the oral route, growth in monolayer cultures of brown adipose tissue, and sensitivity to lipid solvents (Sulkin *et al.*, 1960; Sims *et al.*, 1967; Correa-Giron *et al.*, 1970). In a study of the natural differences between these strains of rabies virus, it was found that certain characteristics of the strains could be altered by serial passage through selected tissues of suckling mice (Sims, 1969). Passage of the neurotropic canine strain through brown fat tissue gradually produced a virus line which possessed characteristics similar to the original lipotropic bat strain in that affinity for brown fat was greatly increased, infectivity for cultured brown fat was enhanced, and sensitivity to chloroform was increased significantly. Serial passage of the lipotropic bat strain through brain tissue resulted in a virus strain which showed less affinity for brown fat tissue coupled with an increased neurotropism, was less infective for brown fat *in vitro*, and was less sensitive to chloroform, thus resembling the original neurotropic canine strain of rabies virus. These observations indicate that the growth of rabies virus in different tissues can result in strains which vary in certain characteristics and suggest that during development host cell material is incorporated into the rabies virus virion. It may be concluded that changes in the lipid content or alterations in the type of lipid the virion contains may contribute to certain differences among strains of rabies virus.

The interaction of rabies virus and bat brown adipose tissue cells was studied in more detail in *in vitro* experiments (Allen *et al.*, 1964a,b). The ability of bat brown fat to grow in explant and monolayer cultures could be correlated with seasonal variations in the physiologic activity of this tissue, suggesting that the major portion of the tissue culture populations were derived from brown fat cells rather than from a minority cell type. Also, it was shown that insulin added to the tissue culture medium stimulated the synthesis of glycogen in monolayer cultures of brown adipose tissue, in a manner similar to that reported by Sidman for organ cultures of rat brown fat (Sidman, 1956) and analogous to the action of insulin on brown adipose tissue in the intact animal (Wertheimer, 1945). The strain of rabies virus isolated from the brown fat of naturally infected bats (Bell and Moore, 1960) proved to be infective for cultured brown adipose tissue on first passage; cultures supported the growth of the virus at 37°C for at least 2 months with no observable degenerative changes (Allen *et al.*, 1964a). Rabies virus was demonstrated in the supernatant of cultures by mouse inoculation; the fluorescent antibody technique was used to detect virus antigen in the cells. Infected cultures contained both cells with diffuse fluorescence and cells with more intense fluorescence, the latter appearing in sharply outlined aggregations of various sizes and shapes in the cytoplasm. The aggregations which fluoresced specifically as rabies virus antigen could be stained by the May–Grünwald–Giemsa technique, and then appeared as definite inclusion bodies surrounded by halos. Similar intracytoplasmic inclusion bodies have been observed by other investigators in studies on the growth of rabies virus in a variety of tissue culture systems (Atanasiu and Lépine, 1959; Kissling and Reese, 1963; Love *et al.*, 1964). In a cytochemical study of monolayer cultures of hamster brown fat infected with rabies virus, various staining techniques revealed the presence of ribonucleic acid, protein, and certain protein-bound groups within the inclusion bodies (Leonard *et al.*, 1967). Certain differences observed in the staining of the inclusion bodies and the surrounding cytoplasm indicated that the ribonucleic acid within the inclusions was unlike that of the cytoplasm, and represented either viral ribonucleic acid or altered cytoplasmic ribonucleic acid.

The differences observed in the degree of lipotropism exhibited by the canine and bat strains of rabies virus in the intact bat (Sulkin *et al.*, 1960) was reflected in a comparison of the infectivity of these two strains for cultured brown fat (Sims, 1969). Cultures infected with the bat strain exhibited specific fluorescence in 90–100% of the cells, often in the form of large, bizarre shaped inclusion bodies, whereas only about 10% of the cells in cultures infected with the canine strain showed evidence of infection consisting of small, discrete, intracytoplasmic inclusion bodies. The respective infectivity of these two strains of rabies virus for cultured brown adipose tissue could be reversed by serial passage of the bat strain through the brains of suckling mice, and by adaptation of the canine strain to growth in mouse brown fat *in vivo* (Sims, 1969).

Since it was found that explant and monolayer cultures of bat brown fat could be stored for prolonged periods at 8°C, the persistence of rabies virus in this tissue culture system at low temperature was studied. Previous studies had shown that rabies virus multiplies at a very slow rate or not at all in bats maintained in simulated hibernation, but the virus remains viable in this suppressed state for weeks or even months, and multiplication is initiated or increased when the animals are transferred to a warmer environment (Sulkin *et al.*, 1960). Determination of specific sites of rabies virus sequestration in the hibernating bat was difficult, since virus could be detected in only a small percentage of inoculated animals sacrificed from the cold. *In vitro* models of rabies virus infection in bat brown fat subjected to long periods at low temperature provided evidence that this tissue might sustain this agent in the hibernating bat (Allen *et al.*, 1964b). Cultures of brown fat retained rabies virus infection for more than 4 months at 8°C, supporting the hypothesis that rabies virus particles present in the interscapular brown adipose tissue of the intact bat would remain viable throughout periods of hibernation. Conclusive evidence of virus multiplication at 8°C was not obtained, although there was a suggestion that some level of viral activity was maintained in the cold. Transfer of infected cultures from 8° to 37°C resulted in rapid virus multiplication. Since the brown fat of the bat has been shown to function in producing the heat necessary for arousal from hibernation (Smith and Horwitz, 1969), it is suggested that the metabolic activity associated with thermogenesis, together with the resultant increase in body temperature, would serve to activate dormant rabies virus particles in this tissue.

Since the initial observations on the growth of coxsackieviruses, polioviruses, and rabies virus in brown adipose tissue, investigators have shown increasing interest in the lipotropic characteristics of neurotropic viruses. Additional studies have explored the growth of Group B coxsackieviruses in brown fat of ground squirrels, bats, and mice, and have included experiments concerning the influence of cold exposure on virus-induced necrosis in this tissue (Grodums and Dempster, 1959, 1962, 1970; Dempster *et al.*, 1961). Studies on the role of bats in the epidemiology of certain arboviruses have demonstrated the presence of these agents in brown adipose tissue of experimentally and naturally infected bats, and the growth of a variety of other viruses in bat brown fat *in vivo* and *in vitro* has also been reported (cf. Sulkin and Allen, 1974).

Acknowledgment

Studies conducted in the authors' laboratory were supported by USPHS Grant AI02316 and NSF Grant GB-12611.

References

Allen, R., Sims, R. A., and Sulkin, S. E. (1964a). *Amer. J. Hyg.* **80**, 11.

Allen, R., Sims, R. A., and Sulkin, S. E. (1964b). *Amer. J. Hyg.* **80**, 25.

Aronson, S. M., and Shwartzman, G. (1956). *Amer. J. Pathol.* **32**, 315.

Aronson, S. M., Teodoru, C. V., Adler, M., and Shwartzman, G. (1954). *Proc. Soc. Exp. Biol. Med.* **85**, 214.

Atanasiu, P., and Lépine, P. (1959). *Ann. Inst. Pasteur, Paris* **96**, 72.

Beauregard, M. (1969). *Can. J. Comp. Med.* **33**, 220.

Bell, J. F., and Moore, G. J. (1960). *Proc. Soc. Exp. Biol. Med.* **103**, 140.

Bell, J. F., Moore, G. J., Raymond, G. H., and Tibbs, C. E. (1962). *Amer. J. Pub. Health* **52**, 1293.

Bell, J. F., Lodmell, D. L., Moore, G. J., and Raymond, G. H. (1966). *Pub. Health Rep.* **81**, 761.

Correa-Giron, E. P., Allen, R., and Sulkin, S. E. (1970). *Amer. J. Epidemiol.* **91**, 203.

Dalldorf, G. (1950). *Bull. N. Y. Acad. Med.* **26**, 329.

Dempster, G., Grodums, E. I., and Spencer, W. A. (1961). *Can. J. Microbiol.* **7**, 587.

Fawcett, D. W. (1952). *J. Morphol.* **90**, 363.

Girard, K. F., Hitchcock, H. B., Edsall, G., and MacCready, R. A. (1965). *N. Engl. J. Med.* **272**, 75.

Godman, G. C., Bunting, H., and Melnick, J. L. (1952). *Amer. J. Pathol.* **28**, 223.

Grodums, E. I., and Dempster, G. (1959). *Can. J. Microbiol.* **5**, 595.

Grodums, E. I., and Dempster, G. (1962). *Can. J. Microbiol.* **8**, 105.

Grodums, E. I., and Dempster, G. (1970). *Can. J. Microbiol.* **16**, 833.

Hook, W. E., and Barron, E. S. G. (1941). *Amer. J. Physiol.* **133**, 56.

Johansson, B. (1959). *Metab., Clin. Exp.* **8**, 221.

Kissling, R. E., and Reese, D. R. (1963). *J. Immunol.* **91**, 362.

Kuroshima, A., Konno, N., Doi, K., and Itoh, S. (1968). *Jap. J. Physiol.* **18**, 446.

Leonard, L. L., Allen, R., and Sulkin, S. E. (1967). *J. Infec. Dis.* **117**, 121.

Lindberg, O., ed. (1970). "Brown Adipose Tissue." Amer. Elsevier, New York.
Love, R., Fernandes, M. V., and Koprowski, H. (1964). Proc. Soc. Exp. Biol. Med. 116, 560.
Menschik, Z. (1953). Anat. Rec. 116, 439.
Pappenheimer, A. M., Daniels, J. B., Cheever, F. S., and Weller, T. H. (1950). J. Exp. Med. 92, 169.
Rasmussen, A. T. (1923). J. Morphol. 38, 147.
Remillard, G. (1958). Ann. N. Y. Acad. Sci. 72, 3.
Shwartzman, G., and Aronson, S. M. (1954). Proc. Soc. Exp. Biol. Med. 86, 767.
Sidman, R. L. (1956). Anat. Rec. 124, 723.
Sidman, R. L., and Fawcett, D. W. (1954). Anat. Rec. 118, 487.
Sims, R. A., Allen, R., and Sulkin, S. E. (1962). Proc. Soc. Exp. Biol. Med. 111, 455.
Sims, R. A., Allen, R., and Sulkin, S. E. (1963). J. Infec. Dis. 112, 17.
Sims, R. A., Allen, R., and Sulkin, S. E. (1967). J. Infec. Dis. 117, 360.
Sims, R., (1969). Ph. D. Diss. The University of Texas Southwestern Medical School, Dallas, Texas.
Smith, R. E. (1961). Physiologist 4, 113.
Smith, R. E., and Horwitz, B. A. (1969). Physiol. Rev. 49, 330.
Stulberg, C. S., Schapira, R., and Eidam, C. R. (1952). Proc. Soc. Exp. Biol. Med. 81, 642.
Sulkin, S. E. (1962). Progr. Med. Virol. 4, 157.
Sulkin, S. E., and Allen, R. (1974). "Viral Infections in Chiroptera," Monogr. Virol. Vol. 8, Karger, Basel.
Sulkin, S. E., Krutzsch, P. H., Wallis, C., and Allen, R. (1957). Proc. Soc. Exp. Biol. Med. 96, 461.
Sulkin, S. E., Krutzsch, P. H., Allen, R., and Wallis, C. (1959). J. Exp. Med. 110, 369.
Sulkin, S. E., Allen, R., Sims, R. A., Krutzsch, P. H., and Kim, C. (1960). J. Exp. Med. 112, 595.
Tuerkischer, E., and Wertheimer, E. (1942). J. Physiol. (London) 100, 385.
Villa-R., B., and Alvarez-L., B. (1963). Zoonoses Res. 2, 77.
Wertheimer, E. (1945). J. Physiol. (London) 103, 359.
Wertheimer, E., and Shapiro, B. (1948). Physiol. Rev. 20, 451.

CHAPTER 17

Latency and Abortive Rabies

J. Frederick Bell

I. Definition and Historical Background

I shall use the term "infection" in the broad sense of mere presence of virus as suggested by McDermott (1961); "'latent infection' is reserved for situations in which the presence of the microbes cannot be demonstrated by any method now available, and the fact that infection is present can only be demonstrated in retrospect by the emergence of overt disease. . . ." (McDermott, 1959). "Abortion" will refer to cessation of adverse effects of virus upon the host. La-

331

tency and abortion are not always clearly distinguishable from masked, inapparent, chronic, and recrudescent infection, eclipse, long incubation periods, and the carrier state (Walker *et al.*, 1958).

In 1762 Layard remonstrated against the practice of euthanasia as a reaction to the assumed hopelessness of rabies infection in man and "went to some pains to try to prove that clinical cases need not necessarily prove fatal" (Pugh, 1962). Pasteur, in 1882, stated uniquivocally that dogs can sicken and recover from rabies. In 1930, Koch betrayed some exasperation that the idea of the certainty of death from rabies continued to be held: "In spite of the fact that Pasteur had already observed . . . that dogs can sicken and recover from rabies, there occurs in the literature a curious agreement in the views on the 'unhealability' of rabies." Since that time much additional information on recovery from rabies has been published (see reviews by Martin, 1963; Bell, 1966; Kraut, 1966; Nilssen, 1970). Nevertheless, the orthodox concept of inexorable death from rabies still has widespread popularity, and claims for recovery thus need to be exceptionally well documented to be convincing. Unfortunately, the severe classic case of rabies is the one most likely to be correctly diagnosed, especially where the disease is uncommon, and is probably the one most likely to end fatally. Even in an area where rabies is common, diagnosis is often made postmortem or retrospectively (Sanmartín *et al.*, 1967). Moreover, as has been emphasized repeatedly (e.g., Hurst and Pawan, 1932; Shiraki *et al.*, 1962), differential diagnosis between rabies and postvaccinal encephalitis in humans is most difficult; the presence of rabies antibodies in both conditions adds to the difficulties. "Spontaneous" occurrences of the syndromes of Landry-Guillain Barré, multiple sclerosis, and even "psychopathological syndromes" (Neves, 1970) in a population must also be differentiated. Because of the *a priori* conclusion that rabies is always fatal after a short illness, survival or long illness have been considered adequate bases for elimination of rabies in differential diagnosis (Waterman, 1959; Cereghino *et al.*, 1970).

Although Cereghino *et al.* (1970) state that "There are no readily available reliable tests for the diagnosis of rabies in the human prior to death," recent developments afford techniques that have been reliable in animals, and should be equally applicable to man retrospectively (Bell *et al.*, 1972) and during active infection (Schneider, 1969a).

II. Criteria and Evidence

A. LATENCY

The incubation period of rabies, especially the occasional very long incubation period, could be considered as latency as defined by McDermott (1959). Characteristically, incubation periods of rabies are extremely variable with reliable records of more than 7 months in a naturally infected bat (Moore and Raymond, 1970), 611 days in an experimentally infected cow (Abelseth and Lawson, 1972), minimum periods of more than 4 months in 7 of 30 quarantined dogs (Hole, 1969), and as long as 120 days in experimentally infected mice (Baer and Cleary, 1972). In the infected mice, amputation of the inoculated limb—even up to the eighteenth day after inoculation—significantly lowered mortality, and it seems fair to infer from those data that virus may remain infective at or near the site of inoculation during long incubation periods. Many long incubation periods, some much longer but perhaps less well documented, especially in man, have been recorded (see reviews by Dean, 1963; Wang, 1956; Lépine, 1951). Paresthesia limited to the inoculation site, a common premonitory symptom even after long incubation periods, and first paralysis in inoculated limbs, must also imply that the infecting virus remained during that period either at the site of inoculation or somewhere in the innervating tract. Evidence for virus in "eclipse" was obtained by Baer *et al.* (1965) who elicited antibody formation in rats injected with sciatic nerves taken from limbs of other rats 48 hours after inoculation; it was not until 72 hours that viable virus could be demonstrated in the nerves of rats given a similar virus dose. Wiktor *et al.* (1972) interpreted their observations of persistent degeneration of the nerve accompanied by Schwann cell proliferation in monoplegic mice a year or more after onset of illness as a persistent active infectious process even though no virus could be isolated. The authors did not attempt to demonstrate hypergammaglobulinemia or persistent high levels of antibody which might be expected to occur with chronic infection.

Presumably some of the inoculum is removed by lymphatic drainage (Dean *et al.*, 1963a), but there is no good evidence to indicate that virus can remain latent in lymph nodes, visceral sites such as liver and spleen, or in nerve cells as does herpesvirus (Stevens and Cook, 1971), and then be mobilized to produce infection.

Although Sulkin *et al.* (1957) believe that "brown fat may serve as a depot for the storage of virus . . . ," Fischman and Schaeffer (1971) opine that "the reported isolations of rabies virus from brown-fat tissue may represent merely a manifestation of the centrifugal neural spread of virus to brown-fat tissue because of its proximity to spinal nerves rather than any special predilection for virus growth in such tissue."

Baer and Cleary (1972) concluded that strictly localized peripheral infections may occur under certain conditions, and Murphy *et al.* (1973) demonstrated increase of rabies virus antigen in myocytes at the site of inoculation in 4-day-old Syrian hamsters 36 to 40 hours after injection of virus isolated from a vampire bat. Extrapolation of the findings in neonatal hamsters to events in other systems may not yet be justified. Krause (1966) and Webb (1969) believe that peripheral propagation is always a necessary antecedent to CNS invasion, a view not commonly held.

B. BREAK OF LATENCY (ACTIVATION)

The prolonged period sometimes noted between exposure and onset of clinical rabies may be due to latency at the site of inoculation (Baer and Cleary, 1972) rather than indolent progressive "slow virus" infection. Late occurrence of rabies probably also differs from the "reactivated" infections of herpes simplex and herpes zoster, although relapse or recurrence (reactivation) of signs of rabies has been reported (Pasteur, 1882; Webster, 1937; Thiery, 1960), and Lépine (1951) states that "In those cases which incubate for more than 70 days, the virus persists in the brain in a latent state of development. . . ." There is little evidence (other than reports of "carrier states") that a tolerated, persistent infection may occur as in lymphocytic choriomeningitis (Traub, 1936).

Apparent reactivation of rabies occurred in a cat that suffered paresis and partial paralysis in the hind legs after experimental infection with low-passage virus of bat origin (Bell, J. F. and Moore, G. J., unpublished). About 10 weeks after onset of illness the neutralizing antibody titers in serum and CSF were 1920 and 256 respectively, and the disability seemed stabilized. Subsequently the serum and CSF titers dropped as low as 1024 and 140, but the decrease was followed by a gradual increase in both titers to maximums of 8960 and 1120, respectively. Because of steadily deteriorating condition the cat was killed 126 weeks after inoculation. Postmortem studies have not yet been completed.

The mechanisms of activation of infection are as obscure as the status of the virus during latency. Soave *et al.* (1961) reported "reactivation" of infection by repeated inoculations of ACTH in one of six guinea pigs that had survived inoculation of street virus 5 months earlier. Similarly, when guinea pigs were treated with corticosteroid, Soave (1964) again reported "reactivation" of infection in 1 of 10 guinea pigs 8½ months after inoculation (attributed to the stress of crowding). But an even longer incubation period in a guinea pig (373 days) was reported by Nilssen (1968), without cortisone administration or crowding. Moore and Raymond (1970) noted an incubation period of at least 209 days in a naturally infected bat kept under uniform conditions. Koprowski (1952) mentions that bacterial pneumonia has been held responsible for activation of rabies in man, and Lépine (1951) states that "any adjuvant conditions such as central nervous disease, trauma or toxic action may convert a latent case of rabies into an active one or may appreciably shorten the incubation period."

Brown fat has been incriminated as a storage site for rabies virus in bats (Sulkin *et al.,* 1957) and it was theorized that because gravid bats are more susceptible to infection than nongravid animals, activation of virus from a latent state in brown fat may occur during pregnancy (Sulkin *et al.,* 1957). Sulkin (1962) also suggests that latent virus may be aroused by fluctuations of ambient temperatures during hibernation which, it should be noted, is not a constant state of dormancy (Bell *et al.,* 1966b).

C. NONFATAL RABIES

To document recovery from rabies it is necessary to establish that active rabies infection has occurred. Circumstantial evidence can be convincing when large numbers of animals are inoculated and some become ill and die, whereas others, with simultaneous and identical signs of illness, recover and survive (Jacotot and Nguyen-Dinh-Lam, 1947; Crandell, 1965). Confirmatory evidence of several kinds is, nevertheless, desirable.

Pasteur (1882) considered resistance to reinoculation a strong indication of previous abortive infection; others have used the same technique for confirmation (Remlinger and Bailly, 1941; Martin, 1963). We also consider it good evidence, but only when the challenge inoculum is into the central nervous system (CNS), since peripheral inoculation often gives irregular results. When such tests are done, it is essential to use control animals identical in respect to age and other characteristics with the test animals because of rapid increase of resistance to peripheral inoculation with age (Casals, 1940; Dean *et al.*, 1963b; Bell, 1966). It is also essential to realize that the antigenic stimulus of the primary inoculation may make the test animals less vulnerable than the control animals, even though the former have not suffered active infection.

Perhaps the most commonly used criterion of nonfatal infection is the isolation of virus from saliva, brain, or other tissues of animals that appear normal, yet it should be emphasized that virus may be present in the CNS and salivary glands well before onset of illness (Wright, 1956; Schneider, 1969a), and isolation of virus from saliva of normal appearing animals is significant only when the animals can be held for observation to see whether they will die — and this has been done repeatedly (see reviews by Van Rooyen and Rhodes, 1940b; Martin, 1963; Bell, 1966; Bell *et al.*, 1971). Virus has been found in saliva of dogs 3 days (Vaughn *et al.*, 1965) and of skunks 5 days (Sikes, 1962) before onset of illness in experimentally infected animals. Konradi (1916) stated that a dog bite may be infectious as long as 14 days before appearance of signs of illness, and Jonnesco and Teodasiu (1928) isolated virus from saliva 7 days before appearance of signs of illness. Baer and Bales (1967) isolated virus from the saliva of an experimentally infected bat 12 days before onset of signs, and Bell *et al.* (1969) demonstrated transmission of rabies by bite of a naturally infected bat 24 days before its death. Virus was present in the brain and brown fat but not in the salivary glands at death; neutralizing antibody, however, could not be demonstrated in any tissue tested. Nevertheless, Delpietro *et al.* (1972) isolated rabies virus from saliva and brown fat of two vampire bats that did not have demonstrable virus in the brain; this finding warrants confirmation and clarification.

Biopsies of both salivary glands and brain tissue for virus isolation have been taken to confirm a diagnosis in human patients who have survived apparent rabies infection (Hattwick *et al.*, 1972). Apart from the rigor of the operation, advisability of the procedure is questionable because virus is not likely to be isolated from either tissue late in infection (Levaditi *et al.*, 1928); a brain tissue neutralization test has, however, been shown to be of diagnostic value for demonstration of past CNS infection in animals (Bell *et al.*, 1966a). But that test can be done as well on the more easily obtained cerebrospinal fluid (CSF) (Bell *et al.*, 1972). It should be emphasized that rabies antigen can often be detected in brain after isolation of virus is no longer possible (Lodmell *et al.*, 1969) and in this regard frozen tissue sections appear to be better than smears for the fluorescent antibody (FA) technique, probably because the interfering CNS antibody has less opportunity to react with the antigen (Atanasiu *et al.*, 1970).

Antibodies in sera of trapped or killed wild animals have been found more commonly in enzootic than in noninfected areas (Scatterday, 1954; Burns *et al.*, 1956; Sikes, 1962; Constantine *et al.*, 1968b; Sodja *et al.*, 1971; Delpietro *et al.*, 1974). But rabies virus neutralization by serum is not always attributable to antibodies, and nonspecific virus-neutralizing substances, clearly not the result of prior or current rabies infection, have been found in the blood of apparently normal animals of several species (Steele, 1965; Ercegovac and Pima-Kostoglou, 1968; Veeraraghavan, 1965). Theoretically, at least, neutralizing antibodies could occur as a result of infection by known or as yet unidentified related viruses (Shope *et al.*, 1970). Another antiviral substance, interferon, can be found in mouse blood and brain with peaks at 10 hours and 3 or 4 days, respectively, after intracerebral (i.c.) inoculation of attenuated rabies virus (Wiktor *et al.*, 1972).

In our experience, presence of CNS antibodies (Kubes and Gallia, 1943) in high titer, and without demonstrable virus or virus antigen, has been reliable evidence of prior rabies encephalitis (Bell *et al.*, 1966a). Specific antibody in brain has been found in other virus infections of the CNS (Fox, 1943; Payne *et al.*, 1969) and in CNS syphilis (Duncan and Kuhn, 1972), and Theiler (1937) found that resistance to mouse poliovirus given i.c. was contingent on prior development of viral encephalitis.

Abortive rabies has been demonstrated most frequently in white mice (Jenkins and Wamberg, 1960; Bell, 1964; Crandell, 1965; Bell *et al.*, 1966a), although signs of illness are at times difficult to assess in that species. For statistical purposes, in our experiments a mouse that does not die in the first 10 days after onset is considered a "survivor-cum-sequelae" (SCS; Fig. 1), while mice that do not show signs of illness within a month after inoculation are called "normal survivors" (NS; Bell, 1964). As a test of the validity of diagnosis, mice in NS and SCS groups, as well as previously uninoculated mice, are given i.c. inoculations of about 10^3 or 10^4 LD_{50} of fixed virus. Results of challenge of these mice as well as controls (in the 10 most recent experiments) were as follows: All of 354 previously uninoculated mice, 998 of 1048 NS mice, but only 18 of 125 SCS mice died. The difference in mortality between NS (95%) and SCS (14%) groups is highly significant. Resistance to challenge of 5% of

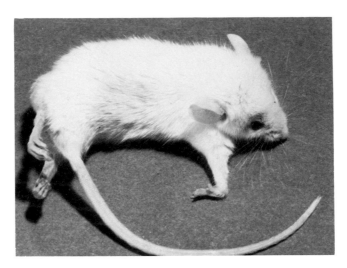

Fig. 1. Residual paralysis 1 month after onset of experimental rabies in a mouse.

NS mice is ascribed to subclinical primary infection, i.e., abortion of infection short of patency; susceptibility of 14% of SCS mice is ascribed to overzealous diagnosis, such as selection because of ruffled fur.

Previously, we had demonstrated good correlation between high titers of neutralizing antibodies in the CNS and resistance to i.c. challenge (Bell *et al.*, 1966a), and, therefore, those tests are considered of equal value as confirmatory criteria of abortive rabies.

Stamm *et al.* (1956) found Negri bodies in the brain of a bat that survived experimental inoculation and Cytoplasmic inclusions with microstructure compatible with Negri bodies have been identified in the brains of paralyzed mice one and one-half years after abortive infections (Perl *et al.*, 1975).

D. RECOVERY

Our impression gained from observation of mice with abortive rabies had been that recovery from paralysis, especially severe paralysis, does not occur in mice (Fig. 1). However, recovery from paralysis to a normal state has been reported in dogs (Johnson, 1948), mules (Badiali and Abou-Youssef, 1968; Ferris *et al.*, 1968), insectivorous bats (Constantine, 1967), and man (Hattwick *et al.*, 1972). We have subsequently seen essentially complete recovery in five experimentally inoculated dogs (Bell *et al.*, 1971, 1972), and survival of a cat with minor sequelae (J. F. Bell and G. J. Moore, unpublished). Crandell (1965) inoculated "Arctic" street virus i.c. into rabbits, and one animal survived with paralysis for months after onset of acute illness. Wiktor *et al.* (1972) believe that "permanent monoplegia, paraplegia or quadriplegia" is evidence of chronic infection of the CNS "in a way similar to that by which other neurotropic agents become involved in the so-called slow virus diseases." However, in our experience, paralysis of limbs is not progressive; mice either die of the infection or reach a rather steady state of paralysis within 10 days after onset (Fig. 1).

In the present state of knowledge of pathogenesis of rabies, conclusions regarding the cause of paralysis and recovery from paralysis are largely stochastic. Hummeler and Koprowski (1969) state "rabies infected neurones seem to remain structurally intact, and, in the absence of neuronolysis and neuronophagia, it is difficult to understand the nature of the damage inflicted on a cell by rabies." Miyamoto and Matsumoto (1967) found that nerve cells infected with street virus appear relatively well preserved, whereas a variety of signs of degeneration were seen in neurons undergoing fixed virus infection. Johnson (1965) also refers to the paucity of neuronophagia and absence of cytopathogenic effect of cell lysis in mouse brain. If the structure remains completely intact recovery of function could be expected, but others (Johnson, 1952; Thiery, 1960; Lépine, 1961; see Van Rooyen and Rhodes, 1940a) describe neuronophagia as concomitant to rabies encephalitis. Atanasiu (1970) suggests that neuronal damage, when it occurs, is a result not of virus growth but of the immune reaction as described in lymphocytic choriomeningitis and herpes infections (Oldstone and Dixon, 1970; Brier *et al.*, 1971) and in rabies-infected cells in tissue culture (Wiktor *et al.*, 1968). Thus the lack of neuronophagia noted by Johnson (1965) might be attributable to failure of the immature mice to mount appreciable immune reaction in the "race between virus and host defenses" (Nathanson and Cole, 1970). Formation of new connections as described by Wall and Egger (1971) could also explain reestablishment of function.

However, an assumption that paralysis is a direct result of infection of the respective innervating neurons may not be valid (Johnson, 1965). It is possible, instead, that temporary dysfunction may at times be a manifestation of allergic edema that extends to the area or areas adjacent to infected cells (Schneider, 1969b), a phenomenon that can be observed best in superficial virus infections such as vaccinia (Roberts, 1962). As infection subsided, edema would be reduced and cells entrained in those reactions, but not infected, might recover quickly and fully.

III. Mechanisms of Abortion

In a review of mechanisms of recovery from viral infection, Baron (1963) in accordance with Lwoff (1959), concluded that "If . . . virus does succeed in establishing an infection within an organ . . . the mechanism by which recovery occurs appears to be nonimmunological. Some of the individual factors which comprise the nonimmune recovery mechanisms are interferon, the febrile response, and local acidity and low oxygen tension caused by the inflammatory reaction."

A. FEVER

The yield of rabies virus in tissue culture is consistently higher at 33°C than at 37°C (Kissling and Reese, 1963), and inactivation of rabies virus in tissue culture fluid occurs rapidly at 37°C (Depoux, 1964). The temperature is usually raised in human rabies, "especially before death" (Van Rooyen and Rhodes, 1940a), and it is rational to assume some inimical effect of pyrexia upon survival of virus. J. F. Bell and G. J. Moore (1974) found that temperatures of mice at onset of illness were lower than normal. Increased body temperature in a high thermic ambience (35°C) during the incubation period was associated with decreased mortality, frequent abortive infections, and delayed onset; but exposure to high ambient temperature after onset of patent illness did not affect the course of the disease. In poikilothermic bats, Sadler and Enright (1959) noted nil mortality at 4°C as compared with 82% and 79% at 22° and 37°C, respectively. Incubation periods were shortened at 37°C. They concluded that daily hibernation does not play a role in survival of the animals but that prolonged seasonal hibernation may do so. Experimentally, Sulkin (1962) demonstrated quiescence of infection in brown fat of bats in hibernation, and progressive infection upon their awakening. His data also suggest that an initial period of latency results in a higher percentage of salivary glands infected.

B. INTERFERON

Rabies virus evokes interferon in the CNS as well as in somatic organs (Stewart and Sulkin, 1966). Protection from rabies by interferon has been inferred from the increased survival of rabbits inoculated with either poly I–poly C (Fenje and Postic, 1970) or bovine parainfluenza #3 virus (Fayaz *et al.*, 1970), at suitable intervals before or after inoculation of rabies virus. Fenje and Postic (1970) entertained the possibility that potentiation of the immune response may have accounted for the results with poly I–poly C. Recent evidence (Wiktor *et al.*, 1972) indicates that interferon elicited by i.c. inoculation of attenuated rabies virus can cause abortion of infection by virulent street virus at the stage of ascent of the nerve. This subject is discussed in detail in Chapter 18.

C. ANTIBODIES

If, in spite of contrary opinion (Lwoff, 1959; Baron, 1963), we grant that specific immune mechanisms may play a part in aborting infections, they could, theoretically, be divided into three categories: cellular, humoral, and cell mediated (delayed hypersensitivity).

When rabies antiserum is given to experimental animals after virus inoculation, it may either hold the virus in abeyance or it may completely inactivate the virus. We have tried to activate possible latent infections by X-ray treatments and by single injections of cortisone into inoculated mice resistant to infection because of maternal antibodies. Patent infections did not develop (Bell *et al.*, 1965, 1970) and virus could not be demonstrated by blind passage (Bell *et al.*, 1965). However, Baer and Cleary (1972) have demonstrated that passive antibody can mask the virus or cause temporary latency with later spontaneous activation similar to that occurring in canine hepatitis (also called fox encephalitis; Green *et al.*, 1935). Bindrich and Schmidt (1958) were convinced, as a result of their experiments, that vaccination is conducive to development of a carrier state in dogs, but we (Bell *et al.*, 1971, 1972) could not find a carrier form of infection in more than 500 intensively studied dogs in an enzootic area in Argentina where large numbers of dogs were vaccinated and prevalence of the disease was declining.

Buchnev and Nikolaeva (cited by Buchnev, 1960) claimed to have prevented appearance of signs of illness and effected a "cure" after onset in dogs experimentally infected and then given massive doses of serum intracerebrally, and Koprowski (1966) states that antiserum given at any time after exposure is therapeutically effective. In at least 5 published articles persons are reported to have survived clinically diagnosed and laboratory-proven rabies, presumably as a result of blood transfusions from donors recently immunized against rabies (Kraut, 1966). However, Gonzalez *et al.* (1956), adduced no evidence of therapeutic efficacy of hyperimmune serum inoculated into the carotid arteries and intrathecally in five rabies patients, and a preponderance of evidence (Chapter 10) indicates that rabies virus is secure once it enters the nerve on its way to the CNS.

Regardless of whether active and progressive infections occur in systems other than the CNS, it is the outcome of the race between infectious encephalomyelitis and host defense (Nathanson and Cole, 1970) that probably determines life or death of the host. Levaditi *et al.* (1928) were the first to report a condition in which the host would die, obviously of rabies or other infectious encephalitis, but virus could not be isolated from the CNS (autosterilization). In the light of results of subsequent studies (Kubes and Gallia, 1943; Constantinescu and Birzu, 1958; Wilsnack and Parker, 1966; Bell *et al.*, 1966a; Lodmell *et al.*, 1969), that phenomenon can be interpreted as due to reaction of antibodies with virus in the CNS, i.e., *in vivo* neutralization of virus at a late stage of pathogenesis. In fact, there is a possibility, if not a likelihood, that the immune reaction to infection, rather than the infection itself, may at times be detrimental or even fatal (Koprowski and Cox, 1948; Bell, 1966; Nathanson and Cole, 1970; Clark and Koprowski, 1971).

Antibodies may be found in serum on the first day of patency (Bell, 1966; Lodmell *et al.*, 1969), but their presence prior to onset is more difficult to substantiate, especially in naturally infected animals. That is, however, a possible explanation of the occurrence of antibodies in normal appearing animals (Sikes, 1962; Johnson, 1964; Ercegovac and Pima-Kostoglou, 1968).

In recovered animals, titers of serum-neutralizing antibodies gradually rise to high levels and are consistently high (Bell *et al.*, 1971, 1972), whereas in those that have received an identical inoculum of street virus without ensuing patent infection, high titers are the exception (Bell *et al.*, 1966a; Lodmell *et al.*, 1969). We construe those observations to signify that, under the conditions extant, little or no proliferation of virus (i.e., active infection and antigenic stimulation) takes place in adult animals outside the CNS prior to infection of that system.

High serum-neutralizing antibody titers from peripheral vaccination with either live or killed rabies vaccines are not accompanied by high titers in the CNS (Kubes and Gallia, 1943; Wilsnack and Parker, 1966; Bell *et al.*, 1966a). Lodmell *et al.* (1969) noted a decreasing titer of virus in the brains of rabid mice for about 5–7 days after onset of illness. Thereafter antibody appeared and increased in the CNS, but viable virus could not be found. However, intracellular antigen could be found even up to a few days later when brain sections were stained by the FA technique. Moreover, at the time of transition, CNS antibody in low titer could be demonstrated in the presence of viable virus, and conversely, virus could be isolated in the presence of appreciable titers of neutralizing antibody by special techniques (Bell *et al.*, 1966a). Decrease of virus as antibody increases does not necessarily imply a cause and effect relationship, although solid long-term resistance to intracerebral challenge after infection (Bell *et al.*, 1966a) would seem to be explainable best on that basis.

Appearance of rabies antibody in brain parenchyma lags several days behind its appearance in the blood of experimentally infected mice, but the final titers are high and more or less equivalent (Lodmell *et al.*, 1969). Since both lymphocytes and plasma cells are abundant in the brains of surviving animals (Schindler, 1961; Shiraki *et al.*, 1962) local antibody production certainly appears possible.

It is noteworthy that, once established, titers of antibody in the CNS remain high for very long periods (Bell *et al.*, 1966a), similar to titers in the blood of recovered animals. The parallel decline of titers in the CNS and in the serum (Bell *et al.*, 1966a) suggests that antibodies produced in the CNS are "leaked" into the circulation (Paterson, 1966), but it has been established (Schneider, 1969a; Fischman and Schaeffer, 1971) that virus is also being propagated peripherally in later stages of infection.

We have found that all of the *in vitro* virus-neutralizing capacity of brain tissue can quite easily be eluted in the cell-free state (Bell *et al.*, 1966a); furthermore, the CSF titer approximates that of brain eluate (Bell *et al.*, 1971), and the popular concept of a few years ago that immune mechanisms had little to do with recovery from primary virus infection is thus succumbing to evidence to the contrary (Nathanson and Cole, 1970, 1971).

Wilsnack and Parker (1966) demonstrated a rabies-inhibiting substance (RIS) in brains and salivary glands of foxes and skunks dying of rabies. We consider RIS identical to neutralizing antibody in the CNS (Lodmell *et al.*, 1969). Failure of RIS to interfere with immunofluorescence (Wilsnack and Parker, 1966) can be explained by the fact that adequate conditions for reaction of antibody and antigen do not ordinarily occur when brain tissue smears are made and quickly fixed or dried, or when frozen sections are prepared.

Perl *et al.* (1975) recently adduced evidence that abortion of rabies infection may occur at the level of the spinal ganglion. In mice inoculated in the footpad, some survived with residual spastic paralysis of the limb. At necropsy about a year later Negri bodies and vacuolization of neurons were found in the dorsal spinal ganglia. Failure of CNS invasion is suggested by the fact that brain antibody titers were very much lower than serum titers.

D. OTHER FACTORS (INTERFERENCE)

A novel mechanism of abortion of infection has been suggested by Johnson (1964) who states that virus may be "neutralized" *in vivo* by inactive virus. Autointerference by rabies virus in tissue culture (Yoshino, 1966) and *in vivo* (Wiktor *et al.*, 1972) has been demonstrated. Infection by another virus (vaccinia) has been shown to interfere with street virus infection (Vieuchange, 1961).

Johnson (1964) also suggests that antibodies elicited in response to "related myxoviruses" may be responsible for amelioration of rabies infection. Viruses serologically related to rabies virus have been discovered recently in Africa (Shope *et al.*, 1970) and Europe (Sodja *et al.*, 1971) (see Chapter 8).

IV. Conditions Conducive to Nonfatal Infection

There are few facts known about the causes of naturally occurring nonfatal rabies infections. Bell (1964), Constantine *et al.* (1968a), and Correa-Giron *et al.* (1970) have noted the lack of correlation between intracerebral titers of virus and their invasiveness by peripheral routes. Constantine (1971) believes that strains of very different lethality have evolved by natural selection in various kinds of mammals, even within the order Chiroptera. Johnson (1966) obtained naturally "attenuated" virus from a striped skunk; adult mice were much less susceptible to the virus than infant mice when inoculated i.c., and one of the latter recovered after 7 days of paralysis. Presumably an enhancement of virulence would be required, by a mechanism yet unknown, if an epizootic were to be initiated by a virus of that low virulence. Experimental infections caused by temperature-sensitive conditional lethal mutants of fixed rabies virus have been found to cause either death or nonfatal infection (Clark and Koprowski, 1971).

Previous exposure to antigenically related viruses has already been mentioned. There is also abundant reason to believe that prior vaccination will permit survival and recovery even after CNS challenge (Bell *et al.*, 1971, 1972).

Survival after onset of signs of illness is often seen in mice challenged i.c. with dilutions of virus after vaccination in the Habel test, and we have used vaccination to produce a high proportion of abortive infections with recovery (but not a carrier state) in dogs (Bell *et al.*, 1972). Some chronic virus infections, normally acute, are thought to be a consequence of infection during the period of declining immunity derived from the mother (Fenner, 1962; Brody and Detels, 1970). However, we could not detect evidence of latent or chronic infection in offspring of immune female mice after inoculation of fixed virus into the CNS or peripherally (Bell *et al.*, 1965, 1970).

Various routes of inoculation may cause nonfatal infection under experimental conditions. Even the intracerebral route will cause nonpatent or nonfatal encephalitis when attenuated virus is inoculated (Johnson, 1948; Johnson, 1966; Badiali and Abou-Youssef, 1968). However, in repeated experiments, abortive infection occurs more commonly in mice after i.p. inoculations than after inoculation by the subcutaneous or intramuscular routes, even though infectivity is often lower and higher, respectively, by those routes (Bell, 1966).

Among animals extensively studied it has been noted that susceptibility to peripherally inoculated rabies virus decreases with age. That resistance may be overcome, at least partially, by inoculation of virus of greater virulence (Bell, 1966). In laboratory studies of abortive rabies we have found it desirable to balance age of mice against virulence of inoculum to achieve about 40–75% patent infections. Higher incidence as a result of animal susceptibility or virus virulence causes proportionate decrease in survival of affected animals; lower incidence yields few survivors with sequelae because few become ill. In our experience the original animal and geographic sources of virus have not been as important to survival as subsequent manipulation of virus in the laboratory (Bell, 1966). Conjecture that small doses of virus may be responsible for development of a carrier state in wild animals (Parker, 1962) has not received support from experimental infections.

When we inoculated mice i.p. with low-passage virus of bat origin, incubation periods ordinarily ranged from 8 days to several weeks, with a peak at about 9–10 days; in one experiment we noted 59 abortive infections among 500 mice, there being a steep downward trend in mortality for incubation periods up to 10 days, but no significant change thereafter (J. F. Bell and D. W. Alling, 1965, unpublished data). We have also confirmed, in dogs, the apparent importance to survival of a sufficiently long incubation period after i.p. inoculation (Bell et al., 1971, 1972).

V. Implications of Nonfatal Infection (The Carrier State)

Although the World Health Organization Expert Committee on Rabies (1957) in their third report stated that "Because of the inevitably fatal outcome of rabies infection in man, investigations of any possible method of therapy should be encouraged," it is doubtful, for reasons stated elsewhere, that lethality is inevitable in man or in other species, and perhaps the more useful attitude would be to admit that recovery does occur and to explore the conditions conducive to it. But the greatest potential importance of survival and especially the carrier state is in the epizootiology of the disease.

A. TERRESTRIAL WILDLIFE

Webster (1937) noted that virus had been isolated from skunks that appeared normal, and inferred that the species might be a reservoir which could account for sporadic rabies in dogs. Kantorovich et al. (1957) inferred the same regarding rabies in Arctic foxes, but later (Zazlonov and Kantorovich, 1963) came to the conclusion that the normal appearing foxes were in the incubation period of the disease. In an analysis of the epizootiology of rabies in foxes in Germany, Wittman and Kokles (1967) concluded that latency of infection is not necessary to explain endemicity of infection in that species. Johnson (1966) records the isolation of rabies virus from a long-tailed weasel in Alaska, and sporadic occurrence of rabies in spotted skunks in California and elsewhere, and believes that Mustelidae and Viverridae constitute the "true carriers" in their respective environment, but Lessman (1971) found no support for that concept in intensive studies of wildlife rabies in Germany.

B. BATS

It is now commonly held that vampire bats have special status in regard to rabies infection with "recovery from rabies and development of the carrier state," a belief that dates from de Queiroz-Lima (1934) and Pawan (1936). The latter reported that the "virus may produce furious rabies in vampire bats from which there can be complete recovery, the bats remaining normal and apparently healthy, though still capable of transmitting rabies to susceptible animals." He concludes that "The virus in bats is therefore of low virulence but of high infectivity." Recent reports of isolation of virus from the brown fat and saliva of vampires that had no detectable virus in brain support the concept of a carrier state in the species (Delpietro *et al.*, 1974). However, the subject needs critical reexamination and study (Constantine, 1971).

Constantine's (1967) extensive investigation of bat rabies in southwestern United States revealed that some bats would survive experimental inoculation with or without signs and sequelae. He (Constantine, 1971) has concluded that there are "at least two kinds of bat species-specific cycles — one that usually does not kill the bat and another that does." Burns *et al.* (1958) found rabies-neutralizing antibodies in serums, and virus in brains, of normal appearing insectivorous bats and interpreted those findings as evidence of nonfatal rabies.

In our Montana area we have found 51 naturally infected colonial and solitary bats, but even so have been unable to detect neutralizing antibody in the brains of 313 and salivary glands of 163 normal bats from the same area (J. F. Bell and G. J. Moore, unpublished results), indicating a very low incidence (if any) of recovery among naturally infected northern bats. Salivary swabs from 1308 bats have yielded no positive specimens in bats that survive, and thus far, in fact, we have not found evidence of recovery, of chronic rabies, or of a carrier state in any bat, although we recovered virus from the saliva of one big brown bat 24 days before death (Bell *et al.*, 1969), and Moore and Raymond (1970) observed an incubation period of 7 months in another bat.

Johnson (1959) believes that the disease can persist in insectivorous bats only by reintroduction of infection by carnivores. On the other hand, transmission of virus by bat bite has been described repeatedly (Bell, 1959; Constantine, 1966; Bell *et al.*, 1969). All naturally infected bats that transmitted by bite later succumbed to infection.

C. Dogs

A possible role for the carrier state in the epidemiology of human rabies has been suggested by a recent survey of the 236 cases of human rabies that occurred in the United States between 1946 and

1965, in which Held *et al.* (1967) found that the source of infection was known in only 149 (63%); Sanmartín *et al.* (1967) found a similar ratio in Colombia. A number of explanations could account for failure to identify infectious sources of the remaining cases, among them prepatent infection in vector species that eventually would die with the disease, or even, theoretically, a carrier state. Remlinger and Bailly (1946) quote "impeccable" histories of people succumbing to rabies while the shedding dog remained alive (see also Svet-Moldavskaya, 1958; Broz and Phan-Trinh, 1961; Yurkovsky, 1962). Nevertheless, stronger evidence is needed, and apparently positive evidence has been supplied by studies of Remlinger and Bailly (1946), Andral and Serié (1957), Fekadu (1969), and Veeraraghavan *et al.* (1969), who recovered virus from saliva samples of normal appearing dogs for a long period. Numerous reports of experimentally induced rabies in dogs (see reviews by Martin, 1963; Bell, 1964; Nilssen, 1970; Bell *et al.*, 1972) attest to the occurrence of infection with recovery (Starr *et al.*, 1952; Markus *et al.*, 1969; Arko *et al.*, 1973) and relapsing forms (Pasteur, 1882; Webster, 1937) as well as the carrier state. Although Andral and Sérié (1957) believe nonfatal forms to exceed classic forms in prevalence in Ethiopia, Remlinger and Bailly (1946) regard the carrier state as rare, of relatively minor importance in epidemiology and a phenomenon that should not enter into consideration in public health practices. The experiences of Clemmer *et al.* (1970) in Colombia and our own experiences (Bell *et al.*, 1971, 1972) are consonant with the latter conclusion. However, most reports of the carrier state in dogs originated from Asia and Africa and those occurrences, together with the occurrence of Oulou fato (Thiery, 1960), an attenuated form of rabies in that general area, may imply accommodation between host and virus. The repeated attacks on people by certain wolves in enzootic areas in Europe (Clarke, 1971) may be comparable to those seen in dogs with chronic rabies as described by Thiery (1960) and Broz and Phan-Trinh (1961).

D. RODENTS

Nikolitsch (1965) postulated that rodents may serve as a reservoir of rabies in Europe by virtue of nonfatal rabies among them. Recently Sodja *et al.* (1971) isolated 13 strains of rabies or rabies-like viruses from a variety of rodents in Europe, and neutralizing antibodies were demonstrated in 22.5% of sera of *Microtus arvalis* from enzootic areas and in 12.8% in "rabies-free" areas. In experimentally infected mice Schneider (1969a) found that 62.5% of the animals had virus in salivary glands (also see Svet-Moldavskaya, 1958), and Winkler *et al.* (1972) observed aggressive behavior as well as infective salivary glands in four species of wild rodents and in white rats experimentally infected with street virus from diverse sources; they reported no instance of chronic rabies or recovery. There is no convincing evidence, however, that rodents constitute a significant reservoir of infection in the western hemisphere (Winkler, 1966) and only circumstantial evidence of nonfatal infections and a reservoir role in other areas. The experience of the California State Department of Public Health (CDC Vet. Pub. Health Notes, Oct. 1971) is rather typical. A fox squirrel was found rabid after it attacked several people; it was the first infected animal of 24,000 rodents and lagomorphs examined for rabies in California since 1950. Irwin (1970) discusses the evidence for a rabies cycle involving ground squirrels in Africa, and the existing local belief that nonfatal rabies (Oulou fato) in dogs is acquired from those species.

VI. Conclusions

The established concept is that rabies is "always fatal," sometimes modified to "always fatal in man." However, the scientific literature from the time of Pasteur to the present constantly reports exceptions (Kraut, 1966; Hattwick *et al.*, 1972).

Perhaps the anomaly can best be explained by wide variations in definitions and criteria. In some instances animals are said to have suffered nonfatal infections if they were inoculated with virulent virus and survived without signs of illness; in other instances, presence of virus in saliva or brains, or antibodies in sera of normal appearing animals is considered factual evidence for the occurrence. But, as we have seen, those phenomena are subject to other interpretations and their recognized fallibility as separate phenomena may have weakened rather than strengthened the case against inexorable infection.

What, then, would constitute "proof" of abortive infection? I believe there are three: (1) high titer of neutralizing antibody in CSF, (2) a positive corneal test in an animal that does not succumb, and (3) isolation of virus from saliva of an animal that does not succumb. "Proof" (1) has the advantage that it can be applied for retrospective diagnoses, is easily done, and useful for survey of prevalence of abortive infection.

Ruegsegger *et al.* (1961) found heat-stable antibodies prior to vaccination in 6% of 230 students and faculty members of a veterinary school. Prospective and retrospective inquiry failed to disclose known antecedent contact with rabies virus in either attenuated or killed form. They concluded that "their findings lend support to a thesis that there are subclinical infections due to attenuated strains of rabies virus."

In the period 1961–1970 there were 16 cases of rabies reported in the United States (K. D. Kappus, personal communication, 1971). Four of the patients died after long periods of illness (R. A. Good, personal communication, 1963; Rubin *et al.*, 1970). The latter authors stated that the intensive care received by their patient was probably responsible for prolonged survival and "it is suggested that such care may allow some rabies victims to survive." Vindication of that position has been afforded by the subsequent well-attested survival of a boy in Ohio (Hattwick *et al.*, 1972). Perhaps even more significant is the fact that the child has recovered from paralysis.

References

Abelseth, M., and Lawson, K. (1972). Personal Communication.

Andral, L., and Serié, C. (1957). *Ann. Inst. Pasteur, Paris* **93**, 475.

Arko, R. J., Schneider, L. G., and Baer, G. M. (1973). *Am. J. Vet. Research* **34**, 937.

Atanasiu, P. (1970). *Bull. Inst. Pasteur, Paris* **68**, 2047.

Atanasiu, P., Guillon, J. C., and Vallée, A. (1970). *Ann. Inst. Pasteur, Paris* **119**, 260.

Badiali, L., and Abou-Youssef, M. (1968). *Vet. Ital.* **19**, 807.

Baer, G. M., and Bales, G. L. (1967). *J. Infec. Dis.* **117**, 82.

Baer, G. M., and Cleary, W. F. (1972). *J. Infec. Dis.* **125**, 520.

Baer, G. M., Shanthaveerappa, T. R., and Bourne, G. H. (1965). *Bull. WHO* **33**, 783.

Baron, S. (1963). *Advan. Virus Res.* **10**, 39.

Bell, J. F. (1959). *Science* **129**, 1490.

Bell, J. F. (1964). *J. Infec. Dis.* **114**, 249.

Bell, J. F. (1966). *Symp. Ser. Immunobiol. Stand.* **1**, 167.

Bell, J. F., Moore, G. J., and Raymond, G. H. (1965). *Arch. Inst. Pasteur Tunis, No. 1–2,* 47.

Bell, J. F., Lodmell, D. L., Moore, G. J., and Raymond, G. H. (1966a). *J. Immunol.* **97**, 747.

Bell, J. F., Lodmell, D. L., Moore, G. J., and Raymond, G. H. (1966b). *Pub. Health Rep.* **81**, 761.

Bell, J. F., and Moore, G. J. (1974). *Infection and Immunity* (Sept. 1974).

Bell, J. F., Moore, G. J., and Raymond, G. H. (1969). *Amer. J. Trop. Med. Hyg.* **18**, 61.

Bell, J. F., Moore, G. J., and Raymond, G. H. (1970). *Amer. J. Vet. Res.* **31**, 1055.

Bell, J. F., Gonzalez, M., Díaz, A. M., and Moore, G. J. (1971). *Amer. J. Vet. Res.* **32**, 2049.

Bell, J. F., Sancho, M. I., Díaz, A. M., and Moore, G. J. (1972). *Amer. J. Epidemiol.* **95**, 190.

Bindrich, H., and Schmidt, U. (1958). *Arch. Exp. Veterinaermed.* **12**, 202.

Brier, A. M., Wohlenberg, C. R., and Notkins, A. L. (1971). *Fed. Proc., Fed. Amer. Soc. Exp. Biol.* **30**, 353, Abstr. No. 906.

Brody, J. A., and Detels, R. (1970). *Lancet* **2**, 500.

Broz, O., and Phan Trinh, D. (1961). *J. Hyg., Epidemiol., Microbiol., Immunol.* **5**, 403.

Buchnev, K. N. (1960). *Tr. Kaz. Nauch.-Issled. Vet. Inst.* **10**, 321 (Transl.).

Burns, K. F., Farinacci, C. J., Murnane, T. G., and Shelton, D. F. (1956). *Amer. J. Pub. Health* **46**, 1089.

Burns, K. F., Shelton, D. F., and Grogan, E. W. (1958). *Ann. N. Y. Acad. Sci.* **70**, 452.

Casals, J. (1940). *J. Exp. Med.* **72**, 445.

Cereghino, J. J., Osterud, H. T., Pinnas, J. L., and Holmes, M. A. (1970). *Pediatrics* **45**, 839.

Clark, H F., and Koprowski, H. (1971). *Virology* **7**, 295.

Clarke, C. H. D. (1971). *Natur. Hist., N. Y.* **80**, 44.

Clemmer, D. I., Thomas, J. B., Vaughn, J. B., Escobar, E., and Sanmartín, C. (1970). *Bol. Of. Sanit. Panamer.* **69**, 212.

Constantine, D. G. (1966). *Amer. J. Vet. Res.* **27**, 20.

Constantine, D. G. (1967). *Pub. Health Rep.* **82**, 867.

Constantine, D. G. (1971). *In* "Rabies" (Y. Nagano and F. M. Davenport, eds.), pp. 253–262. Univ. Park Press, Baltimore, Maryland.

Constantine, D. G., Solomon, G. C., and Woodall, D. F. (1968a). *Amer. J. Vet. Res.* **29**, 181.

Constantine, D. G., Tierkel, E. S., Kleckner, M. D., and Hawkins, D. M. (1968b). *Pub. Health Rep.* **83**, 303.

Constantinescu, N., and Birzu, N. (1958). *Ann. Inst. Pasteur, Paris* **94**, 739.

Correa-Giron, E. P., Allen, R., and Sulkin, S. E. (1970). *Amer. J. Epidemiol.* **91**, 203.

Crandell, R. A. (1965). *Acta Pathol. Microbiol. Scand.* **63**, 587.

Dean, D. J. (1963). *N. Y. State J. Med.* **63**, 3507.

Dean, D. J., Evans, W. M., and McClure, R. C. (1963a). *Bull. WHO* **29**, 803.

Dean, D. J., Sherman, I., and Thompson, W. R. (1963b). *Amer. J. Vet. Res.* **24**, 614.

Delpietro, H., Díaz, A. M. O., Fuenzalida, E., and Bell, J. F. (1972). *Bol. Of. Sanit. Panamer.* **63**, 222.

Depoux, R. (1964). *Can. J. Microbiol.* **10**, 527.

de Queiroz-Lima, E. (1934). *Rev. Dep. Nac. Prod. Anim., Brazil* **1**, 1–165.

Duncan, W. B., and Kuhn, U. S., III. (1972). *J. Infec. Dis.* **125**, 61.

Ercegovac, D., and Pima-Kostoglou, M. (1968). *Delt. Hellen. Kten. Hetair.* **19**, 146 (Transl.).

Fayaz, A., Afshar, A., and Bahmanyar, M. (1970). *Arch. Gesamte Virusforsch.* **29**, 159.

Fekadu, M. (1969). "Scientific Group on Rabies Research," Background Doc. No. 44. World Health Organ., Geneva.

Fenje, P., and Postic, B. (1970). *Nature (London)* **226**, 171.

Fenner, F. (1962). *In* "The Problems of Laboratory Animal Disease" (R. J. C. Harris, ed.), pp. 39–55. Academic Press, New York.

Ferris, D. H., Badiali, L., Mamdouh, A-Y., and Beamer, P. D. (1968). *Cornell Vet.* **58**, 270.

Fischman, H. R., and Schaeffer, M. (1971). *Ann. N. Y. Acad. Sci.* **177**, 78.

Fox, J. P. (1943). *J. Exp. Med.* **77**, 487.

Gonzalez, H., Agulleiro Moreira, J. M., Moreau, E. J., and Tchoulamjan, A. (1956). *Med. Panamer.* **7**, 265.

Green, R. G., Ziegler, N. R., Green, B. B., Shillinger, J. E., Dewey, E. T., and Carlson, W. E. (1935). *Amer. J. Hyg.* **21**, 366.

Hattwick, M. A., Weis, T. T., Stechschulte, C. J., Baer, G. M., and Gregg, M. B. (1972). *Ann. Intern. Med.* **76**, 931.

Held, J. R., Tierkel, E. S., and Steele, J. H. (1967). *Pub. Health Rep.* **82**, 1009.

Hole, N. H. (1969). *Nature (London)* **224**, 244.

Hummeler, K., and Koprowski, H. (1969) *Nature (London)* **221**, 418.

Hurst, E. W., and Pawan, J. L. (1932). *J. Pathol. Bacteriol.* **35**, 301.

Irwin, A. D. (1970). *Vet. Rec.* **87**, 333.

Jacotot, H., and Nguyen-Dinh-Lam, N. (1947). *Bull. Acad. Vet. Fr.* **20**, 430.

Jenkins, M., and Wamberg, K. (1960). *J. Amer. Vet. Med. Ass.* **137**, 183.

Johnson, H. N. (1948). *Amer. J. Hyg.* **47**, 189.

Johnson, H. N. (1952). *In* "Viral and Rickettsial Infections of Man" (T. M. Rivers, ed.), 2nd ed., pp. 267-299. Lippincott, Philadelphia, Pennsylvania.

Johnson, H. N. (1959). *Proc. 63rd Annu. Meet. U. S. Livestock Sanit. Ass.* p. 267.

Johnson, H. N. (1964). *In* "Diagnostic Procedures for Viral and Rickettsial Diseases" (E. H. Lennette and N. J. Schmidt, eds.), 3rd ed., Chapter 10, pp. 356–380. Amer. Pub. Health Ass., Inc., N. Y.

Johnson, H. N. (1966). *In* "National Rabies Symposium Proceedings National Communicable Disease Center," Atlanta, Georgia. May 5–6, pp. 25–30.

Johnson, R. T. (1965). *J. Neuropathol. Exp. Neurol.* **24**, 662.

Jonesco, D., and Teodasiu, T. (1928). *C. R. Soc. Biol.* **97**, 983.

Kantorovich, R. A. (1957). *Acta Virol. (Prague), Engl. Ed.* **1**, 220.

Kissling, R. E., and Reese, D. R. (1963). *J. Immunol.* **91**, 362.

Koch, J. (1930). *In* "Handbuch der pathogenen Mikroorganismen" (W. Kolle and A. von Wasserman, eds.), **8**, Part I, pp. 547–694, Fischer, Jena.

Konradi, D. (1916). *Ann. Inst. Pasteur, Paris* **30**, 33.

Koprowski, H. (1952). *Ann. N. Y. Acad. Sci.* **54**, 963.

Koprowski, H. (1966). *Symp. Ser. Immunobiol. Stand.* **1**, 423.

Koprowski, H., and Cox, H. R. (1948). *J. Immunol.* **60**, 533.

Krause, W. W. (1966). *Symp. Ser. Immunobiol. Stand.* **1**, 153.

Kraut, J. J. (1966). *J. Amer. Med. Ass.* **197**, 224.

Kubes, V., and Gallia, F. (1943). *Bol. Inst. Invest. Vet., Maracay, Venez.* **1**, 105, reprinted in H. S. Banks ed. *Can. J. Comp. Med. Vet. Sci.* **8**, 48 (1944).

Lépine, P. (1951). *In* "Modern Practice in Infectious Fevers," (H. S. Banks, ed.) Second Volume p. 724. Butterworth, London.

Lépine, P. (1961). *FAO Agr. Stud.* **25**, 215–225.

Lessman, F-J. (1971). Dissertation, Tierärztlichen Fakultät der Ludwig-Maximilians-Universität München.

Levaditi, C., Sanches-Bayarri, V., and Schoen, R. (1928). *C. R. Soc. Biol.* **98**, 911.

Lodmell, D. L., Bell, J. F., Moore, G. J., and Raymond, G. H. (1969). *J. Infec. Dis.* **119**, 569.

Lwoff, A. (1959). *Bacteriol. Rev.* **23**, 109.

McDermott, W. (1959). *Pub. Health Rep.* **74**, 485.

McDermott, W. (1961). *Bacteriol. Rev.* **25**, 173.

Markus, H. L., Jobim, G. O., and Jobim, G. B. (1969). *Bol. Of. Sanit. Panamer.* **67**, 101.

Martin, L. A. (1963). *Maroc Med.* **42**, 467.

Miyamoto, K., and Matsumoto, S. (1967). *J. Exp. Med.* **125**, 447.

Moore, G. J., and Raymond, G. H. (1970). *J. Wildl. Dis.* **6**, 167.

Murphy, F. A., Bauer, S. P., Harrison, A. K., and Winn, W. C. (1973). *Laboratory Investigation* **28**, 361.

Nathanson, N., and Cole, G. A. (1970). *Advan. Virus Res.* **16**, 397.

Nathanson, N., and Cole, G. A. (1971). *Fed. Proc., Fed. Amer. Soc. Exp. Biol.* **30**, 1822.

Neves, J. (1970). *Rev. Ass. Med. Minas Gerais* 21, 13.

Nikolitsch, M. (1965). *Blue Book, Hoechst, Frankfurt* 10, 7.

Nilsson, M. R. (1968). *An. Congr. Bras. Vet. Niteroi, 11th, 1968* Vol. 1, p. 248.

Nilsson, M. R. (1970). *Bol. Of. Sanit. Panamer* 68, 180.

Oldstone, M. B. A., and Dixon, F. J. (1970). *J. Exp. Med.* 131, 1.

Parker, R. L. (1962). *Proc. 65th Annu. Meet. U. S. Livestock Sanit. Ass.* p. 273.

Pasteur, L. (with the collaboration of M. M. Chamberland, E. Roux, and L. Thuillier). (1882). *C. R. Acad. Sci.* 95, 1187.

Paterson, P. Y. (1966). *Advan. Immunol.* 5, 131–208.

Pawan, J. L. (1936). *Ann. Trop. Med. Parasitol.* 30, 401.

Payne, F. E., Baublis, J. V., and Itabashi, H. H. (1969). *N. Engl. J. Med.* 281, 585.

Perl, D., Van Orden, A., and Baer, G. M. (1975). In preparation.

Pugh, L. P. (1962). *Vet. Rec.* 74, 486.

Remlinger, P., and Bailly J. (1941). *Bull. Acad. Med., Paris* 124, 389.

Remlinger, P., and Bailly, J. (1946). *Arch. Inst. Pasteur Alger.* 24, 289.

Roberts, J. A. (1962). *Brit. J. Exp. Pathol.* 43, 462.

Rubin, R. H., Sullivan, L., Summers, R., Gregg, M. B., and Sikes, R. K., (1970). *J. Infec. Dis.* 122, 318.

Ruegsegger, J. M., Black, J., and Sharpless, G. R. (1961). *Amer. J. Pub. Health* 51, 706.

Sadler, W. W., and Enright, J. B. (1959). *J. Infec. Dis.* 105, 267.

Sanmartín, C., Correa, P., Duenas, A., and Muñoz, N. (1967). *Mem. Semin. Nac. Sobre Rabia, 1st, Medellín, Colombia 1967,* pp. 155–161.

Scatterday, J. E. (1954). *J. Amer. Vet. Ass.* 124, 125.

Schindler, R. (1961). *Bull. W. H. O.* 25, 119.

Schneider, L. G. (1969a). *Zentralbl. Veterinaermed, Reihe B* 16, 24.

Schneider, L. G. (1969b). *Zentralbl. Bakteriol., Parasitenk., Infektionskr. Hyg., Abt. I: Orig.* 212, 1.

Shiraki, H., Otani, S., Tamthai, B., Chamuni, A., Chitanondh, H., and Charuchinda, S. (1962). *World Neurol.* 3, 125.

Shope, R. E., Murphy, F. A., Harrison, A. K., Causey, O. R., Kemp, G. E., Simpson, D. I. H., and Moore, D. L. (1970). *J. Virol.* 6, 690.

Sikes, R. K. (1962). *Amer. J. Vet. Res.* 23, 1041.

Soave, O. A. (1964). *Amer. J. Vet. Res.* 25, 268.

Soave, O. A., Johnson, H. N., and Nakamura, K. (1961). *Science* 133, 1360.

Sodja, I., Lim, D., and Matouch, O. (1971). *J. Hyg., Epidemiol., Microbiol., Immunol.* 15, 271.

Stamm, D. C., Kissling, R. E., and Eidsen, M. E. (1956). *J. Infec. Dis.* 98, 10.

Starr, L. E., Sellers, T. F., and Sunkes, E. J. (1952). *J. Amer. Vet. Med. Ass.* 121, 296.

Steele, J. H. (1965). "Rabies Survey." Territory of Papua, New Guinea (unpublished report).

Stevens, J. G., and Cook, M. L. (1971). *Science* 173, 843.

Stewart, W. E., and Sulkin, S. E. (1966). *Proc. Soc. Exp. Biol. Med.* 123, 650.

Sulkin, S. E. (1962). *Amer. J. Pub. Health* 52, 489.

Sulkin, S. E., Krutzsch, P. H., Wallis, C., and Allen, R. (1957). *Proc. Soc. Exp. Biol. Med.* 96, 461.

Svet-Moldavskaya, I. A. (1958). *Acta Virol. (Prague) English Ed.* 2, 228.

Theiler, M. (1937). *J. Exp. Med.* 65, 705.

Thiery, G. (1960). *Rev. Elevage Med. Vet. Pays Trop.* [N. S.] 13, 259.

Traub, E. (1936). *J. Exp. Med.* 63, 533.

Van Rooyen, C. E., and Rhodes, A. J. (1940a). In "Virus Diseases of Man," Chapter 49, p. 642. Oxford Med. Publ., London.

Van Rooyen, C. E., and Rhodes, A. J. (1940b). *In* "Virus Diseases of Man," Chapter 51, pp. 656–680. Oxford Med. Publ., London.

Vaughn, J. B., Gerhardt, P., and Newell, K. W. (1965). *J. Amer. Med. Ass.* **193**, 363.

Veeraraghavan, N. (1965). "Coonoor Scientific Report," p. 82. Pasteur Institute of Southern India, Coonoor, Tamilnadu, India.

Veeraraghavan, N., Gajanana, A., Rangsami, R., Oonnunni, P. T., Saraswathi, K. C., Devaraj, R., and Hallan, K. M. (1969). "Coonoor Scientific Report," p. 66. Pasteur Institute of Southern India, Coonoor, Tamilnadu, India.

Vieuchange, J. (1961). *C. R. Soc. Biol.* **160**, 2278.

Walker, D. L., Hanson, R. P., and Evans, A. S., eds. (1958). "Latency and Masking in Viral and Rickettsial Infections." Burgess, Minneapolis, Minnesota.

Wall, P. D., and Egger, M. D. (1971). *Nature (London)* **232**, 542.

Wang, S. P. (1956). *J. Formosan Med. Soc.* **55**, 8.

Waterman, J. A. (1959). *Carib. Med. J.* **21**, 46.

Webb, H. D. (1969). *In* "Virus Diseases and the Nervous System" (C. W. M. Whitty, J T. Hughes, and F. O. MacCallum, eds.), pp. 169–177. Blackwell, Oxford.

Webster, L. T. (1937). *N. Engl. J. Med.* **217**, 687.

Wiktor, T. J., Kuwert, E., and Koprowski, H. (1968). *J. Immunol.* **101**, 1271.

Wiktor, T. J., Koprowski, H., and Rorke, L. B. (1972). *Proc. Soc. Exp. Biol. Med.* **140**, 759.

Wilsnack, R. E., and Parker, R. L. (1966). *Amer. J. Vet. Res.* **27**, 39.

Winkler, W. G. (1966). *Proc. Nat. Rabies Symp.*, 1966 pp. 34–36.

Winkler, W. G., Schneider, N. J., and Jennings, W. L. (1972) *J. Wildl. Dis.* **8**, 99.

Wittman, W., and Kokles, R. (1967). *Arch. Exp. Veterinaermed.* **21**, 165.

World Health Organization Expert Committee on Rabies. (1957). *World Health Organ., Tech. Rep. Ser.* **121**.

Wright, G. P. (1956). *Guy's Hosp. Rep.* **105**, 57.

Yoshino, K. (1966). *Proc. Soc. Exp. Biol. Med.* **123**, 387.

Yurkovsky, A. M. (1962). *J. Hyg., Epidemiol. Microbiol., Immunol.* **6**, 73.

Zazlonov, M. S., and Kantorovich, R. A. (1963). *Veterinariya (Moscow)* **40**, 13.

CHAPTER 18

Interferon and Rabies Virus Infection

S. Edward Sulkin* and Rae Allen

The discovery of interferon occurred during the course of investigations of the phenomenon of viral interference (Isaacs and Lindenmann, 1957). It is generally agreed that viral interference was first demonstrated experimentally in the studies of Hoskins (1935) and of Magrassi (1935) and definitely established by Findlay and MacCallum (1937), who ruled out the question of the role of specific immunity in the phenomenon by demonstrating interference between antigenically unrelated viruses. However, the prejudiced eye, viewing the literature in retrospect, can find examples of what might have been the interference phenomenon in reports which appeared much earlier (cf. Findlay, 1948; cf. Henle, 1950; cf. Lennette, 1951). With regard to rabies virus there is a statement by Pasteur (1888) to the effect that small doses of virus induce rabies in rabbits more frequently than the administration of larger amounts of virus. This observation may be viewed as a classic example of autointerference. Several years before the phenomenon of viral interference was described and long before the discovery of interferon, observations suggestive of interference between different strains of rabies virus, and between rabies virus and an unrelated virus, also appeared in the literature; these were the studies of Levaditi *et al.* (1926) who observed what they termed "antagonism" between strains of fixed and street rabies virus, and also demonstrated the

* Deceased.

suppressive effect of vaccinia virus on the development of rabies infection in rabbits. Despite these early references to homologous and heterologous interference with rabies virus there have been relatively few truly definitive studies devoted to this subject compared with the vast literature concerning interference and the interferon system with other viral agents. However, sufficient evidence has accumulated to establish that rabies virus is capable of inducing interferon *in vivo* and *in vitro* and is sensitive to this substance in both endogenous and exogenous form. Thus it may be assumed that, in the light of present-day knowledge, suppression of virus growth in past studies was in all probability due, at least in part, to interferon mediated interference even when the mechanism of the observed inhibition has not been fully characterized.

I. Homologous and Heterologous Interference with Rabies Virus

Studies demonstrating interference between strains of rabies virus and between rabies virus and unrelated viruses are listed in Table I. Subsequent to the early references cited above (Pasteur, 1888; Levaditi *et al.*, 1926) no other reports suggestive of homologous or heterologous interference with rabies virus appeared until almost 20 years after the phenomenon had been described (Hoskins, 1935; Magrassi, 1935; Findlay and MacCallum, 1937). During development of egg-adapted Flury rabies virus vaccines the resistance noted in hamsters inoculated with high egg passage (HEP) Flury virus appeared to result from a mixed population consisting of a small proportion of particles still pathogenic for animals, and a larger proportion which had lost pathogenic properties through adaptation to the egg embryo (Koprowski *et al.*, 1954). The presence of an interfering fraction in HEP Flury virus was demonstrated by using suspensions of this virus as diluent in titrating low egg passage (LEP) virus which still retained pathogenic properties. The titer of a stock suspension of LEP virus in hamsters was significantly lower when dilutions were made in a suspension of chick embryo cells (CEC) infected with HEP virus, as opposed to a suspension of normal CEC. Hamsters were used as the test animals for the intracerebral (i.c.) titrations. No interference between HEP virus and street or rodent fixed strains of rabies virus was demonstrated in titrations carried out by the i.c. inoculation of 21-day-old mice. The ability of an egg-adapted strain of rabies virus to interfere with the growth of an unrelated virus in mouse brain was demonstrated by Kanazawa and Ohtomi (1958) who

Table I

Homologous and Heterologous Interference with Rabies Virus

Interfering virus	Host system	Suppressed virus	Investigators
Rabies	Rabbits	Rabies	Pasteur, 1888
Rabies (rabbit brain fixed Pasteur)	Rabbits	Rabies (street)	Levaditi et al., 1926
Rabies (high egg passage Flury)	Hamsters	Rabies (Low egg passage Flury)	Koprowski et al., 1954
Rabies (high egg passage Nishigahara)	Mice	Poliovirus Type II (MEFl)	Kanazawa and Ohtomi, 1958
Rabies (mouse brain fixed CVS)	Chick embryo cells	Western equine encephalitis	Kaplan et al., 1960
Rabies (high egg passage Flury)	Human diploid cells (WI-38)	Rabies (rabbit brain fixed Pitman-Moore) Poliovirus Type I (Chat) Eastern equine encephalitis	Wiktor et al., 1964
Rabies (mouse brain fixed CVS)	Rabbit endothelial cells	Rabies (rabbit brain fixed Pitman-Moore) Rabies (mouse brain fixed CVS) Vesicular stomatitis	Fernandes et al., 1964
Rabies (high egg passage Flury)	Chick embryo cells	Western equine encephalitis Pseudorabies Sendai Newcastle disease ("M") Vaccinia (WR)	Selimov et al., 1965
Rabies (high egg passage Flury)	Chick embryo cells	Rabies (High egg passage Flury) Western equine encephalitis Vaccinia (Dairen I)	Yoshino et al., 1966
Rabies (Fermi vaccine, live-fixed)	Chicks	Rous sarcoma (Schmidt-Ruppin)	Kravchenko et al., 1967
Rabies (rabbit brain fixed Paris)	Chicks	Rous sarcoma (Bryan Master)	Desai, 1970
Rabies (20S particle of low egg passage Flury)	Baby hamster kidney cells (BHK21)	Rabies (low egg passage Flury)	Crick and Brown, 1974
Vaccinia	Rabbits	Rabies (street, rabbit brain fixed Pasteur)	Levaditi et al., 1926; Vieuchange et al., 1966, 1967; Vieuchange, 1968

357

showed that i.c. inoculation of a strain of high egg passage fixed rabies virus significantly reduced mortality rates in mice given poliovirus Type II via the same route.

Kaplan *et al.* (1960) showed that monolayer cultures of CEC infected with the CVS strain of rabies virus (which is noncytocidal in this tissue culture system) were resistant to superinfection with Western equine encephalitis (WEE) virus. Since WEE virus produced a cytopathic effect in normal CEC monolayers this observation provided a method for quantitating rabies virus based on plaque inhibition. These investigators also demonstrated that medium from rabies virus infected CEC monolayers was capable of interfering with WEE virus. Treatment of CEC monolayers with rabies virus-infected culture media (centrifuged twice at 40,000 *g* for 1½ hours, then treated with rabies virus antiserum to neutralize any residual live virus) induced resistance to subsequent infection with WEE virus, although the inhibition was less than when media containing live virus was used. The authors referred to this inhibition as being due to interferon, but the inhibitor was not fully characterized as such. In subsequent studies with CEC monolayers infected with HEP Flury virus it was found that these cultures, in addition to being resistant to superinfection with WEE virus, were also resistant to Newcastle Disease, vaccinia, Sendai, and pseudorabies viruses (Selimov *et al.*, 1965). The interference phenomenon was observed only in cultures inoculated 48 hours or more after infection with doses of rabies virus sufficient to induce virus replication, and was not apparent in cultures first inoculated with rabies virus inactivated by heating, UV irradiation, or antiserum treatment. The investigators made no effort to determine if this observed interference was due to interferon production.

In studies on the growth of rabies virus in a variety of tissue culture systems it was found that human diploid cells (WI-38) and rabbit endothelial cells infected with HEP Flury or CVS strains of rabies virus were resistant to superinfection with other strains of rabies virus, as well as to a number of unrelated agents (Fernandes *et al.*, 1964; Wiktor *et al.*, 1964). The degree of resistance to various viruses was a function of the number of rabies virus-infected cells in a culture as demonstrated by the fluorescent antibody technique; resistance to superinfection was complete in cultures in which all cells contained rabies virus antigen. It was not possible to demonstrate an interferonlike substance in fluids from these cultures. Subsequently, this group of investigators reported that cultures of hamster fibroblasts (stable line Nil-2) and baby hamster kidney (BHK21) cells infected with rabies virus were resistant to homologous and heterologous challenge and an inhibitor with interferon-like properties was recovered from the culture fluids (Wiktor and Koprowski, 1967; Wiktor and Clark, 1972).

Yoshino and associates (1966), in demonstrating that HEP Flury virus formed plaques in primary chick embryo fibroblasts, noted that suspensions containing high concentrations of virus failed to form plaques, indicating that autointerference was occurring. Interference was also observed when attempts were made to plaque vaccinia virus or WEE virus on rabies virus-infected monolayers, though to a lesser extent than with homologous virus; no resistance to superinfection with Sindbis virus was observed. An acid stable interferonlike inhibitor, active against vaccinia virus, was demonstrated in fluids from rabies virus-infected cultures.

Kravchenko *et al.* (1967) demonstrated interference between antirabies vaccine (Fermi) and the Schmidt-Ruppin strain of Rous sarcoma virus (RSV) when the vaccine was inoculated into the wing web of chicks 2 days prior to, simultaneously with, or 1 day after the injection of RSV; inoculation of a live fixed strain of rabies virus also suppressed tumor formation. Three other strains of RSV were not inhibited by either the vaccine or fixed rabies virus. Similarly, Desai (1970) blocked tumor formation in the wing webs of white Leghorn chickens by the Bryan Master strain of RSV using the Paris strain of live, fixed rabies virus (Semple vaccine strain); ultraviolet-irradiated rabies virus was a less effective inhibitor.

Recently, Crick and Brown (1974) reported that BHK21 cells infected with the LEP strain of rabies virus produce a shortened particle which contains RNA and interferes with the multiplication of the virus. Heterologous interfering activity against the Indiana serotype of vesicular stomatitis virus could not be demonstrated with preparations of the 20S component.

In some of the studies listed in Table I it is assumed that interferon mediated the suppressive effect that rabies virus had on superinfection of the host systems with rabies virus or unrelated agents, yet the inhibitor was not fully characterized as interferon in any instance. Rabies virus-induced interferon was, however, demonstrated and fully characterized in an investigation of the role of this substance in rabies virus infection in hamsters (Stewart and Sulkin, 1966); the inhibitor fitted the various criteria which serve to distinguish interferon from other viral inhibitors (Larke, 1966). When weanling hamsters were inoculated intramuscularly with the CVS strain of rabies virus interferon was first detected in brain tissue, then blood, and then simultaneously in spleen, lung, kidney, and brown fat. Levels of interferon were highest in brain tissue, the most active site for virus replication, and lower in the other tissues. No evidence of the growth of rabies virus in the liver was obtained, nor was interferon demonstrated in this tissue. Thus, in this system, interferon production could be taken as an index of virus multiplication, and the appearance of interferon in the various organs demonstrated that replication of CVS rabies virus induces interferon in several tissues of the hamster. The ability of street strains of rabies virus to induce interferon *in vivo* was also studied. Two strains were used, one of canine origin and one isolated from the interscapular brown fat of a naturally infected bat, previously shown to differ from each other in several characteristics, including infectivity for hamsters and mice by intramuscular inoculation (Sulkin *et al.*, 1960; Sims *et al.*, 1967; Chapter 6, Volume II, this treatise; and Chapter 16, this volume). The canine strain, administered intramuscularly, infected hamsters and induced interferon in a manner similar to that observed with the CVS strain (S. E. Sulkin and R. Allen, unpublished observation). The bat strain of rabies virus, on the other hand, does not produce disease in hamsters or mice when inoculated intramuscularly, and did not induce demonstrable levels of interferon in animals given virus by this route. The bat strain is infective by intracerebral inoculation, however, and induced levels of brain interferon comparable to those measured in brains of hamsters infected with the CVS strain (Stewart and Sulkin, 1966).

In addition to demonstrating interference between strains of fixed and street rabies virus, Levaditi *et al.* (1926) also showed that rabbits did not develop rabies when vaccinia virus was inoculated simultaneously with rabies virus (Table I). If, however, rabies virus was given first and administration of vaccinia virus was delayed 24 hours or longer, the animals were not protected from rabies. It seems unfortunate, in the light of the demonstration of the phenomenon of viral interference in 1937 (Findlay and MacCallum, 1937), and the discovery of interferon in 1957 (Isaacs and Lindenmann, 1957), that the observations of Levaditi and his associates (1926) were not reinvestigated earlier. Forty years elapsed before their experiments were repeated and extended to show that intradermal inoculation of vaccinia virus prevented rabbits from developing rabies when the former virus was injected 1–5 days prior to intradermal inoculation of either fixed or street strains of rabies virus (Vieuchange *et al.*, 1966, 1967; Vieuchange, 1968). The studies which were designed to determine whether the observed interference between vaccinia and rabies virus was interferon mediated are discussed below.

II. Inhibition of Rabies Virus Infection by Exogenous Interferon

A limited number of studies have investigated the effect of exogenous interferon on the growth of rabies virus; those which have provided some evidence of inhibition of rabies virus infection by interferon are listed in Table II. Interferon was one of several biologics used in studies on local treatment of wounds to prevent rabies (Kaplan *et al.*, 1962); the effect of two different interferon preparations was determined by local infiltration into rabies virus-infected wounds in guinea pigs. When interferon of guinea pig origin was inoculated into the wounds, 3 of 10 animals died as compared to 6 of 10 control pigs; interferon of monkey kidney tissue culture origin

Table II

Inhibition of Rabies Virus Infection by Exogenous Interferon

Preparation of interferon		Experimental host	Administration of interferon[a]	Rabies virus strain (route)	Investigators
Host system	Inducer				
Guinea pig kidney monolayers	Newcastle disease virus	Guinea pigs	1 hour after (infiltrated under wound)	Fixed CVS (wound)	Kaplan *et al.*, 1962
Rabbits	Vaccinia virus	Rabbits	24 hours before (intradermal)	Fixed and street (intradermal)	Vieuchange, 1967, 1969
Rabbits	Newcastle disease virus	Rabbits	Concurrently (intravenous or intramuscular or both)	Street	Postic and Fenje, 1971
Dog submaxillary gland monolayers	Influenza virus (W.S. strain)	Dog submaxillary gland monolayers	For 24 hours before	Fixed CVS	Depoux, 1965
Mice	West Nile virus	Mouse ependymoma monolayers	For 24 or 12 hours before	Fixed	Barroeta and Atanasiu, 1969
Primary hamster kidney monolayers	Newcastle disease virus	Baby hamster kidney (BHK) monolayers	For 18 hours before	Fixed ERA	Wiktor *et al.*, 1972b
Human leukocyte cultures	Sendai virus	Primary human embryonic fibroblast monolayers	For 18 hours before	Fixed ERA	Wiktor *et al.*, 1972b

[a] Time in relation to rabies virus inoculation.

used in the same way was completely ineffective in protecting guinea pigs.

Vieuchange (1967, 1969) tried to determine whether the previously discussed interference between vaccinia virus and rabies virus in rabbits was interferon mediated; it was shown that rabbits did not develop rabies when crude interferon preparations (20% suspensions of rabbit skin or brain tissue infected with vaccinia virus, centrifuged, and filtered to remove live virus) were administered intradermally 24 hours before intradermal inoculation of rabies virus at an adjacent site. Little success was achieved in preventing rabies in rabbits when preparations were administered after rabies virus injection (Vieuchange and Fayaz, 1969). Although these experiments suggest that the original demonstration by Levaditi and his associates (1926) of an "antagonism" between rabies virus and vaccinia virus was in truth interferon mediated, failure to use a fully characterized vaccinia virus-induced interferon preparation leaves room for doubt, especially since some antirabies activity was noted with normal rabbit tissue in certain experiments (Vieuchange, 1967).

Postic and Fenje (1971) studied the effect of interferon on rabies infection in rabbits; the interferon had been induced in rabbits inoculated with Newcastle Disease virus, and was characterized by biologic and physicochemical methods. Four groups of six rabbits each were injected with 80 rabbit intramuscular LD_{50} of a street strain of rabies virus and, concurrently, given varying doses of interferon by various routes. The maximum total dose of interferon (6.4 × 10^6 units/rabbit) administered in three equal injections (two intramuscular and one intravenous) protected all six rabbits in one group. Intramuscular inoculation of a smaller dose (1.6 × 10^6 units/rabbit) at the site of virus inoculation protected three of six rabbits in another group; no protection was noted in the two groups given either an intramuscular inoculation of the same dose of interferon into the opposite leg, or intravenous injection of a larger dose (3.2 × 10^6 units/rabbit).

Depoux (1965) reported that the growth of CVS rabies virus in dog submaxillary gland tissue cultures was inhibited by interferon induced in this tissue by the W.S. strain of influenza virus. Inhibition was noted when monolayers were treated 24 hours prior to inoculation of rabies virus, but when cultures were treated just 1 hour before inoculation no inhibition was observed. Barroeta and Atanasiu (1969), using interferon prepared in mice, also demonstrated the inhibition of the growth of a fixed rabies virus strain adapted to mouse ependymoma tissue culture. Cells treated with 1000 units of interferon 12–24 hours before, or simultaneously with, inoculation of virus were completely resistant to infection, while 100 units of interferon resulted in partial protection; 10 units had no effect. Treatment of cells with 10,000 units of interferon, even 12 hours *after* inoculation with rabies virus, inhibited growth of the virus completely.

Wiktor *et al.* (1972b) demonstrated the inhibition of rabies virus infection by exogenous interferon in cells of hamster and human origin. Treatment of baby hamster kidney (BHK) cells with 100 units of homologous interferon for 18 hours prior to inoculation with a strain of fixed rabies virus decreased significantly the number of cells showing the presence of rabies-specific fluorescent antigen. Similar results were obtained in human embryonic fibroblast monolayers using interferon induced in human leukocyte cultures by Sendai virus. Experiments with vesicular stomatitis virus (VSV) were included in these studies to monitor interferon activity, and rabies virus appeared to be as sensitive to the inhibitory effect of interferon as VSV.

III. Inhibition of Rabies Virus Infection by Endogenous Interferon

Studies in which some degree of inhibition of rabies virus has been demonstrated by treatment of animals with various endogenous interferon inducers are listed in Table III. In experiments in which a synthetic interferon inducer, a double-stranded ribopolynucleotide, polyinosinic-polycytidylic acid (poly I:C) was used, partial to complete protection of mice and rabbits from rabies has been reported. Nemes *et al.* (1969) demonstrated some evidence of protection in groups of mice treated with poly I:C intraperitoneally 3 hours prior to inoculation of CVS fixed rabies virus. In other studies in mice, poly I:C was shown to be effective in preventing rabies in animals challenged with a street strain of rabies virus; multiple doses of the compound beginning 3 hours after virus inoculation afforded almost complete protection, and a single dose administered into the site of virus injection prevented rabies in some mice even when given as long as 67 hours after virus inoculation (Janis and Habel, 1972). In experiments with rabbits, investigators have demonstrated complete protection of animals against street and fixed strains of rabies virus by multiple doses of poly I:C administered intravenously or intramuscularly into the site of virus inoculation (Fenje and Postic, 1970, 1971; Janis and Habel, 1972). Interferon was demonstrated in

Table III

Inhibition of Rabies Virus Infection by Endogenous Interferon

Inducer	Administration of Inducer		Experimental host	Rabies virus strain (route)	Investigators
	Route	Time[a]			
Poly I:C[b]	Intraperitoneal	3 hours before	Mice	Fixed CVS (intraplantar, intracerebral)	Nemes et al., 1969
Poly I:C	Intravenous, intramuscular	24 hours before to 3 hours after	Rabbits	Street (intramuscular)	Fenje and Postic, 1970, 1971
Poly I:C	Intravenous, intramuscular	24 hours before to 3 hours after	Rabbits	Fixed, street (intramuscular)	Janis and Habel, 1972
	Intramuscular, intraperitoneal	3–67 hours after	Mice	Street (intramuscular)	
Bovine parainfluenza, Type 3	Intravenous	24 hours before to 10 min after	Rabbits	Street (intradermal)	Fayaz et al., 1970
Newcastle disease virus	Intravenous	24 hours before to 3 hours after	Rabbits	Street (intradermal)	Vieuchange et al., 1970
Newcastle disease virus	Intraperitoneal	24 hours before	Rabbits, hamsters	Fixed CVS (intramuscular)	Atanasiu et al., 1970

[a] Time of single injection or first of a series of injections in relation to time of virus inoculation.
[b] Double stranded ribopolynucleotide, polyinosinic-polycytidylic acid (Field et al., 1967).

sera of poly I:C-treated rabbits, and levels were higher in animals inoculated intravenously than in those inoculated intramuscularly.

Viruses which have been used as inducers of endogenous interferon in studies on rabies virus infection in animals include bovine parainfluenza Type 3 (BPI3) virus and active and inactive Newcastle disease virus (NDV). In a study by Fayaz et al. (1970) rabbits were protected against rabies by the intravenous injection of BPI3 virus, either 24 hours before or 10 min after the intradermal inoculation of a street strain of rabies virus; virus given 24 hours later had no effect. Mice were not protected from rabies by intraperitoneal inoculation of BPI3 virus before or after infection with fixed rabies virus. Vieuchange et al. (1970) demonstrated that intravenous inoculation of NDV 24 hours prior to injection of street rabies virus in rabbits prevented rabies from developing; increased amounts of NDV gave some evidence of protection even when given 10 min, 1 hour, and 3 hours after inoculation of rabies virus. The serum interferon levels, however, were not determined at the time the rabbits were challenged with rabies virus. Other investigators (Atanasiu et al., 1970) demonstrated the induction of high levels of endogenous interferon in mice, hamsters, and rabbits by intravenous or intraperitoneal inoculation of inactive NDV. Hamsters and rabbits were resistant to subsequent challenge with fixed CVS rabies virus, but mice were not protected. In subsequent studies these investigators found that NDV induced interferon could protect immunosuppressed hamsters from the increased susceptibility to rabies virus which they exhibited following treatment with cyclophosphamide (Tsiang and Atanasiu, 1973).

IV. Rabies Virus Strain Differences and Sensitivity to Interferon

Negative results have been noted in some of the studies investigating the effect of exogenous or endogenous interferon on rabies virus infection. All of these were done using the CVS strain of fixed rabies virus in mice, and investigators have reasoned that these failures were due to the rapid spread of fixed virus in the mouse, and the failure of administered or induced interferon to reach those cells of the central nervous system in which infection is initiated (Finter, 1967; Baron, 1967; Soave, 1968; Fayaz *et al.*, 1970). It has also been suggested, in view of the varying sensitivities of certain viruses to the action of different animal interferons (Stewart *et al.*, 1969), that rabies virus, while sensitive to rabbit and hamster interferons, may not be inhibited by mouse interferon (Atanasiu *et al.*, 1970). Turner (1972) reported that hamsters but not mice were protected by poly I:C-induced interferon against lethal challenge with CVS rabies virus.

However, as discussed above, Nemes *et al.* (1969) demonstrated partial protection of mice against infection with the CVS strain of rabies virus by treatment with poly I:C, and the sensitivity of a fixed strain of rabies virus to mouse interferon in an *in vitro* system (mouse ependymoma cell monolayers) had also been reported (Barroeta and Atanasiu, 1969). Janis and Habel (1972), in discussing their success in demonstrating partial protection of mice against a street strain of rabies virus by poly I:C treatment, reiterate the point made by Finter (1967) that street and fixed strains of virus may differ in their sensitivity to interferon. Studies in the authors' laboratory have explored possible differences in the sensitivities of strains of rabies virus to interferon by comparing the influence of poly I:C induced interferon in mice on the course and outcome of infection with a number of street strains isolated from various domestic and wild animal hosts. Data accumulated indicate that rabies virus strains do differ in sensitivity to the action of poly I:C induced interferon in mice. In general, highly invasive strains which are infective by peripheral routes of inoculation are less sensitive to interferon than are strains which do not infect by peripheral routes or are low titered when administered intramuscularly or via the footpad (S. E. Sulkin and R. Allen, unpublished observations).

V. Induction of Interferon by Rabies Vaccines

Although the mechanism responsible for the protection afforded by Pasteur treatment has never been fully defined, there is evidence which indicates that factors other than the neutralizing antibody response of an individual animal play a role in preventing death from rabies. The above-mentioned experimental work suggesting that interferon may play a role in inhibiting rabies infection prompted recent studies using animal models to evaluate the protective activity of rabies virus vaccines. Baer and Cleary (1972) compared the interferon-inducing capacity of duck embryo vaccine (DEV) and a concentrated, inactivated rabies vaccine prepared from tissue culture fluids from baby hamster kidney (BHK) cells infected with Pitman-Moore (PM) fixed rabies virus by the technique of Wiktor *et al.* (1969). One dose of the latter vaccine (PM-BHK) induced measurable levels of interferon in serum of mice for 3–32 hours following treatment, whereas no interferon could be demonstrated in the serum of mice inoculated with DEV. The difference in interferon-inducing capacity of the two vaccines correlated with the difference in mortality rates between groups of animals receiving the two vaccines 24 hours following footpad inoculation of a street strain of rabies virus; only 1 of 36 mice treated with PM-BHK vaccine died of rabies whereas 10 of 35 mice given DEV succumbed. However, the PM-BHK vaccine had a higher antigenic value than DEV and produced higher and more persistent levels of neutralizing antibodies against rabies virus in mice, which also could have been a factor in protecting some of the animals. In studies in the authors' laboratory attempts were made to demonstrate interferon in serum samples obtained from a limited number of individuals receiving DEV following exposure to rabid animals; no evidence was obtained of interferon induction during or following the courses of immunization (S. E. Sulkin and R. Allen, unpublished observations). Wiktor *et al.* (1972a) demonstrated that a chronic infection of the central nervous system of adult mice could be induced when HEP Flury virus was administered along with otherwise lethal doses of fixed or street rabies virus. Since the sparing effect of the HEP virus was not eliminated by irradiating the animals it seemed unlikely that neutralizing antibodies were involved and assays demonstrating serum interferon and brain interferon 7 and 14 hours, respectively, after intracerebral injection of HEP virus suggested that this mechanism was responsible for arresting the spread of the virulent strains of rabies virus. The most extensive study to date on the role of interferon induction in the protective activity of rabies vaccines is that of Wiktor *et al.* (1972b). Using a hamster model system these investigators correlated the protective effect of pre- and postexposure administration of different rabies vaccines with neutralizing antibody levels and the induction of interferon. Inactivated rabies virus vaccines of tissue culture origin administered shortly before or immediately after challenge with street rabies virus prevented death in significant numbers of animals. Similar results were obtained when animals received either Kern Canyon virus or influenza virus vaccine at or near the time of challenge with rabies virus. However, when vaccination preceded the challenge by 5 days or more only animals which received homologous (rabies) vaccine were protected. Since all vaccines induced interferon in hamsters, these results suggested that, depending on time of administration of vaccine in relation to exposure to rabies virus, interferon may play a role in protecting animals. Additional evidence favoring this hypothesis was obtained by demonstrating that hamsters pretreated with bacterial endotoxin and given rabies vaccine 24 hours before challenge produced less interferon and were not as well protected. Also, rabies vaccines with good antigenic values but which failed to induce interferon in animals (presumably due to loss of a factor during long-term storage) protected those given rabies virus 2 weeks after vaccination but not those challenged just 24 hours after treatment. In comparing different types of rabies vaccines for their capacity to induce interferon in hamsters and protect against rabies virus challenge it was found that all preparations which induced interferon were protective when given 24 hours before challenge. When treatment was administered 2 hours after challenge, however, no direct correlation could be established between levels of interferon and degrees of protection. In other experiments to obtain data relating to interferon and rabies vaccines it was demonstrated that concentrated rabies virus vaccines also induced interferon in rabbits and in rabbit kidney cell and human embryonic fibroblast cultures. Live virus vaccines were found to induce more interferon than inactivated preparations both *in vivo* and *in vitro*, but even live HEP virus vaccine failed to induce interferon in rabies-immune rabbits. Turner (1972) reported the failure of several different rabies vaccines (Fermi, Semple, modified Semple, duck embryo, and tissue culture vaccine) to induce interferon in rabbits, mice, or hamster, nor were any animals afforded immediate protection against lethal challenge with CVS rabies virus.

Although certain of the studies discussed above provide evidence that interferon may play a role in the protective activity of rabies vaccine they also indicate that other mechanisms are involved. It seems likely that so long as rabies vaccines remain the crude biologics they are at present, their mode of action in preventing rabies will remain an enigma; the most effective way to use them will not be understood, and treatment failures will continue to occur. However, the advent of the new, more purified rabies vaccines of tissue culture origin will not only provide a more effective tool for the prevention of rabies but will also simplify research on mechanisms of their protective activity.

Acknowledgment

Studies conducted in the authors' laboratory were supported by USPHS Grant AI02316 and NSF Grant GB-30775X.

References

Atanasiu, P., Barroeta, M., Tsiang, H., and Favre, S. (1970). *Ann. Inst. Pasteur, Paris* **119**, 767.
Baer, G. M., and Cleary, W. F. (1972). *J. Infec. Dis.* **125**, 520.
Baron, S. (1967). *Interferon; Ciba Found. Symp.* pp. 215–216.
Barroeta, M., and Atanasiu, P. (1969). *C. R. Acad. Sci., Ser. D* **269**, 1353.
Crick, J., and Brown, F. (1974). *J. Gen. Virol.* **22**, 147.
Depoux, R. (1965). *C. R. Acad. Sci.* **260**, 354.
Desai, S. M. (1970). *Nature (London)* **228**, 460.
Fayaz, A., Afshar, A., and Bahmanyar, M. (1970). *Arch. Gesamte Virusforsch.* **29**, 159.
Fenje, P., and Postic, B. (1970). *Nature (London)* **226**, 171.
Fenje, P., and Postic, B. (1971). *J. Infec. Dis.* **123**, 426.
Fernandes, M. V., Wiktor, T. J., and Koprowski, H. (1964). *J. Exp. Med.* **120**, 1099.
Field, A. K., Tytell, A. A., Lampson, G. P., and Hilleman, M. R. (1967). *Proc. Nat. Acad. Sci. U. S.* **58**, 1004.
Findlay, G. M. (1948). *J. Roy. Microsc. Soc.* [3] **68**, 20.
Findlay, G. M., and MacCallum, F. O. (1937). *J. Pathol. Bacteriol.* **44**, 405.
Finter, N. B. (1967). *Interferon; Ciba Found. Symp.* pp. 204–215.
Henle, W. (1950). *J. Immunol.* **64**, 203.
Hoskins, M. (1935). *Amer. J. Trop. Med.* **15**, 675.
Isaacs, A., and Lindenmann, J. (1957). *Proc. Roy. Soc., Ser. B* **147**, 258.
Janis, B., and Habel, K. (1972). *J. Infec. Dis.* **125**, 345.
Kanazawa, K., and Ohtomi, Y. (1958). *Virology* **6**, 571.
Kaplan, M. M., Wecker, E., Forsek, Z., and Koprowski, H. (1960). *Nature (London)* **186**, 821.
Kaplan, M. M., Cohen, D., Koprowski, H., Dean, D., and Ferrigan, L. (1962). *Bull. WHO* **26**, 765.
Koprowski, H., Black, J., and Nelsen, D. J. (1954). *J. Immunol.* **72**, 94.
Kravchenko, A. T., Voronin, E. S., and Kosmiadi, G. A. (1967). *Acta Virol.* **11**, 145.

Larke, R. P. B. (1966). *Can. Med. Ass. J.* **94,** 23.

Lennette, E. H. (1951). *Annu. Rev. Microbiol.* **5,** 277–294.

Levaditi, C., Nicolau, S., and Schoen, R. (1926). *Ann. Inst. Pasteur, Paris* **40,** 973.

Magrassi, F. (1935). *Z. Hyg. Infektionskr.* **117,** 501.

Nemes, M. M., Tytell, A. A., Lampson, G. P., Field, A. K., and Hilleman, M. R. (1969). *Proc. Soc. Exp. Biol. Med.* **132,** 776.

Pasteur, L. (1888). *Ann. Inst. Pasteur, Paris* **1,** 1.

Postic, B., and Fenje, P. (1971). *Appl. Microbiol.* **22,** 428.

Rytel, M. W., and Kilbourne, E. D. (1966). *J. Exp. Med.* **123,** 767.

Selimov, M. A., Chuprikova, M., Kalinina, L., and Sharova, Z. (1965). *Acta Virol. (Prague),* Engl. Ed. **9,** 445.

Sims, R. A., Allen, R., and Sulkin, S. E. (1967). *J. Infec. Dis.* **117,** 360.

Soave, O. A. (1968). *Amer. J. Vet. Res.* **29,** 1507.

Stewart, W. E., and Sulkin, S. E. (1966). *Proc. Soc. Exp. Biol. Med.* **123,** 650.

Stewart, W. E., Scott, W. D., and Sulkin, S. E. (1969). *J. Virol.* **4,** 147.

Sulkin, S. E., Allen, R., Sims, R. A., Krutzsch, P. H., and Kim, C. (1960). *J. Exp. Med.* **112,** 595.

Tsiang, H., and Atanasiu, P. (1973) *C. R. Acad. Sci. (D), Paris* **276,** 1085.

Turner, G. S. (1972), *J. Hyg.* **70,** 445.

Vieuchange, J. (1967). *Arch. Gesamte Virusforsch.* **22,** 87.

Vieuchange, J. (1968). *Bull. Acad. Nat. Med., Paris* [3] **152,** 234.

Vieuchange, J. (1969). *Bull. Acad. Nat. Med., Paris* [3] **153,** 374.

Vieuchange, J., and Fayaz, A. (1969). *C. R. Acad. Sci., Ser. D* **268,** 991.

Vieuchange, J., Chabaud, M. A., and Vialat, C. (1966). *C. R. Soc. Biol.* **160,** 2278.

Vieuchange, J., Chabaud, M. A., and Vialat, C. (1967). *Bull. Acad. Nat. Med., Paris* [3] **151,** 33.

Vieuchange, J., Fayaz, A., and de Lalun, E. (1970). *C. R. Acad. Sci., Ser. D* **271,** 734.

Wiktor, T. J., and Clark, H. F. (1972). *Infection and Immunity* **6,** 988.

Wiktor, T. J., and Koprowski, H. (1967). *Bacteriol. Proc.* p. 166.

Wiktor, T. J., Fernandes, M. V., and Koprowski, H. (1964). *J. Immunol.* **93,** 353.

Wiktor, T. J., Sokol, F., Kuwert, E., and Koprowski, H. (1969). *Proc. Soc. Exp. Biol. Med.* **131,** 799.

Wiktor, T. J., Koprowski, H., and Rorke, L. B. (1972a). *Proc. Soc. Exp. Biol. Med.* **140,** 759.

Wiktor, T. J., Postic, B., Ho, M., and Koprowski, H. (1972b). *J. Infec. Dis.* **126,** 408.

Yoshino, K., Taniguchi, S., and Arai, K. (1966). *Proc. Soc. Exp. Biol. Med.* **123,** 387.

PART III

Diagnosis

CHAPTER 19

Animal Inoculation and the Negri Body

P. Atanasiu

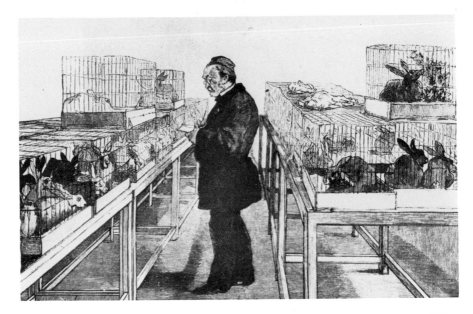

Pasteur in his laboratory. *Science Illustrée* 15 September 1888. By courtesy of The Pasteur Museum, Paris.

I. Introduction

Long before Pasteur's time it was shown that rabies could be transmitted to rabbits and dogs by infecting cutaneous wounds with saliva (Zinke, 1804), but later investigators including Galtier (1879) were not able to transmit the disease with any regularity by this method. Galtier had selected the rabbit as an experimental animal, but subcutaneous or intravenous inoculations either gave irregular results or produced extremely long incubation periods. Duboué (1879), during the same period, had realized that after a bite the virus must travel from the peripheral nerves toward the nerve centers, a supposition which was later confirmed by DiVestea and Zagari (1887).

Proper experimentation on rabies began with Pasteur's conclusion

---

Fig. 1. (A) Street virus in human brain. Many typical Negri bodies showing internal structure. (Hematoxylin and Eosin stain, ×1000.) (B) Street virus in cat brain. (Mann stain, ×1000.) (C) Street virus in dog brain. (Mann stain, ×1000.) (D) Street virus in suckling mouse brain. (Hematoxylin and Eosin stain, ×1000.) (E) Street virus in a bovine brain. (Hematoxylin and Eosin stain, ×1000.) (F) Street virus in the brain of a Fox. (Hematoxylin and Eosin stain, ×1400.) Courtesy of P. Atanasiu and J. Sisman, Institut Pasteur, Paris. (See facing color plate.)

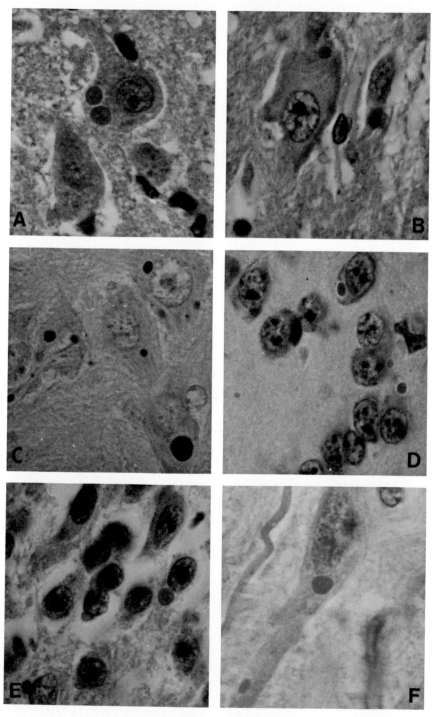

Fig. 1.

that rabies virus cannot be grown outside the nervous system; Pasteur had inoculated it intracerebrally, thus obtaining its multiplication and regular transmission. A short note on rabies, "Note sur la rage" was presented by Pasteur (1881), presenting the first results on the transmission of the disease by the intracerebral inoculation in rabbits.

In a second note (1882) Pasteur reported that all the forms of rabies were due to the same organism, located in the brain and that "submeningeal" inoculation infallibly transmitted the disease. Somewhat later Pasteur (1885) became the first to immunize animals by injecting them with rabbit medullas in which the virus had been attenuated by desiccation.

In early research, vaccine production, and diagnosis, the rabbit played an important role; later on mice and rats (Babes, 1887; Remlinger, 1904; Jonnesco, 1934; Webster and Dawson, 1935; Johnson and Leach, 1940) played an equally significant role in experimental research, diagnosis and, recently, vaccine production (Fuenzalida and Palacios, 1955; Svet-Moldavskaja and Svet-Moldavsky, 1959).

The histologic diagnosis of rabies evolved in three steps. The first was the histologic study of the neuraxis in man and animals succumbing to rabies, and the description of specific lesions called Babes nodules (Babes, 1892). Research then concentrated on proliferative and infiltrative lesions, and in particular upon their localization in the spinal ganglia (Van Gehuchten, 1900), but they were soon found to be nonspecific, and often were observed in toxic conditions and other viral diseases.

The second period began with the description by Negri (1903) of inclusion bodies in the cytoplasm of certain nerve cells infected with street rabies (see Fig. 1). The third and last period is characterized by the specific identification of the rabies antigen by specific immunologic techniques: immunofluorescence (Goldwasser and Kissling, 1958), the immunoperoxidase technique (Atanasiu *et al.*, 1971a) (Fig. 2A and B) and the ferritin technique by electronic microscopy (Atanasiu *et al.*, 1963b; Hummeler *et al.*, 1968).

This chapter summarizes the inoculation of laboratory animals susceptible to rabies virus, the rapid histologic diagnosis, and, finally, the new immunoperoxidase technique.

II. Animal Inoculation

Several laboratory animals can be used to isolate and identify rabies virus, especially the mouse, rabbit, guinea pig, and hamster.

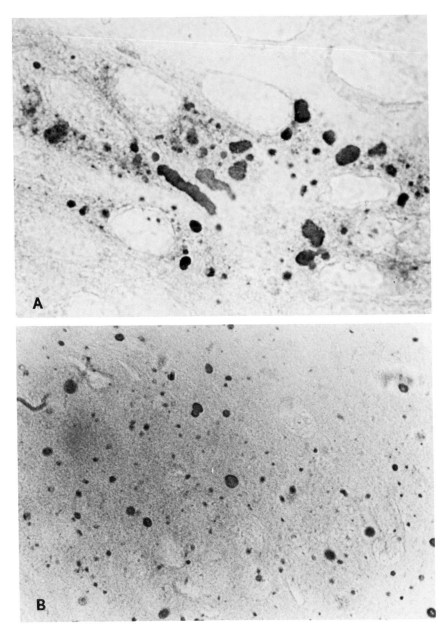

Fig. 2. A: Fixed virus in tissue culture. Note the many specific inclusions in the cytoplasm. B: Street virus brain impression. (A and B: Immunoperoxidase stain. Courtesy of Sisman, Dragonas, Tsiang, Harbi, and Atanasiu.)

The intracerebral inoculation technique is identical for all animals. We will present the clinical signs of the disease in rabbits, guinea pigs, and hamsters, and will also give a detailed description of inoculation of mice.

A. RABBIT

The first to work with this animal was Galtier (1879). Pasteur (1881) selected it as the most suitable animal for the passage and transmission of the virus, as well as for production of antirabies vaccine.

Signs of rabies in the rabbit vary according to whether street or fixed virus is inoculated. In experimental infections one has to consider the weight of the animal, the method of inoculation, dose, and nature of the virus employed. If, for example, one inoculates the Pasteur fixed virus intracerebrally and sacrifices an animal every day, virus can be detected from the third day in the brain stem and brain.

1. Infection with Fixed Virus

The clinical signs of fixed rabies infection begin to appear about the sixth or seventh day and are characterized by weight loss, temperature rise, and change in behavior, followed by cerebellar and meningeal signs: chewing and grinding of the teeth, trembling of the head, intermittent lack of coordination in the hind legs (one after the other), then paralysis of the hindquarters and rapidly generalized paralysis. In the following days the animal lies on its side with its head stretched out, and dyspnea is noted. Weight loss continues and the animal reacts to stimuli with epileptic fits. This "death-throes" stage lasts a long time and the only sign of life is the rhythmic movement of the thorax. The respiration becomes intermittent and death apparently comes from asphyxia. The signs last from 1 to 4 days.

2. Infection with Street Virus

When isolates from the brain or salivary glands of rabid dogs are inoculated into rabbits the furious form of the disease is rarely produced. Galtier (1879) described the usual paralytic form in detail. The incubation period varies greatly, depending on the virus isolate used, but generally does not exceed 2–3 weeks. The animals lose weight and invariably pass through a premonitory febrile period before manifestation of the disease; the signs are identical with those of fixed rabies. Street viruses may be found whose incubation periods are short and identical to that of fixed rabies.

It should be noted that the incubation period of fixed virus may vary according to the species or route of inoculation employed. The Sassari (Fermi) strain, for example, produced clinical signs 4 days after intracerebral inoculation in rabbits, but, after subcutaneous inoculation, kills mice in 7–10 days.

B. MOUSE AND RAT

As early as 1887 Babes had insisted on the susceptibility of mice and rats to rabies. The albino mouse has been selected as the most suitable animal for rabies diagnosis (Jonnesco, 1934; Webster and Dawson, 1935), for the immunologic study of "strains" of rabies virus and the testing of antirabies vaccines (Habel, 1940). After intracerebral inoculation of the mouse or rat with street virus, signs are usually noted 9–12 days later, and these may vary but often include paralysis. The mouse can exhibit either furious, pruritic, or spasmodic forms, with sudden death after a short period of agitation. Remlinger (1904) noted a bilateral serous conjunctivitis in this species even before paralysis. It has been shown that the cornea of the rabbit contains Negri bodies (Levaditi and Schoen, 1936). In mice, too, specific rabies antigen has been found in the superficial cells of the cornea (Schneider, 1969). Street rabies may rarely provoke the furious form in mice or rats, in which they attack people and objects. These animals should be regarded as dangerous since they eliminate the virus by the salivary glands, transmitting the disease to animals which they bite (Galli-Valerio, 1906). In mice, the virus may also be excreted in the skin of the nose, the tongue papillae, and the intestines (Atanasiu *et al.*, 1970; Fischman and Schaeffer, 1971).

The age of mice is an important factor in their susceptibility to rabies. Flury strains rabies virus, high egg passage (HEP), for instance, kills 2- to 3-day-old suckling mice by the intracerebral route, but the same virus inoculated in adult mice does not produce illness (Koprowski, 1954). Some rabies isolates from wild animals are more pathogenic to suckling mice than adults. Many workers in rabies diagnosis and isolation prefer the suckling mouse because it appears to be more susceptible than the adult (Webster and Dawson, 1935; Johnson, 1964; Nilsson *et al.*, 1968). It should be noted that weanling mice, however, are routinely used in almost all diagnostic laboratories that perform mouse inoculation.

The clinical disease in mice or rats lasts from 1 to 3 days, but the incubation period usually varies from 7 to 20 days, according to the method of inoculation; suckling animals commonly sicken 1 or 2 days earlier.

C. Guinea Pig

Pasteur (1884) and Marie (1930) drew attention to the susceptibility of these animals. Pasteur (1884) and Babes (1912b) claimed that the guinea pig may be even more susceptible to rabies than the rabbit. Street virus inoculated intracerebrally produces the disease in 10–20 days. The incubation period for fixed virus is about 6 days. The disadvantage of inoculating guinea pigs with street virus is that manipulation of sick animals is very dangerous: they become very restless and frightened at the least noise, jump about in the cage, squeal, quarrel with their companions, bite them and show abnormal sexual excitement. Paralysis follows and death ensues very quickly. The guinea pig may also be used for testing attenuated veterinary vaccines (Koprowski, 1967).

D. Hamster

The Syrian hamster (*Mesocricetus auratus*) is as susceptible to rabies as the mouse when inoculated intracerebrally. It is considered as the most sensitive laboratory animal when inoculated parenterally (Koprowski, 1949). The clinical signs are identical to those in mice. It is rarely used in diagnosis but is often used in immunologic research.

Primary hamster kidney cells are used for the preparation of antirabies vaccines (Kissling and Reese, 1963), and the BHK_{21} S13 cell line is often used in rabies research, including investigations into the physicochemical properties of the rabies virion (Atanasiu *et al.*, 1963a; Fernandes *et al.*, 1963).

The Chinese hamster (*Cricetulus griseus*) is susceptible to fixed rabies virus, with the production of Negri bodies in Ammon's horn. This animal is also susceptible to street virus inoculated intracerebrally, intramuscularly, and subcutaneously (Yen, 1936).

III. The Mouse Inoculation Technique

For the usual diagnosis of rabies the susceptible and inexpensive weanling mouse is chosen. The inoculation technique has been summarized by Koprowski (1967).

A. ANIMALS

In order to obtain reliable results in a diagnostic laboratory, a reproducible technique should be followed which does not vary and is performed by the same inoculators. The animals used should originate from a known breed and be free of latent viruses [especially mouse poliomyelitis (Theiler, 1934) and lymphocytic choriomeningitis (Armstrong and Lillie, 1934)], ectoparasites, or *Salmonella*. Runts or animals showing ruffled hair, diarrhea, or excessive weakness must be eliminated. If the animals have been shipped they should be observed for 3 days before inoculation. All strains of mice appear to be equally susceptible to rabies. The gray mouse should be avoided simply because it is difficult to manipulate.

The 9- to 15-g albino mouse (21 to 31 days old) is used, regardless of sex, since both sexes appear to be equally susceptible. If mice are to be held for long periods of time, females are preferred since they do not fight as much as males.

B. SPECIMEN FOR INOCULATION

The brain or salivary glands are usually used for diagnosis. The virus is often found in all parts of the brain examined; preference is given to certain parts, such as the Ammon's horn, the cerebellum, and the medulla and cortex. The submaxillary glands, considered the richest in rabies virus when they are infected, are increasingly used.

The saliva and throat swab from patients with rabies are a source of virus. The saliva is collected near the parotid duct opening or under the tongue with a syringe, Pasteur pipette, or moistened cotton swab, then is placed in 1–2 ml buffered saline solution with serum (10%) and antibiotics. It is also important to swab the nasal mucosa and eyes of suspect human rabies cases.

C. GRINDING

The specimen taken for inoculation should be finely ground. Pieces from various parts of the brain (usually Ammon's horn, cerebellum and brain stem) are mixed together to give 3 to 4 grams of material, and these are then ground with a mortar and pestle or a small Waring or Ten Broeck blender. The size of the grinder depends on the quantity of material to be ground. Sterile sand (alundum) may be added as an abrasive, especially for the submaxillary glands which are very resistant to crushing.

D. Dilution and Centrifugation

The material must be diluted for grinding. The diluent used is basically an isotonic solution, or simply sterile distilled water plus 2% (rabbit, horse, or calf) inactivated serum (56°C for 30 min). The serum should of course be free of rabies antibodies. If the specimen is to be frozen, 10% serum should be added. All the diluents should contain antibiotics (2 mg streptomycin and 500 IU penicillin/ml), but if mice die of contamination (with brain abscesses) one should double that concentration or add other antibiotics. It should be emphasized that bacteria or other viruses, especially lymphocytic choriomeningitis, may produce symptoms identical to rabies.

Usually 10–20% nerve tissue is inoculated, but this dilution is increased when, on rare occasions, difficulties are found in isolating the virus because of interference phenomena, self-sterilizing neuroinfections, or inhibiting factors (Levaditi *et al.*, 1928; Parker and Sikes, 1966). The suspension is centrifuged in the cold for 5 min at 1000 rpm to get rid of large particles. The inoculum should be cool or cold throughout all these procedures.

E. Inoculation Technique

For intracerebral inoculations 0.25 ml (tuberculin) syringes should be used, using 0.03 ml for a single mouse dose. Either 26 or 27 gauge needles (0.40–0.45 mm) ¼ to ⅜ inch (1–1.5 cm long) should be used.

The mice are anesthetized by ether inhalation before inoculation. A glass jar with a piece of cotton inside is used for anesthesia; some ether is poured on the cotton and a wire mesh is placed inside the jar over the cotton.

The anesthetized mouse is laid on its left side, its legs toward the inoculator, who puts his left thumb under the lower jaw and his index finger on the top of the skull, pulling the skin lightly from the head, thus fixing the head firmly, and taking care not to suffocate the animal (Fig. 3A).

The syringe is held in the right hand in a position perpendicular to the head, is forced rapidly 1–2 mm through the brain case, 2 mm from the frontal arch, in the direction of the median line; 0.03 ml is injected and the needle is withdrawn. The mice are then checked and any dead animals are replaced by others inoculated with the same specimen, care being taken to use a fresh syringe for each diagnostic case.

The possibility of transmission of rabies by aerosol should be

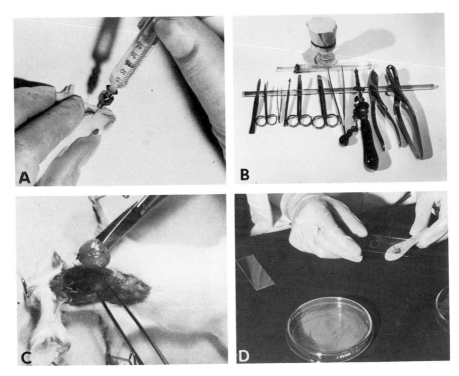

Fig. 3. Mouse inoculation test. A: Intracerebral inoculation of mice. B: Old and new instruments for inoculation and removal of dog and mouse brains. C: Removal of a mouse brain. D: Impression slide preparation of mouse brain.

borne in mind (Atanasiu, 1965). The inoculated animals should not be mixed with healthy ones, and the syringes should be handled with care when air bubbles are forced out; this latter should be done inside a sterile tube or in a sterile gauze in order to avoid aerosol production. The syringes should be rinsed and sterilized after inoculation.

F. OBSERVATION OF ANIMALS

A serial number is given to each mouse, either in a notebook or on the type of card suggested by the World Health Organization (Koprowski, 1954). The mice are observed daily. The signs noted are humping, trembling, incoordination of the hind legs, paralysis, and prostration. The same signs are manifested in the suckling mouse; in this age animal the first sign noted may be the lack of milk in the stomach. The death of the animal before the fifth day is regarded as nonspecific, due, perhaps, to another virus, bacteria, or trauma during inoculation.

The signs of rabies are very characteristic, but other viral or bacterial infections may produce similar ones. In order to confirm that death was due to rabies one may sacrifice one mouse daily (or take a dead mouse) from the fifth or the sixth day and examine its brain by immunofluorescence; if it is found that the animals have died of bacterial infection in spite of the antibiotics present, the cerebral material should be filtered, the antibiotic concentration increased, or other antibiotics added.

G. EXTRACTION OF THE BRAINS

From the fifth day on, any prostrate mouse may be killed with chloroform. The brain is taken in order to find Negri bodies by Sellers' technique, or rabies antigen by immunofluorescence. The head of the dead mouse is pinned to a dissecting board. The legs and tail are pinned down as well as the muzzle, which is stretched forward. The skin over the head is first disinfected with alcohol, then cut with scissors to expose the skull. Disinfection is repeated, the ocular orbits are fixed with forceps, and the skull is then cut open with curved scissors, cutting first at the level of the orbits and then back along the sides, following which the brain case is folded back and the brain is cut at the brain stem, removed (Fig. 3C), and placed in a sterile Petri dish. The chiasma is turned upward. The brain is rapidly sectioned at the posterior third. The posterior part is transferred to a tongue depressor (or paper towel) with the cut section facing upward. Clean microscopic slides are then pressed lightly against the cut surface of the section to obtain impressions (Fig. 3D), to be stained either by Sellers' stain, or with conjugate for the immunofluorescence technique. One part of the brain may then be fixed for histologic examination, and the other part held at −70°C (or in glycerol) to conserve the virus.

IV. Negri Body Diagnosis

A. HISTOLOGIC EXAMINATION

In the histologic study of rabies, two types of lesions are to be distinguished, the inflammatory lesions common to all viral infections of the nervous system, and the specific inclusions that may be identified by histologic and immunologic techniques. The histologic examination of the nervous system reveals diffuse encephalitis and ganglionic and cellular lesions.

1. Rabies Encephalitis

The systematic histologic studies of rabies went on between 1872 and 1900 with the help of the following investigators: Meynert (1872), Benedikt (1875), Kolesnikoff (1875), Schaeffer (1887), Coats (1877), Gamaleia (1887), Babes (1892), and Van Gehuchten (1900). The mere names of Babes and Van Gehuchten evoke all the important works on the subject.

The encephalitic lesions had been described in full by Babes (1892). In rabies, at different levels of the neuraxis, he had verified a marked hyperemia followed by diapedesis and formation of perivascular nodules. All these characteristics constitute what we commonly call an "encephalitic focus" in which various types of mononuclear cells (lymphocytes, monocytes, and plasmocytes) can be seen (Fig. 4A–C). These nodules are usually found in neuronophagic areas. The presence of the nodules led Babes to conceive of the idea of a histologic diagnosis confirmed by intracerebral rabbit inoculation of the suspect material.

Babes' histologic technique (1912b) consisted in cutting brain and medulla sections, fixing them rapidly in absolute alcohol, and staining them with methylene blue or Löffler's fuchsin.

2. Ganglionic Lesions

Van Gehuchten and Nelis (1900) have described histologic lesions which they considered specific, at least by their ganglionic localization. These lesions consist of an endothelial cell proliferation arising from the capsule of the spinal or sympathetic nerve ganglia. The normal nerve cells are gradually replaced by clusters of small round cells. The few remaining nerve cells undergo alterations in their structure and in the shape of their cytoplasm and nucleus. These lesions vary in intensity according to the species considered and from one animal to another as well. Significant lesions are found in the dog, but in rabbit and human beings they are of lesser intensity. The fact that they invariably occur led Van Gehuchten to recommend that they be observed for a rapid diagnosis (Fig. 5A–D).

Fig. 4. Street rabies virus in rabbit brain. A: A field rich in inflammatory foci (Babes) with meningitis, × 350. B and C: Hyperemia and perivascular nodules. D: Pyramidal cells with Negri bodies in Ammon's horn. Mann stain, × 1500.

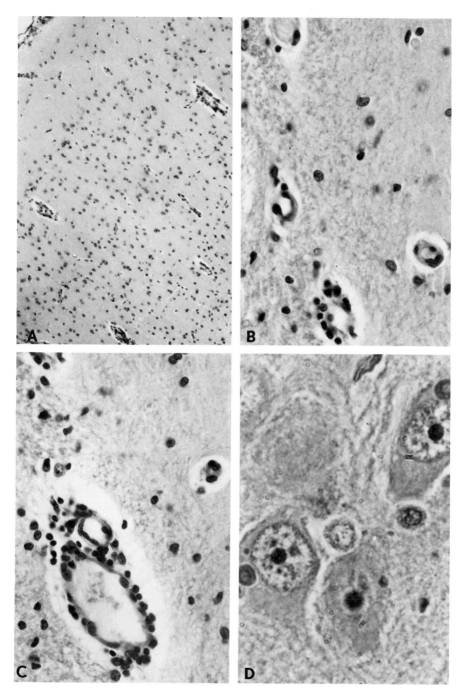

Fig. 4.

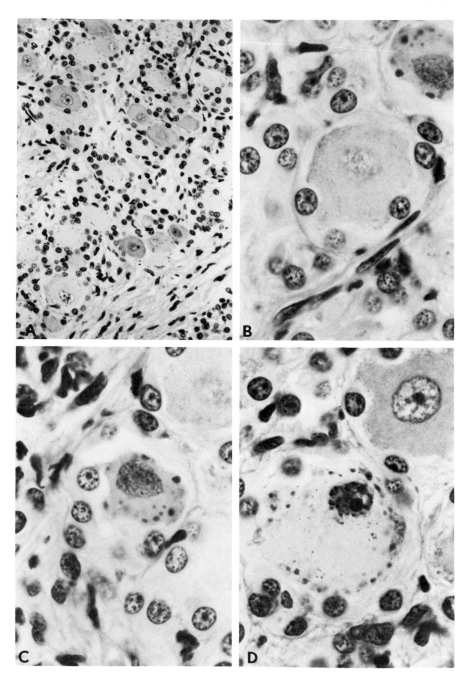

Fig. 5.

The nodules have the same characteristics as the lesions described by Babes, but their absence does not exclude a positive diagnosis of rabies.

3. Cellular Lesions

Before Negri's discovery, the description of histologic lesions only pointed out inflammatory processes due to neurotropic viruses in general. Golgi (1894) found that, in fixed rabies infection, the nerve cells become thinner and the nucleus smaller, with accompanying karyolysis, vacuolization of the cytoplasm, complete disappearance of Nissl's body and hypertrophy, followed by degeneration and neurofibrils (Schaeffer, 1889; Ramon y Cajál and Dalmacco-Garcia, 1904).

Babes described intracytoplasmic hyalin corpuscles in nerve cells which stained well with aniline dyes. These corpuscles or inclusions are identical with those described later on by Negri; Babes, however, did not give them any significance (Fig. 6).

In 1903 Negri demonstrated the corpuscles pathognomonic for rabies. At present it may be said that the histologic lesions of rabies are of two types: Negri bodies in street rabies infection and nuclear alterations in fixed rabies infection.

4. Negri Bodies

Other investigators had noted intracellular formations in rabies (Babes, 1892; Di Vestea, 1894), but homage is to be paid to Negri, the first to give a complete description of the bodies and of their relationship to rabies infection. Negri bodies have been described as being invariably intracytoplasmic formation,* round, ovular, or oblong, varying in size, and mainly localized in the pyramidal cells of Ammon's horn, in the Purkinje cells of the cerebellum, and in the cells of the medulla and various ganglia. In nerve cell prolongations they are oblong. The size of the Negri bodies ranges from 0.25 to 27 μm (Fig. 1 and 5D). They are very small in the neurons of salivary glands and tongue (Manouelian, 1906).

The abundance of Negri bodies varies according to the animal, the

* In impressions or smears the mechanical manipulation of the nervous tissue often results in their being outside the cell.

Fig. 5. Monkey inoculated with street virus. A: Invasion of Gasserian ganglia with inflammatory cells, lesion of the van Gehuchten type, ×250. B: Beginning of neuronophagic process followed by cell chromatoysis. C and D: Negri body in cytoplasm of ganglia cells. B–D, ×1000.

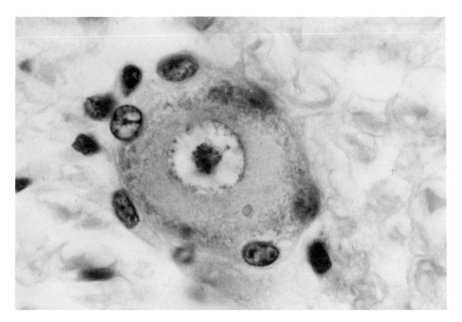

Fig. 6. Fixed virus infection in a rabbit (Babes) showing early infiltration of Gasserian ganglia and hyalin corpuscles in cytoplasm, × 1500. (Courtesy of Gamet and Atanasiu.)

virus isolate, and the passage of the virus. In the dog they may also be found in the neuraxis of the plexiform ganglia and, in the rabbit, in the Gasserian ganglia. In cows they may be very large, at times reaching macroscopic size.

5. Nuclear Lesions

In fixed rabies Lentz (1909) had noticed some nuclear lesions which later have been called "passage corpuscles." Lépine and Sautter (1936) gave a pathognomonic significance to those nuclear lesions in fixed rabies. In the median part of the external zone of Ammon's horn a small number of ovular hyperchromic corpuscles replace the nucleus of some cells. This oxyphilic degeneration of the nucleus is constant in fixed rabies (Fig. 7A and B).

B. Technique of Studying Negri Bodies

The histologic diagnosis of rabies depends on the rapid detection of Negri bodies as well as the demonstration of an encephalitis with intracytoplasmic inclusions in histologic sections. Satisfactory decap-

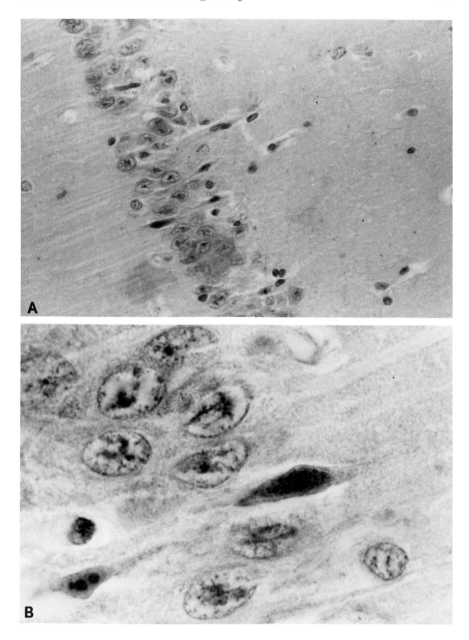

Fig. 7. Fixed virus in rabbit brain. A: Localization of lesions in Ammon's horn, × 350. B: Hyperchromic corpuscles replace the nucleus of some neurons, × 1500.

itation of the dead or killed animals and the rapid delivery of heads to the laboratory contribute greatly to the success of the diagnosis and of the isolation of the virus. Animals should not be destroyed by shooting them through the skull.

If the fluorescent antibody technique is not available for diagnosis and Sellers' stain is the only means of rapid staining, the animals should not be killed since it is thought that the development of Negri bodies is related to the period of illness before death.

The whole head (or the brain only, in the case of bovines) should be sent to the nearest diagnostic laboratory as early as possible and in the best conditions for preservation. Fifty percent glycerol in neutral saline is employed for shipping specimens (Roux, 1887). The World Health Organization recommends that the head or the brain be placed in a metal tin which, in turn, is put into a larger one containing ice. Freezing should be avoided. The small tin may be replaced by a plastic bag. The package should be clearly labeled, giving the following information: species and breed of the animal; whether it died, or, if killed, the means used for destroying it, as well as the signs noted; whether it has bitten somebody or has been in contact with other animals; whether and when it was vaccinated against rabies (Tierkel, 1967).

In the diagnostic laboratory the autopsy should be carried out in a room used for that purpose only. All precautions, including the use of protective glasses for the eyes, should be taken to prevent the infection of persons carrying out the opening of the tins and the removal of the animal brains. Preexposure vaccination of the staff is advisable (Tierkel and Sikes, 1967; Lépine et al., 1971). To insure bacterial sterility and protect the operator when the brain is extracted, rubber autopsy gloves should be used.

1. Removal of the Brain

It is important not to damage the brain and the medulla when they are removed from the skull. The heads of carnivores should be held firmly on an autopsy table, either by grasping them with large forceps which immobilize the jaw, or by using a clamp. A midline incision is made on the top of the head. The skull is then exposed by dissecting away the aponeurosis and temporal muscles and reflecting them laterally. The skull is sawed by cutting the occipital bone, then the temporal bones, and finally joining these two lateral cuts by a last incision just above the eyes. The calvarium is lifted off with the aid of a bone chisel. The meninges are then cut on each side of the longitudinal sinus with sterile rat tooth forceps and sharp pointed scissors. Another incision, perpendicular to the first, reveals the brain. After severing the medulla as far back as possible and then cutting the optic nerves, the brain is transferred to a large Petri dish.

The cerebellum of bovine brains may be removed through the foramen magnum as suggested by Schleifstein and Tompkins (1951).

2. Removal of the Salivary Glands

The salivary glands may contain large quantities of virus. In most animals they are situated subcutaneously on either side of the median line of the lower jaw. The dog's submaxillary gland is just behind the posterior border of the lower jaw; the glands are elliptical in shape, about 5 cm long and 3 cm wide, light pink to gray in color, and covered by a fibrous capsule.

3. Dissection of the Brain and Salivary Glands

The specific inclusions, the Negri bodies, have most often been found in Ammon's horn in the pyramidal cells of the cortex, in the Purkinje cells of the cerebellum, in the pons, and, less frequently, in the spinal cord and ganglia, cornea, adrenals, and other organs. The Ammon's horn is commonly thought of as being the best area for finding Negri bodies and also for rabies antigen by the FA technique. Ammon's horn is the select site for histologic diagnosis and mouse inoculation; in order to locate it in the dog, cat, or fox, a longitudinal incision is made into the dorsal surface at the rear of each cerebral hemisphere, 2 cm to either side of the midline. The incisions are made in the region of occipital lobe and extended 5–6 cm forward, depending on the size of the animal. After having first cut through the gray matter and then the white matter, the operator reaches the top of the lateral ventricle. By widening the incised hemisphere a white, glistening, semicylindrical body is exposed on the floor of the ventricle; this is Ammon's horn, identified by sectioning transversally to show the characteristic dark outer and lighter inner zones.

Transverse sections are made at various points on both sides so as to make histologic sections and impressions to be stained by Sellers' stain or examined by immunofluorescence. Some fragments are kept for mouse inoculation.

C. Histologic Techniques

Negri bodies may be detected by several procedures. The choice of the technique varies, but for rapid diagnosis, Sellers' stain or the

Ira Van Giesen stain (1906) are preferred. Both may be performed in a few minutes.

1. Sellers' Rapid Technique (Impression or Smear)

Sellers' rapid staining technique (1927, 1967) appears to be the simplest and most economical. Staining requires two stock solutions: one of methylene blue, another one of basic fuchsin; these are stored, without filtration, in screw-capped bottles and are kept refrigerated and protected from light. Two parts of methylene blue are mixed with one part of basic fuchsin for staining. The stain usually improves with time. The staining procedure is simple. Small sections of Ammon's horn, cortex, cerebellum, or medulla are cut for making impressions or smears, using two slides for each specimen. Each smear or impression must be made immediately before staining, since they must remain moist until they are immersed for 1–5 sec in the stain; this fixes and stains them at the same time. After being rinsed with running water and dried at room temperature, the preparations are examined under low power to find an area rich in nerve cells, then under oil immersion.

The best results are obtained with fresh, well-spread material. The cytoplasm of the nerve cell stains blue or purplish-blue, the nuclei and nucleoli strong blue, the interstitial tissue rose pink, nerve fibers deeper pink, and the erythrocytes copper red. Negri bodies are found in the cytoplasm of the large neurons, or between the membrane and the nucleus, or in the cell axon or dendrite. When smears or impressions are prepared the Negri bodies are most often seen outside the cells. The diameter is ordinarily more than 10 μm and the shape is oval, spherical, or elongated. One neuron may contain several inclusions, variable in size. The Negri body ground substance takes the fuchsin stain and appears magenta red or cherry red. Negri bodies, to be specific for rabies, must contain blue staining granules or inner bodies. These corpuscles, with a diameter of 0.2–0.5 μm, are arranged in concentric layers. The small bodies do not demonstrate evident inner corpuscles, and when the large bodies are absent it may not be possible to make a diagnosis of rabies. Out of 771 routine brain animal specimens found rabies positive by mouse inoculation, only 10.5% failed to show Negri bodies (Johnson, 1964). In Kazakhstan (USSR) rabies in common in foxes; in general no Negri bodies are noted in the brains of these rabid foxes, nor in the animals they bite (Kolomakin et al., 1968). Schaaf (1968) detected 2572 cases of rabies (in wild and domestic animals) by mouse inoculation: in 2469 cases (96%) he found Negri bodies by Sellers' stain.

Table I

Comparative Results Obtained by Three Diagnostic Methods in Wild and Domestic Animals[a]

Diagnostic method	Results[b]						Positive results for each method	Percent positive
Immunofluorescence	0	+	+	0	0	+	161	90.4
Histology	0	+	0	+	0	+	155	87.6
Mouse inoculation	0	+	+	+	+	0	177	99.1
NUMBER OF CASES	1926	147	13	7	10	1		

[a] Performed at the Pasteur Institute, Paris (Levaditi *et al.*, 1971).
[b] Total number of cases examined: 2104; total found positive by at least one test: 178.

Levaditi *et al.* (1971) compared the three methods (mouse inoculation, FA, and histology) for 2104 diagnostic specimens; 147 cases were positive by the three tests and 1926 negative. In spite of the disparity between the results of the tests used, 31 more cases were found to be rabies positive (Table I) by only one or two of the techniques.

If the results obtained by Sellers' staining are doubtful or negative, the immunofluorescence (or immunoperoxidase) techniques must be done, although the classic histologic method still remains available.

2. Fixation and Embedding

In the first work Negri proposed the following histologic technique: fix some fragments of Ammon's horn in Zenker's fluid; embed them in paraffin, and, after sectioning, proceed with Mann's stain (1902). This technique is still employed in many areas of the world today. A variant employed in many laboratories is as follows:

The brain or organ fragments are fixed in Susa's liquid:

Solution A:
Distilled water . . . . 800 ml
Sublimate (HgCl₂) . . . . 45 g
Sodium chloride. . . . . 5 g
Solution B:
Formalin 40%. . . . . 200 ml
Acetic acid . . . . 40 ml
Trichloracetic acid . . . . 20 g

Eighty ml of solution A are mixed with 25 ml of solution B.

Thin slides of tissue are fixed for 2 hours. Then the pieces are transferred directly to alcohol so as to eliminate the sublimate, and then, in turn, to a 5% hyposulfite solution, to absolute alcohol, xylol, and finally toluene. If the pieces have been fixed in Bouin's solution, they should be passed in a saturated solution of lithium carbonate and in 80° alcohol.

3. Mann's Stain

This is prepared just before use, as follows:

> 35 ml of an aqueous solution of 1% methylene blue,
> 35 ml of an aqueous solution of 1% eosine,
> 100 ml distilled water.

The sections are left in an alcoholic caustic soda solution for 20 min. They are then treated with the hyposulfite (5%) until they become white. After that, they are washed, rinsed in double distilled water, and later immersed in Mann's stain for 24 hours at room temperature, or for 6 hours at 37°C.

After being washed in distilled water and then rapidly in absolute alcohol, the sections are held for a few minutes in alcoholic caustic soda solution until they stain pink. Next they are washed in absolute alcohol, then with tap water. The section should acquire a sky blue color. They are rapidly treated with a dilute solution of acetic acid with water and then, after dehydration with absolute alcohol, they are passed into xylene and mounted in Canada balsam.

4. Results

When Sellers' staining gives doubtful results (for instance, a few Negri bodies atypical in size) the histologic method may be used. It confirms either a total absence of Negri bodies or their presence with a halo and inner corpuscles in the cytoplasm of nerve cells. With this technique the distemper inclusions (Lentz, 1909), the cytoplasmic inclusions in normal mice (Nicolau et al., 1933), or inclusions in the normal fox (Szlachta and Habel, 1953) can be differentiated from Negri bodies because only the last have inner basophilic bodies.

In rabies brain sections the red blood cells stain pink, the nucleoli of the neurons violet red, the chromatin blue, and the Negri bodies bright red with Mann's stain. In dogs with street rabies, we found a degeneration of the acinar epithelium in salivary glands, and a definite mononuclear cell infiltration in the interstitial tissue; the few Negri bodies seen are small in size.

The rapid methods such as the technique of Stovall and Black (1940) can also be used; fixation in acetone is followed by differential staining (eosin, methylene blue). The Schleifstein modification of Sellers' method (1937) consists of embedding in dioxan, and gives equally good results.

D. Immunofluorescence Technique

This excellent, rapid, and highly specific technique is discussed in the next chapter.

E. Immunoperoxidase Technique

This technique has been recently applied to the diagnosis of rabies (Atanasiu *et al.*, 1971a). Its principle is the same as immunofluorescence. A highly purified serum is conjugated to peroxidase by the means of glutaraldehyde. The evidence of the antigen–antibody reaction is obtained with the help of benzidine. The technique is sensitive, highly specific, and requires only an ordinary light microscope.

We present the technique of purification of rabies antibody by an insoluble rabies polymer, the procedure of conjugating rabies antibody with peroxidase, the direct staining technique, and the results obtained.

1. Preparation of the Immune Adsorbent Rabies Polymer

Four-day-old suckling mice are inoculated intracerebrally with 1000 LD_{50} of fixed virus. The brains are harvested 5 days later by using a pistol-shaped syringe connected to a suction pump.

After emulsification the brains are diluted in an equal volume of distilled water. The suspension is centrifuged for 10 min at 3000 rpm. The proteins are titrated in 10 ml of supernatant liquid by the Biuret method. Bovine albumin is added to these proteins in a ratio of four parts of albumin to one part of the protein antigen. The mixture is then added to 40 ml of an acetate solution, pH 5 (sodium acetate 1.0, acetic acid 1.0). Next, 8 ml of a 2.5% glutaraldehyde solution are added. Two hours later the gel obtained is washed three times with a phosphate buffer solution (PBS). Antirabies serum is slowly added to this gel and is stirred for 1 hour at room temperature. The gel is washed three times with PBS.

The antibodies are eluted by washing the immunoadsorbent with 0.2 *N* HCl–glycine buffer, pH 2.8. The total amount of protein is calculated before neutralization, followed by an overnight dialysis and final concentration.

2. Conjugation of Antirabies Antibody to Peroxidase

Ten to 14 mg of peroxidase RZ 3.6 (Sigma Chemical Company, St. Louis, Missouri) are conjugated to each ml of solution containing 5–7 mg of purified antirabies antibodies; the pH has previously been adjusted to 6.8 with bipotassic buffer (0.1 *M*). To this mixture is added

0.05 ml of 1% glutaraldehyde, and it is stirred for 2 hours at room temperature. The conjugate is then dialyzed overnight against PBS, pH 7.4. The next day it is centrifuged for 15 min at 3000 rpm. This conjugate is diluted 1:10 in physiologic saline before use (Avrameas, 1969).

3. Direct Staining

The fresh specimens (impressions, smears of brains infected with fixed or street virus, infected tissue culture, etc.) are fixed in cold acetone (−20°C) for 10 min.

Once dried, the slides or the coverslips are flooded with a 1:10 dilution of rabies immunoperoxidase conjugate. They are incubated for 3 hours in a humid chamber at room temperature, then washed with distilled water and covered with a benzidine buffer tris solution, pH 7.4 (3,3′-diaminobenzidine tetrachloride, 0.5 mg %). After 5–10 min the slides are again washed and mounted in Elvanol. They are examined with an ordinary light microscope.

4. Results

In tissue culture or organ sections the antigen can be seen in the cytoplasm early, and only later spreads to the other part of the cells, giving a focal appearance. Its size varies from hardly visible to about 10 μm, and stains dark yellowish-brown (Fig. 2A,B).

In impressions of brains infected with fixed virus the rabies antigen is revealed as small and large particles, as well as antigenic dust. With street rabies, on the other hand, the corpuscles are larger and are stained yellowish-brown, darker at the periphery. An internal structure in the form of many dark condensations is seldom seen inside the corpuscles (Fig. 2B).

E. NATURE AND DIAGNOSTIC VALUE OF NEGRI BODIES

From the beginning of his work (1903), Negri had considered that the intracytoplasmic inclusions in street rabies were due to a parasite responsible for the disease, most likely a protozoan.

For Volpino (1904) the Negri bodies were nothing but a reaction of the infected cells. The parasite was found inside the bodies in the form of basophilic corpuscles. The so-called parasitic nature of the Negri body, with its multiple variants such as microsporidia with filtrable elements, etc., provoked many discussions until the biochemical identification of the corpuscles was undertaken.

Marinesco and Stroesco (1938), using the Feulgen technique, had already shown that Negri bodies did not contain DNA and Lépine and Sautter (1946) confirmed the absence of DNA with toluidine blue staining. The confirmation of the nucleic acid nature was obtained by staining rabies-infected brains impressions with acridine orange (Lépine and Atanasiu, 1963) or in cell cultures infected with the virus (Love *et al.*, 1964). This method reveals the Negri bodies stained bright red, i.e., containing RNA. It is also known that in tissue culture rabies virus does not multiply in the presence of 5-fluorouracyl. It appears certain that the matrix of Negri bodies is built of nucleocapsids, and that the rabies virions are of RNA nature (Atanasiu *et al.*, 1963b; Hummeler *et al.*, 1968; Hamparian *et al.*, 1963; Wiktor, 1966; see Chapter 4).

The diagnostic value of Negri bodies was shown by Negri himself: he examined 98 clinical rabid dogs and found inclusions in all of the brains except one (Babes, 1912b). If the presence of Negri bodies confirms the street rabies, however, their absence does not exclude it. Different statistics have shown that, in confirmed rabies cases, the percentage of heads with Negri bodies varies between 66% (Tustin and Smit, 1962) and 93.3% (McQueen, *et al.*, 1960). This explains why, for the diagnosis of rabies, one should use three methods if possible (Atanasiu, 1967; Atanasiu *et al.*, 1968): (1) a rapid staining Sellers' technique; (2) the immunofluorescence (FA) technique; and (3) mouse inoculation.

The comparison of three diagnostic methods: immunofluorescence, a rapid staining, and animal inoculation shows that the animal inoculation technique is most valuable, followed by the immunofluorescence, and then rapid staining (Levaditi *et al.*, 1971). The results obtained by the three methods abolish possible error.

Animal inoculation gives a precise diagnosis, but the animals do not die until 5–10 days after inoculation, and this does not permit a rapid decision for human treatment.

The rapid staining method is very rapid, yet (as already mentioned) the absence of Negri bodies does not necessarily indicate absence of rabies. Nevertheless, it may indicate the existence of an extensive contingent encephalitis.

It is important to recognize that, in cats and rodents, inclusions simulating Negri bodies may be found in the cytoplasm of the nerve cells. They are *not* rabies lesions (Szlachta and Habel, 1953; Nicolau *et al.*, 1933).

Immunofluorescence will give a rapid and specific diagnosis. It must be noted, however, that one may get false negative reactions under conditions of improper brain removal or poor transport conditions. McQueen *et al.* (1960) found animal inoculation and immunofluorescence to be of equal sensitivity, but Wachendörfer (1967) saw false negative results in 1.5% of immunofluorescence tests. Carski *et al.* (1962) found (in wild animals postmortem) rabies antigen by fluorescent antibody staining, while no virus could be isolated by mouse inoculation. Later Wilsnack and Parker (1966) found this phenomenon is due to the presence of "rabies inhibiting substances" (RIS) in the brains of animals with long morbidity periods.

References

Armstrong, G., and Lillie, R. D. (1934). *Pub. Health Rep.* **49,** 1019.
Atanasiu, P. (1965). *C. R. Acad. Sci.* **261,** 277.
Atanasiu, P. (1967). *Semin. Int. Sobre Rabia Para Las Americas, 1st, Buenos Aires, 1967,* p. 195.
Atanasiu, P., Lépine, P., and Dighe, P. (1963a). *C. R. Acad. Sci.* **256,** 1415.
Atanasiu, P., Orth, G., Sisman, J., and Barreau, C. (1963b). *C. R. Acad. Sci.* **257,** 2204.
Atanasiu, P., Gamet, A., and Guillon, J. C. (1968). *Rec. Med. Vet.* **144,** 1083.
Atanasiu, P., Gamet, A., Tsiang, H., Dragonas, P., and Lépine, P. (1970). *C. R. Acad. Sci., Ser. D* **271,** 2434.
Atanasiu, P., Dragonas, P., Tsiang, H., and Harbi, A. (1971a). *Ann. Inst. Pasteur, Paris* **121,** 247.
Atanasiu, P., Gamet, A., Guillon, J. C., Lépine, P., Levaditi, J. C., Tsiang, H., and Vallée, A. (1971b). *Pathol. Biol.* **19,** 207.
Avrameas, S. (1969). *Immunochemistry* **6,** 43.
Babes, V. (1887). *Arch. Pathol. Anat. Physiol. Klin. Med.* **110,** 562.
Babes, V. (1892). *Ann. Inst. Pasteur, Paris* **6,** 209.
Babes, V. (1912a). *In* "Traité de la rage," p. 220. Baillère et Fils, Paris.
Babes, V. (1912b). *In* "Traité de la rage," p. 360. Baillère et Fils, Paris.
Benedikt, M. (1875). *Arch. Pathol. Anat. Physiol. Klin. Med.* **64,** 557.
Carski, T. R., Wilsnack, R. E., and Sikes, R. K. (1962). *Amer. J. Vet. Res.* **30,** 1048.
Coats, J. (1877). *Lancet* **1,** 162.
DiVestea, A. (1894). *Rec. Acad. Med. Chir. (Naples)* **4,** 47.
DiVestea, A., and Zagari, G. (1887). *Rev. Sci.* **40,** 503.
Duboué (de Pau) (1879). *In* "De la physiologie pathologique et du traitement rationnel de la rage" (A. J. Delahaye, ed.), Vol. XIV, p. 269. Paris.
Fernandes, M. V., Wiktor, T. J., and Koprowski, H. (1963). *Virology* **21,** 128.
Fischman, R. H., and Schaeffer, M. (1971). *Ann. N. Y. Acad. Sci.* **177,** 78–97.
Fuenzalida, E., and Palacios, R. (1955). *Bol. Inst. Bacteriol. Chile* **8,** 3.
Galli-Valerio, B. (1906). *Zentralbl. Bakteriol., Parasitenk. Infektionskr., Abt. 1: Orig.* **40,** 318.
Galtier, M. (1879). *C. R. Acad. Sci.* **89,** 444.
Gamaleia, N. (1887). *Ann. Inst. Pasteur, Paris* **1,** 63.
Goldwasser, R. A., and Kissling, R. E. (1958). *Proc. Soc. Exp. Biol. Med.* **98,** 219.
Golgi, C. (1894). *Berlin. Klin. Wochenschr.* **1,** 325.
Habel, K. (1940). *Pub. Health Rep.* **55,** 1619.

Hamparian, V. V., Hilleman, M. R., and Ketler, A. (1963). *Proc. Soc. Exp. Biol. Med.* 112, 1040.

Hideto, U., Taemon, K., Junichi, O., Hajime, M., and Koji, S. (1957). *Amer. J. Vet. Res.* 18, 216.

Hummeler, K., Tomassini, N., Sokol, F., Kuwert, E., and Koprowski, H. (1968). *J. Virol.* 2, 1101.

Johnson, H. N. (1942). *Ill. Med. J.* 81, 382.

Johnson, H. N. (1964). *In* "Diagnostic Procedures for Viral and Rickettsial Diseases" (E. H. Lennette and N. J. Schmidt, eds.), 3rd ed., p. 356. Amer. Pub. Health Ass.

Johnson, H. N., and Leach, C. N. (1940). *Amer. J. Hyg.* 32, 32.

Jonnesco, D. (1934). *C. R. Soc. Biol.* 116, 545.

Kissling, R. E., and Reese, D. R. (1963). *J. Immunol.* 91, 362.

Kolesnikoff, J. (1875). *Zentralbl. Med. Wiss.* 2, 853.

Kolomakin, G. A., Barinova, T. D., Smirnova, M. M., and Timonina, M. S. (1968). *Vop. Virusol.* 13, 470.

Koprowski, H. (1949). *Can. J. Pub. Health* 40, 60.

Koprowski, H. (1954). *Bull. W.H.O.* 10, 109.

Koprowski, H. (1967). *In* "La rage, techniques de laboratoire," Monogr. No. 23, p. 72. OMS, Geneva.

Lentz, O. (1909). *Z. Hyg. Infektionkr.* 62, 63.

Lépine, P., and Atanasiu, P. (1963). *C. R. Acad. Sci.* 256, 4783.

Lépine, P., and Sautter, V. (1936). *Bull. Histol. Tech. Microsc.* 13, 287.

Lépine, P., and Sautter, V. (1946). *Ann. Inst. Pasteur, Paris* 72, 174.

Lépine, P., Atanasiu, P., and Gamet, A. (1971). *J. Ther.* 11, 1.

Levaditi, C., and Schoen, R. (1936). *C. R. Acad. Sci.* 202, 702.

Levaditi, C., Sanches-Bayarri, V., and Schoen, R. (1928). *C. R. Soc. Biol.* 98, 911.

Levaditi, J. C., Atanasiu, P., Gamet, A., and Guillon, J. C. (1971). *Arch. Inst. Pasteur Alger.* (in press).

Love, R., Fernandes, M. V., and Koprowski, H. (1964). *Proc. Soc. Exp. Biol. Med.* 116, 560.

Lucas, A., Carnero, R., Picard, M., Costes, C., and Lahelle, C. M. (1971). *Ecol. Med. Anim.* 12, 297.

Mann, G. (1902). "Physiological Histology," pp. 216, 217. Garandon Press, Oxford.

McQueen, J. L., Lewis, A. L., and Schneider, N. J. (1960). *Amer. J. Pub. Health* 50, 1743.

Marie, A. C. (1930). *C. R. Soc. Biol.* 103, 868.

Marinesco, G., and Stroesco, V. (1938). *Ann. Inst. Babes*, 9, 140.

Manouelian, M. Y. (1906). *C. R. Soc. Biol.* 61, 374.

Meynert, K. (1872). "Hundswut. Eulenburg Realencyclopedie der gesamte Heilkunde" (cited by Babes 1912a).

Negri, A. (1903). *Z. Hyg. Infektionskr.* 43, 507.

Nicolau, S., Kopciowska, L., Galloway, J. A., and Balmus, G. (1933). *C. R. Soc. Biol.* 114, 441.

Nilsson, M. R., Sugay, W., Pasqualin, O. L., and Muller, S. B. K. (1968). *Arq. Inst. Biol. (Sao Paulo)* 35, 43.

Parker, R. L., and Sikes, R. K. (1966). *Pub. Health Rep.* 81, 941.

Pasteur, L. (with the collaboration of Roux, E., Chamberland, C., and Thuillier, L.) (1881). *C. R. Acad. Sci.* 92, 1259.

Pasteur, L. (with the collaboration of Roux, E., Chamberland, C., and Thuillier, L.) (1882). *C. R. Acad. Sci.* 95, 1187.

Pasteur, L. (with the collaboration of Chamberland, C., and Roux, E.) (1884). *C. R. Acad. Sci.* **98**, 457.

Pasteur, L. (1885). *C. R. Acad. Sci.* **101**, 7655.

Ramón y Cajál, S., and Dalmacco-Garcia, D. (1904). *Trab. Lab. Invest. Biol. Univ. Madrid* **3**, 213.

Remlinger, P. (1904). *C. R. Soc. Biol.* **56**, 42.

Roux, E. (1887). *Ann. Inst. Pasteur, Paris* **1**, 87.

Schaaf, J. (1968). *Zentralbl. Veterinaermed. Reihe B* **15**, 241.

Schaeffer, H. (1887). *Arch. Psychiat. Nervenkr.* **19**, 45.

Schaeffer, H. (1889). *Ann. Inst. Pasteur, Paris* **3**, 644.

Schleifstein, J. (1937). *Amer. J. Pub. Health* **27**, 1283.

Schleifstein, J., and Tompkins, V. (1951). *J. A. V. M. A.* **109**, 103–132.

Schneider, L. G. (1969). *Zentralbl. Veterinaermed.* **13**, 16.

Sellers, T. F. (1927). *Amer. J. Pub. Health* **17**, 1080.

Sellers, T. F. (1967). *In* "La rage, techniques de laboratoire," Monogr. No. 23, p. 35. OMS, Geneva.

Stovall, W. D., and Black, C. E. (1940). *Amer. J. Clin. Pathol.* **10**, 1.

Svet-Moldavaskaya, I. A., and Svet-Moldavsky, G. I. (1959). *Acta Virol. (Prague)* **3**, 1.

Szlachta, H. L., and Habel, R. E. (1953). *Cornell Vet.* **43**, 207.

Theiller, M. (1934). *Science* **80**, 122.

Tierkel, E. S. (1967). *In* "La rage, techniques de laboratoire," Monogr. No. 23, p. 18. OMS, Geneva.

Tierkel, E. S., and Sikes, R. K. (1967). *J. Am. Med. Ass.* **201**, 911.

Tustin, R. C., and Smit, J. D. (1962). *J. S. Afr. Vet. Med. Ass.* **33**, 295.

Van Gehuchten, A. (1900). *Bull. Acad. Roy. Med. Belg.* **14**, 389.

Van Gehuchten, A., and Nelis, C. (1900). *Ann. Med. Vet.* **49**, 389.

Van Giesen, I. (1906). *Proc. N. Y. Pathol. Soc.* **6**, 83.

Volpino, G. (1904). *Arch. Sci. Med.* **28**, 153.

Wachendörfer, G. (1967). *Wien. Tieraerztl. Monatsschr.* **54**, 451.

Webster, L. T., and Dawson, J. R. (1935). *Proc. Soc. Exp. Biol. Med.* **32**, 570.

Wiktor, T. J. (1966). *Proc. Nat. Rabies Symp., Center for Disease Control, Atlanta, Georgia, 1966.*

Wilsnack, R. E., and Parker, R. L. (1966). *Amer. J. Vet. Res.* **27**, 39.

Yen, A. C. H. (1936). *Proc. Soc. Exp. Biol. Med.* **34**, 315 and 651.

Zinke, M. (1804). *In* "Neue Ansichten der Hundswut" (C. E. Gabler, ed.), p.180. Fisher, Jena.

CHAPTER 20

The Fluorescent Antibody Test in Rabies

Robert E. Kissling

I. History

The introduction of immunofluorescence to the discipline of microbiology (Coons and Kaplan, 1950) and the development of a stable fluorochrome (fluorescein isothiocyanate) by Riggs and co-workers (1958) placed fluorescent antibody methods within the capability of most microbiologic laboratories. The usefulness of immunofluorescence for identifying rabies antigen in tissues of naturally infected animals was demonstrated soon thereafter (Goldwasser and Kissling, 1958). McQueen (1959) and others (Etchebarne *et al.*, 1960; Lennette *et al.*, 1965; Hurter, 1966; Schneider and Ludwig, 1968; Schaaf, 1968; Nairn, 1969) soon adapted the method for the routine diagnosis of rabies in public health laboratories. Today, because of its increased sensitivity, it largely supplants older staining methods, such as that of Sellers, for the direct microscopic diagnosis of rabies (Dean and Abelseth, 1973).

II. The Principle of the Fluorescent Antibody Technique

In immunofluorescence (fluorescent antibody or FA) procedures a specific antiserum conjugated with a fluorescing dye is used to locate the site of antigenic substances. The fluorescent dye, or fluorochrome, is excited by radiant energy of certain wavelengths and emits energy of a different wavelength in the visible spectrum. The use of an exciting radiation in the long ultraviolet or adjacent part of the visible spectrum permits the largest possible contrast between the exciting and emitted wavelengths. For optimum results to be obtained, the fluorochrome selected for conjugation to the antiserum should have a number of attributes: (a) it should absorb ultraviolet energy and emit a nearly equivalent amount of energy in the form of visible light, (b) the color of the emitted light should be one not usually encountered (for instance, as different as possible from the autofluorescence noted in animal tissues), and (c) the fluorochrome should combine with the antibody molecule in sufficient amounts to produce adequate fluorescence, without hindering the active antibody sites.

III. Selection of the Preferred Fluorochrome

Fluorescein isothiocyanate (FITC) satisfies many of the necessary criteria (Nairn, 1969). It has a maximum absorption peak in the blue range at 490 nm, and its emission peak of 525 nm gives a green fluorescence not commonly encountered in autofluorescence of mammalian tissues, especially when excitation is accomplished with blue wavelengths. The amino group of lysine is probably the site of conjugation of FITC to proteins. Because of its small size, FITC probably does not exert much steric hindrance.

IV. Microscopes and Light Sources Used in the FA Test

A number of satisfactory fluorescent microscopes and light sources are available on the market. High pressure mercury vapor lamps, such as the Osram HBO200, are generally used as a source of excitation energy. Iodine–quartz light sources (Goldman, 1971) give a more continuous spectrum in the desired range, and because of this versatility may eventually replace the mercury lamps. High-pressure xenon arc lamps (Ploem, 1971) also provide more intense energy in the FITC excitation range than do the mercury arc lamps. In general, the intensity of the light should be as great as possible, but it must be consonant with the heat dissipating capacity of the ancillary equipment.

When a primary filter such as the BG12 or the BG22 is inserted between the light source and the exciter filter it transmits UV and blue wavelengths, but absorbs the longer red and infrared radiations and thus protects the exciter filter from heat damage. This exciter filter narrows the band of wavelengths reaching the specimen; it should be selected to permit maximum transmission of the wavelength suitable for excitation of the fluorochrome used, while blocking the wavelengths in its emission spectrum. Corning filter No. 5840 or Zeiss UG2 filters generally prove satisfactory for use with FITC.

A dark-field condenser permits a strong contrast between the specific fluorescing material and the background, and a cardioid darkfield condenser is preferred since it focuses more UV light on the specimen.

The microscope objectives are selected to provide adequate magnification combined with good resolution and satisfactory control of chromatic and spherical aberration. For close examination, a 40× fluorite objective has proven satisfactory. This objective gives better control of aberration than achromatic objectives and also provides a field large enough to permit relatively rapid scanning and a magnification adequate to detect even small accumulations of antigen.

The intensity of the emitted light reaching the eye of the microscopist is greater with a monocular microscope. Binocular fluorescent microscopes are now available, however, that have excellent optics and thus permit adequate viewing intensity with lessened fatigue for the user; for this reason, they are recommended over the monocular instrument.

Barrier (ultraviolet-absorbing) filters that protect the observer's eyes must be inserted between the objectives and the eye of the viewer. These filters should efficiently transmit light in the 500–550 nm wavelength region. A Wratten 2A filter satisfies these criteria.

V. Fluorescent Antibody Techniques

Fluorescent antibody techniques can be varied to (a) directly identify a selected antigen, (b) locate a specific antibody, or (c) detect the presence of complement in an immune complex (Goldwasser and

Shepard, 1958). The direct method, in which a specific antibody to rabies is conjugated with a fluorochrome, is most commonly used for detection of rabies antigen in brain, salivary gland or other tissues. The indirect method is used to detect rabies antibody; in this modification, an antiserum against the serum globulins of the species being tested (human, for example) is conjugated with the fluorochrome and is applied to the rabies antigen–antibody complex to locate the sites of antibody attachment (see Chapter 21). The presence of complement in an antigen–antibody complex can be demonstrated by using a fluorochrome-conjugated antiserum directed against the species (guinea pig, for example) supplying the complement in the test. The direct FA test is recommended for diagnostic examination of rabies antigen in tissue specimens since the limited number of steps reduces the opportunity for technical error, and there is also less opportunity for encountering undesired nonrabies antigen–antibody reactions.

VI. The FA Technique in Rabies

A. PREPARATION OF CONJUGATE

An antiserum must be carefully prepared for conjugation in order to avoid the development of antibodies against those animal tissues used for immunization; this may be accomplished by using an immunizing antigen prepared from the same species as that used for antibody production, by purifying the antigen to rid it of host protein, or by producing the antigen in a species not likely to be examined for rabies. Immunizing antigens are generally obtained from infected brain tissue or from virus grown in tissue culture systems; primary hamster kidney cultures or BHK-21 cells serve particularly well in this latter category. The infectivity of the immunizing antigen should be destroyed, and treatment with β-propiolactone (BPL) at a final concentration of 1:2000 to 1:3000 has been one method commonly used for this purpose. Since the breakdown products of BPL are acidic, the pH must be monitored to prevent acid denaturation of the rabies antigens. Animals may be immunized by any of several schedules generally used for the preparation of immune sera; Freund's adjuvant may aid in producing higher antibody titers.

For reproducible and economical conjugation of an antiserum, it is advisable to fractionate the serum and work with the immunoglobulins only. Immunoglobulins can be precipitated out of the whole serum with ammonium sulfate (Hebert *et al.*, 1972), or they can be largely separated from albumin and other serum components by DEAE chromatography (Riggs *et al.*, 1960). It is important to select a method that does not cause undue denaturation and loss of specific antibody activity. When ammonium sulfate precipitation is used, the serum, precipitated globulins, and the ammonium sulfate are all kept at 0°–4°C. The globulins are precipitated from the whole serum by adding specified amounts of cold saturated NH_4SO_4 (Goldwasser and Shepard, 1958). The precipitate is collected by centrifugation, redissolved in cold water, and once again precipitated with NH_4SO_4. This step is repeated a third time, and the globulin is then dissolved in a quantity of cold water sufficient to restore the original volume of serum. This solution is dialyzed against repeated changes of 0.85% NaCl until tests with barium chloride indicate that there are no SO_4 ions present in the dialysate; sulfate ions interfere with conjugation and must therefore be removed. When small volumes of serum $(1-10$ ml) are fractionated, the use of DEAE column chromatography (Hebert *et al.*, 1972) offers a rapid and mild method for obtaining the immunoglobulins.

Conjugation of the FITC to the immunoglobulin molecules is accomplished by allowing the two to react at 4°–10°C at a pH of 9–10. The ratio of FITC to protein used during the conjugation procedure is generally 1:20, although good results can be obtained with ratios as low as 1:50. If the FITC/protein ratio is too high, the immunoglobulin becomes denatured with concomitant loss of specificity (Goldstein *et al.*, 1961). After conjugation is completed, the unreacted FITC is removed by dialysis or filtration through a Sephadex G-25 column. The column must be tall enough to allow separation of the material into two yellow-colored bands. The conjugated globulin emerges from the column before the band containing the smaller free FITC molecules or any FITC breakdown products. At this stage the conjugate should be tested for specific and nonspecific staining. The conjugate is ready for routine use, but if excessive nonspecific background staining is observed, additional treatment is required. Although adsorption with tissue powders has been recommended to reduce nonspecific staining (Coons and Kaplan, 1950), it is our experience that these powders generally adsorb both specific and nonspecific staining substances.

Nonspecific staining, often due to excessively labeled globulins, can be most efficiently resolved by passage of the conjugated globulins through a DEAE column; various fractions are collected, and those possessing the desired qualities are pooled and used for routine work. Those labeled globulins emerging from the column last display the most nonspecific staining.

B. Staining of Tissue for Rabies Diagnosis

Tissue smears or impressions to be stained with FA should be relatively thin, because thick preparations may adsorb conjugate that cannot then be effectively rinsed off. Fresh tissue is the best material for making smears or impressions, but satisfactory preparations can also be made from frozen or glycerinated tissues (McQueen *et al.*, 1960) or even from the sediment of tissue suspensions. Frozen (and thawed) brain tissue must be handled carefully in order to avoid excessively thick preparations. Glycerinated tissues do not adhere well to the microscope slides unless the tissue fragments are adequately rinsed in saline solutions to remove excess glycerin. Slides that are prepared with the sediment of tissue suspensions used for animal inoculation may be stained by FA (when adequate tissue is not otherwise available) but they are generally much less satisfactory than preparations made directly from tissue.

Rabies virus is unevenly distributed in the brain; therefore, tissue from several areas should be selected for examination, including the thalamus, cerebellar cortex, both hippocampi, and both cerebral cortices. Most diagnostic laboratories that perform many rabies examinations daily usually limit the number of slides per brain, and the hippocampus (Ammon's horn) and cerebellum are the sites most often chosen for FA examination. Histologic orientation is not as important a factor for FA staining as it is for Sellers' staining. Thin, frozen, cryostat sections permit excellent orientation, but extra equipment, effort required, and risk is involved to obtain these preparations and they are not warranted for purely diagnostic purposes.

It has been shown that fluorescent antigen may still be seen in putrid rabies specimens after mouse inoculation and Sellers' stain are no longer effective methods of diagnosis (W. G. Winkler and D. B. Adams, personal communication; Lewis and Thacker, 1974), but one cannot predict at which time each diagnostic method begins to fail.

There are difficulties in preparing salivary gland tissues for fluorescent examination. Insufficient tissue often adheres to the glass slides if impressions are attempted, or material adheres so poorly that it is washed away during subsequent staining and rinsing. The best salivary gland preparations are made by blotting the tissue to remove excess mucoid material, mincing it, and then crushing the fragments onto the slide with the side of a scalpel blade. Moreover, a further difficulty arises from the fact that rabies virus is irregularly distributed throughout the salivary glands, requiring that samples be taken from several areas of the glands. In most species, the submaxillary salivary glands are more likely sources of rabies virus than the parotid or sublingual salivary glands. Corneal smears have also been reported to be a source for demonstration of rabies antigen (Schneider, 1969; Lopez *et al.*, 1970; Cifuentes *et al.*, 1971).

The smears, impressions, or films are permitted to air dry and then are fixed before staining with conjugate. Fixation increases the permeability of tissues, and allows maximum contact between the intracellular rabies antigen and the conjugated antiserum. Although some antigen will be stained even in unfixed preparations (especially when it is present in large amounts), there is a risk of obtaining false negative results in those specimens which contain only small amounts of antigen. Properly fixed preparations fluoresce more brilliantly than unfixed or underfixed preparations. Fixation must be accomplished without denaturation of the viral antigen. Fixation with acetone at −20° to −5°C for 1–4 hours gives good results. Fixation for longer periods, such as overnight, is not harmful, but shorter fixation in acetone at these cold temperatures results in less brilliant and possibly incomplete staining. In emergencies, preparations may be fixed in acetone for short periods (10 min) at room temperature (Martell *et al.*, 1970; Larghi and Jiménez, 1971), although the possibility of antigen denaturation is a disadvantage that should be recognized. Fixing with ethyl alcohol (Fischman and Ward, 1969) results in excessive nonspecific staining, and ethanol gives results inferior to those obtained with cold acetone. It should be emphasized that fixed preparations contain viable virus (Fischman and Ward, 1969) and should be handled accordingly. After fixation, the preparations are air dried and then are ready for staining.

Before the conjugate is added for staining, the fixed slides are ringed with an ether–vaseline mixture or special marking pen to contain the conjugate over the fixed tissue. Staining is accomplished by covering the tissue with appropriately diluted conjugated antibody, and incubating the slide in a humidified chamber at room temperature for 30 min. A moist atmosphere is required during incubation to prevent drying and precipitation of the conjugate. The slides are then rinsed in buffered water to remove unreacted conjugate. A mounting medium of 90% glycerine buffered to pH 8.6 is used, and a coverslip is placed over the smear. The mounting medium must be above pH 8.0 to permit maximum fluoresence (fluorescence of FITC is quenched at low pH values), and should be checked frequently to determine that it is satisfactory.

C. Performing the Rabies FA Test

Several procedures are necessary to properly control the FA test for rabies. Since the control of specificity is very important, an absorption should be included in every run. Two identical smears of the diagnostic specimen are stained on each slide, one with conjugate mixed with equal parts of 20% rabies-infected mouse brain in diluent, the other conjugate mixed with equal parts 20% normal mouse brain in diluent (Fig. 1). The rabies antigen in the infected suspension reacts with conjugated antibody and thus eliminates or greatly reduces the subsequent staining in the diagnostic specimen (Fig. 2).

The use of mouse brain suspensions also helps to reduce nonspecific staining of the diagnostic specimen. Known rabies positive and rabies negative smears, impressions or films *in each run* should also be stained with both preparations of the conjugate.

Accumulations of rabies antigen are found in the cytoplasm of infected cells, which vary in size and shape. The classic Negri body (see Chapter 19) is readily identified by its round to oval shape and smooth contours. The periphery of these bodies often fluoresces with more intensity than the internal portions. In addition to these structures, rabies antigen is also seen as long, irregularly shaped fluorescing masses as well as small, granular, dustlike material. This granular material should be carefully differentiated from precipitated stain, which appears crystalline, has an especially brilliant fluores-

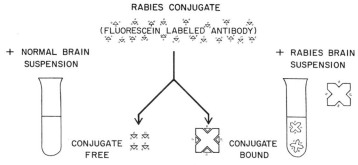

Fig. 1. Basic reactions in the rabies fluorescent antibody technique.

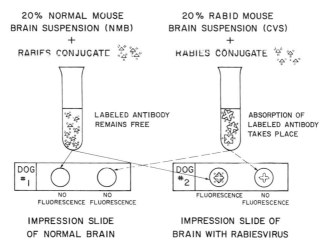

Fig. 2. Detection of rabies virus by the fluorescent antibody technique.

cence, and often has irregular contours. Rabies antigen in salivary gland tissue usually occurs in smaller, more irregular masses than those observed in brain tissue; dustlike antigen is very commonly found.

Examination should begin with the rabies-positive control slide. The smear stained with conjugate mixed with normal brain tissue should show brilliantly fluorescing masses of apple-green antigen (Fig. 3) whereas the smear stained with conjugate mixed with rabies-infected brain should show no fluorescence, or only fluorescence of greatly reduced intensity. If the positive control smears prove satisfactory, the rabies negative control smears should next be examined; no fluorescence should be observed. *Only when both positive and negative controls are satisfactorily stained should the diagnostic specimens be examined.* The smear of the diagnostic tissue stained with conjugate mixed with normal mouse brain should be examined first. If no specific fluorescent material is observed, the specimen is considered negative for rabies antigen. If fluorescing masses typical of rabies antigen accumulations are seen, the adjacent smear, stained with conjugate mixed with rabies-infected mouse brain, should be examined. If typical fluorescence is absent (inhibited) in this preparation, the specimen is considered to be positive for rabies antigen. If fluorescence is observed on the "inhibited" smear, results of the test are considered nonspecific, and the test should be repeated (preferably with another conjugate prepared from a different source of antibody).

Animal tissues normally fluoresce a pale bluish color. Other fluorescing colors may be encountered, such as the bright red of ceroid pigment, or the bright blue of crystals of salts such as sodium chloride. Normal tissue components, however, do not ordinarily autofluoresce with the bright green color of FITC.

Leukocytes will give nonspecifical fluorescence even with adsorbed FITC-conjugated proteins. The diagnostician must learn to differentiate these rare cells from accumulations of rabies antigen, an easy procedure based on morphologic criteria and the fact that fluorescence is observed in both the "inhibited" and "uninhibited" smears.

D. USE OF THE FA TECHNIQUE IN THE RABIES DIAGNOSTIC LABORATORY

Fluorescent antibody procedures for rabies are most widely used for diagnosis in public health laboratories. The FA test has generally supplanted the older staining procedures for the identification of Negri bodies. These older direct staining methods, which only identified up to 80–85% of the rabies-infected brain specimens (see Chapter 19) were, moreover, unsuitable for the identification of infected salivary gland tissues. The FA test for rabies, when performed

---

Fig. 3. *Diagnostic immunofluorescence.* The four figures are of brain impressions from confirmed rabies specimens. They were processed by the standard FITC direct immunofluorescence method, examined in a Zeiss microscope (UG 1 exciter filter, 410 nm barrier filter), and photographed on Kodak High Speed Ektachrome film (daylight) using ESP-1 processing. All magnifications ×350. (Courtesy of F. A. Murphy.) a: Human rabies, Duvenhagé strain, Republic of South Africa (obtained from Dr. C. D. Meredith, Onderstepoort). Impression is from third mouse brain passage of isolate. Modest size aggregates of viral antigen are seen against a background of brown brain tissue; this brown fluorescence is most common in specimens which have been frozen and thawed before making the impressions. b: Skunk rabies, United States. Impression is from first mouse brain passage of isolate. As shown by comparison of frozen sections with impressions from the same specimen, irregular linear specifically antigenic masses actually result from disruption and "dragging" of some large discrete inclusions during the process of making the impression or smear. They do not detract from the diagnostic value of the specimen. c: Human rabies, United States. Large aggregates (Negri bodies) and smaller specifically immunofluorescent forms stand out from the bluish background most typical of optical systems in general use. d: Arctic fox rabies, Alaska. Fluorescent viral antigen masses are relatively small and in high concentration. The apple-green color of the specific reaction product stands out from a brownish background which is also typical of other optical systems in use. (See facing color plate.)

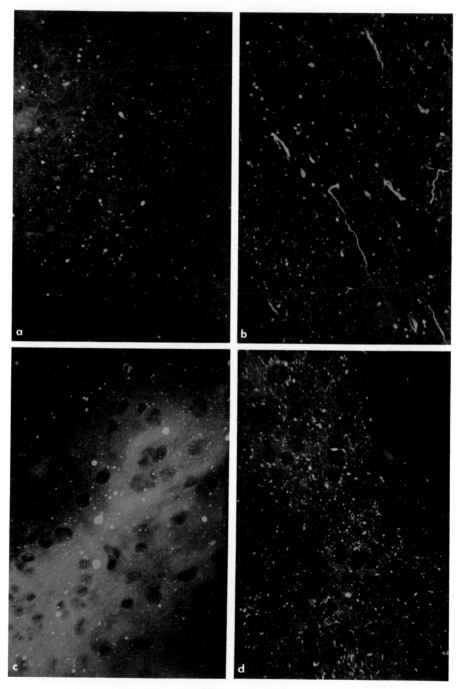

Fig. 3.

Table I

Summary of the False Negative FA Results of Various Authors[a]

Total no. of heads examined	No. of positive cases	Positive brains not diagnosed by FA			References
		No.	Percent of all cases	Percent of positive cases	
825	70	–	–	–	McQueen *et al.* (1960)
14	7	–	–	–	Etchebarne *et al.* (1960)
424	40	–	–	–	Goldwasser *et al.* (1961)
42	42	1	2.4	2.4	Carski *et al.* (1962)
112	85	7	6.25	8.2	Veeraraghavan *et al.* (1963)
59	50	1	1.7	2.0	Selimov *et al.* (1964)
525	216	2	0.4	1.1	Schneider (1964)
224	111	1	0.5	0.9	Schneider and Wachendörfer (1964)
65	20	–	–	–	Guliew (1964)
100	65	3	3.0	4.6	Liebke (1965)
77	18	–	–	–	Jentzsch and Pitzschke (1965)
750	181	8	1.1	4.4	Beauregard *et al.* (1965)
4230	361	2	0.05	0.6	Lennette *et al.* (1965)
640	209	5	0.8	2.4	Pitzschke (1966)
200	62	–	–	–	Winkler and Patzwaldt (1966) (one case FA +, animal inoc. –)
274	10	1	0.4	10.0	Matthias *et al.* (1965) Wachendörfer (1966)
1074 fresh	169	–	–	–	(one case FA +, animal inoc. –)
44 putrid	34	5	14.3	14.7	(five cases FA +, animal inoc.–)
1678	421	10	0.6	2.0	Hurter (1966) (also, 2 cases FA + animal inoc.–)
1284	331	3	0.3	1.0	Schaaf (1968)
557	206	4	0.8	2.0	Zimmerman (1968)
531	15	5	1.0	33.0	Schepky (1971) (3 FA + animal inoc. –)
1427	105	12	0.1	11.4	Atanasiu *et al.* (1971)
10413	321	17	0.2	1.9	Lee and Becker (1973) (also, 13 FA + animal inoc. –)
TOTAL 25569	3049	87	0.34	2.9	

[a] After Jentzsch (1967).

by a competent laboratory worker, identifies at least 98% of rabies-infected brain specimens submitted for diagnosis (see Table I for a comparison of the efficacy of various diagnostic tests).

The mouse inoculation test is a slightly more sensitive diagnostic procedure than the FA test for rabies. When the two tests are performed by competent and experienced laboratory workers, agreement between them is usually 99% or higher, with a few specimens giving negative results by the FA test but positive results by mouse inoculation.

A crucial factor in the use of the FA technique for rabies diagnosis is its sensitivity and reliability; both have been investigated, not only during the development of the test, (McQueen, 1959, McQueen *et al.*, 1960) but afterward also. An extensive review by Jentzsch (1967) (summarized in part in Table I) in which the sensitivity of the FA technique is compared with that of mouse inoculation demonstrates an efficacy of 98% with 30 of 1,537 total positive cases negative by the FA technique, yet confirmed by animal inoculation; there were some cases, however, in which the FA technique was positive and animal inoculation proved negative. (Additional data accumulated after the 1967 article have been added to Jentzsch's table, and the total number of cases reported positive by animal inoculation but not by FA was 87 of 3049, or 2.9%.) Jentzsch concluded that "the fluorescence method . . . is on principle equal to the animal experiment." In order to study the 2% discrepancy, Jentzsch (1967) showed that a titer of $10^{2.45}$ MICLD$_{50}$/0.03 cm^3 is the sensitivity threshold in naturally infected dog brains [$10^{1.33}$ in mice; see also Fabrega and Muller (1970)] but that "these early stages of infection which cannot be diagnosed by . . . fluorescence . . . could under no circumstances actively endanger . . . any contact persons." In other words, any animal whose brain (when submitted as a fresh specimen) is FA negative, even if it is eventually found to be positive by animal inoculation, does not present any danger of infection for man.

The submission of putrid specimens also causes discrepancies between the FA and mouse inoculation results in rabies diagnosis. This problem has been reviewed by Wachendörfer (1966), and his comparison (Table II) clearly indicates that with an increased number of putrid specimens there is greater difficulty in FA diagnosis, and the diagnosis of such specimens must be reviewed very carefully in the diagnostic laboratory in order not to consider a positive (but now decomposed) specimen negative and thus without danger for an exposed individual; treatment in those cases must depend on epidemiologic findings surrounding the exposure, and will very often be initiated in spite of a negative FA finding.

In rare cases animals with long morbidity periods (especially wildlife) develop high levels of antibodies to rabies that interfere with virus isolation by mouse inoculation (Sikes, 1962; Wilsnack and Parker, 1966; Parker and Wilsnack, 1966), and this must be taken into account when a specimen is found positive by the fluorescent antibody test but no virus can be isolated by mouse inoculation; the

Table II

Comparison of the FA Technique and Animal Inoculation in Rabies Diagnosis[a]

Condition of the brains	Fluorescent antibody		Mouse inoculation		
	Results	Number	Negative	Positive	Not examined
1. Fresh, recently removed, excluding severely damaged or putrid brains	Negative	754	471	–	283
	Positive	320	1[b]	169	150
Total		1074	641		433
2. Mummified or altered by autolysis; definitely putrid brains	Negative	18	10	5[c]	3
	Positive	33	5[d]	24	4
Total		51	44		7

[a] After Wachendörfer (1966).

[b] Only 1 of 641 (0.16%) of fresh brains examined was positive by the FA technique but negative by mouse inoculation (none the reverse).

[c] Thus 5 of 44 (11.1%) putrid brains examined were positive by mouse inoculation but negative by the fluorescent antibody technique.

[d] Thus 5 of 44 (11.1%) putrid brains examined were negative by mouse inoculation but positive by the fluorescent antibody technique (equal to the reverse situation in c).

possibility must be considered that the animal might have had virus in the saliva prior to death, although no virus could be isolated from the salivary glands at death. [This has been shown experimentally in skunks (Wilsnack and Parker, 1966), foxes (Carski et al., 1962), and bats (Baer and Bales, 1967).]

Errors in diagnosis of rabies by FA staining can be reduced by careful attention to certain details:

1. Include adequate controls in every run.

2. Make adequate sampling of each specimen. When possible, six different areas of the brain should be examined, including the thalamus, right and left hippocampi, right and left cerebral cortices, and cerebellum. Many diagnostic laboratories routinely examine the Ammon's horn, cerebellum, and brain stem. When salivary glands are examined, several areas should be sampled.

3. Avoid undue exposure of the conjugated antiserum to light. This reagent should be stored refrigerated and in the dark.

4. Avoid exposure of the stained preparation to light, especially ultraviolet light, before examination begins. The energy emitted by fluorescein is significantly reduced after even 1 min of exposure to

UV radiation. Examine the specimen immediately after staining, or hold it in a cold dark place until examination can be made.

5. Maintain the pH of the mounting medium at 8.0–8.6. Fluorescence is lessened at lower pH values; it is 50% lower at pH 6.0 than at 8.0.

6. Use morphologic criteria as well as fluorescence to arrive at a diagnosis. Experience will help the laboratory worker in this regard.

7. Examination should be made promptly in a careful, objective manner. The technician must avoid being influenced by the near-hysterical subjectivity surrounding some specimens submitted to the laboratory for rabies diagnosis.

The counterstaining of FA preparations with dyes such as lissamine rhodamine B has been reported to reduce nonspecific staining (Nairn, 1969). In our experience such treatment also reduces the brilliance of specific staining and therefore cannot be recommended for general use. If high quality conjugates are used and morphologic criteria are carefully noted, problems with nonspecific staining should be drastically reduced.

E. USE OF THE FA TECHNIQUE IN RESEARCH

Fluorescent antibody methods have been useful in various aspects of rabies research. Allen and co-workers (1964a,b; Leonard et al., 1967) have used FA techniques to demonstrate rabies antigen in the brown fat of experimentally infected bats; this finding shows that the antigen persisted without infectivity during periods when the animals were held at low temperatures similar to those which would be experienced during hibernation. When the bats were returned to higher temperatures, infectivity could again be demonstrated.

The cytopathic effect (CPE) of rabies virus on tissue cultures is difficult to detect (see Chapter 9). It does not become obvious until several days after maximum virus production has occurred. Fluorescent antibody staining has proven useful in following the progression of rabies virus and antigen in infected tissue cultures in the absence of readily detectable CPE (Leonard et al., 1967). Fluorescent methods have been instrumental in elucidating many of the events that occur in the pathogenesis of rabies (Carski et al., 1962; Johnson, 1965; Baer et al., 1965; Fischman, 1969; Dierks et al., 1969); some of the details, such as the centripetal progression of infection along peripheral nerves, have escaped detection by both FA and electron microscopy.

The use of conjugates prepared against the several subviral components (Schneider *et al.*, 1973) would seem to be a logical step toward refinement of pathogenesis studies. The FA technique has also been one of the tools used to examine the antigenic relationships among the rabies-related viruses (see Chapter 8).

The major contribution of fluorescent antibody methods to research is the introduction of the capability of simultaneously observing morphology and detecting antigenic specificity. Several major limitations of FA, however, must also be recognized: antigenic masses smaller than those resolvable by light microscopy cannot be detected by FA methods, and quantitation of antigen materials is still difficult and less precise than by alternate immunologic methods.

References

Allen, R., Sims, R. A., and Sulkin, S. E. (1964a). *Amer. J. Hyg.* **80**, 11–24.
Allen, R., Sims, R. A., and Sulkin, S. E. (1964b). *Amer. J. Hyg.* **80**, 25–32.
Atanasiu, P., Gamet, A., Guillon, J. C., Lépine, P., Levaditi, J. C., Tsiang, J., and Vallée, A. (1971). *Pathol. Biol.* **19**, 207–212.
Baer, G. M., and Bales, G. L. (1967). *J. Infec. Dis.* **117**, 82–90.
Baer, G. M., Shanthaveerappa, T. R., and Bourne, G. H. (1965). *Bull. W.H.O.* **33**, 783–794.
Beauregard, M., Boulanger, P., and Webster, W. A. (1965). *Can. J. Comp. Med. Vet. Sci.* **29**, 141–147.
Carski, T. R., Wilsnack, R. E., and Sikes, R. K. (1962). *Amer. J. Vet. Res.* **23**, 1048–1052.
Cifuentes, E., Calderon, E., and Bijlenga, G. (1971). *J. Trop. Med. Hyg.* **74**, 23–25.
Coons, A. H., and Kaplan, M. H. (1950). *J. Exp. Med.* **91**, 1–13.
Dean, D. J., and Abelseth, M. K. (1973). *World Health Organ., Monagr. Ser.* **23**.
Dierks, R. E., Murphy, F. A., and Harrison, A. K. (1969). *Amer. J. Pathol.* **54**, 251–273.
Etchebarne, M., Bernal, P. G., and Leyton, G. R. (1960). *J. Immunol.* **84**, 6–10.
Fabrega, F., and Muller, A. (1970). *Rev. Soc. Med. Vet. Chile* **20**, 29–35.
Fischman, H. R. (1969). *Amer. J. Vet. Res.* **30**, 1213–1221.
Fischman, H. R., and Ward, F. E. (1969). *Amer. J. Vet. Res.* **30**, 2205–2208.
Goldman, M. (1971). *Ann. N. Y. Acad. Sci.* **177**, 407–409.
Goldstein, G., Slizys, S., and Chase, M. W. (1961). *J. Exp. Med.* **114**, 89–110.
Goldwasser, R. A., and Kissling, R. E. (1958). *Proc. Soc. Exp. Biol. Med.* **98**, 219–223.
Goldwasser, R. A., and Shepard, C. C. (1958). *J. Immunol.* **80**, 122–131.
Goldwasser, R. A., Kemron, A., and Nobel, T. A. (1961). *Refuah Vet.* **18**, 208–212.
Guliew, M. A. (1964). *Fortschr. Geb. Tollwut, Moskau* p. 17 (in Russian).
Hebert, G. A., Pittman, B., McKinney, R. M., and Cherry, W. B. (1972). The preparation and physiochemical characterization of fluorescent antibody reagents. U. S. Dept. of Health, Education, and Welfare, Center for Disease Control, Atlanta, Ga.
Hurter, K. P. (1966). *Berlin. Muenchen. Tieraerztl. Wochenschr.* **79**, 289–292.
Jentzsch, K. D. (1967). *Zentralbl. Bakteriol. Parasitenk. Infektionskr. Hyg.* **202**, 307–327.

Jentzsch, K. D., and Pitzschke, H. (1965). *Monetsch. Veterinaermed.* **20**, 17–20.

Johnson, R. T. (1965). *J. Neuropathol. Exp. Neurol.* **24**, 662–674.

Larghi, O. P., and Jimenez, C. E. (1971). *Appl. Microbiol.* **21**, 611–613.

Lee, T. K., and Becker, M. E. (1973). *Pub. Health Lab.* **31**, 149–164.

Lennette, E. H., Woodie, J. D., Nakamura, K., and Magoffin, R. L. (1965). *Health Lab. Sci.* **2**, 24–34.

Leonard, L. L., Allen, R., and Sulkin, S. E. (1967). *J. Infec. Dis.* **117**, 121–128.

Lewis, V. J., and Thacker, W. L. (1974). *Health Lab. Sci.* **11**, 8–12.

Liebke, H. (1965). *Zentralbl. Bakteriol., Parasitenk., Infektionskr. Hyg.* **196**, 371–372.

López, J. H., Alvarez, J., Gil, J. C., and Caballos, C. (1970). *Memorias del Segundo Seminario Nacional Sobre Rabia, Manizales, Colombia 2nd 1970*, pp. 42–48.

McQueen, J. L. (1959). *Proc. 63rd Annu. Meet. U. S. Livestock Sanit. Asso.* pp. 356–363.

McQueen, J. L., Lewis, A. L., and Schneider, N. J. (1960). *Amer. J. Pub. Health* **58**, 1743–1752.

Martell, M., Batalla, D., and Baer, G. M. (1970). *Tec. Pecuar.* (*Mex.*) **14**, 48–50.

Matthias, D., Jakob, W., Herrmann, H. J., and Fuchs, H. W. (1965). *Monatsch. Veterinaermed.* **20**, 462–469.

Nairn, R. C. (1969). "Fluorescent Protein Tracing," 3rd ed. Williams & Wilkins, Baltimore, Maryland.

Parker, R. L., and Wilsnack, R. E. (1966). *Amer. J. Vet. Res.* **27**, 33–38.

Pitzschke, H. (1966). *Monatsch. Veterinaermed.* **21**, 870.

Ploem, J. S. (1971). *Ann. N. Y. Acad. Sci.* **177**, 414–429.

Riggs, J. L., Seiwald, R. J., Burckhalter, J., Downs, C. M., and Metcalf, T. G. (1958). *Amer. J. Pathol.* **34**, 1081–1097.

Riggs, J. L., Loh, P. C., and Eveland, W. C. (1960). *Proc. Soc. Exp. Biol. Med.* **105**, 655–658.

Schaaf, J. (1968). *Zentralbl. Veterinaermed.* **15**, 255–258.

Schepky, A. (1971). *Tieraerztl. Umsch.* **26**, 312–314.

Schneider, L. G. (1964). *Tieraerztl. Umsch.* **19**, 502–509.

Schneider, L. G. (1969). *Zentralbl. Veterinaermed. Reihe B* **16**, 24–31.

Schneider, L. G., and Ludwig, H. (1968). *Wien. Tieraertzl. Monatschr.* **55**, 133–148.

Schneider, L. G., and Wachendörfer, G. (1964). *Berlin. Muenchen. Tieraerztl. Wochenschr.* **77**, 454–458.

Schneider, L. G., Dietzschold, B., Dierks, R. E., Matthaeus, W., Enzmann, P. J., and Strohmaier, K. (1973). *J. Virol.* **11**, 748–755.

Selimov, M. A., Kljujewa, E. W., and Semjonowa, E. W. (1964). *Medizina, Moskau* (in Russian).

Sikes, R. K. (1962). *Amer. J. Vet. Res.* **23**, 1041–1047.

Veeraraghavan, N., Chandrasekhar, D. S., Subrahmanyan, T. P., Rajan, M. A., Hallan, K. M., and David, J. (1963). "Annual Report of the Director 1961 and Scientific Report 1962," pp. 63–67. Pasteur Institute of Southern India, Coonoor, Tamilnadu, India.

Wachendörfer, G. (1961). *Deut. Tieraerztl. Wochenschr.* **68**, 261–268.

Wachendörfer, G. (1966). *Deut. Tieraerztl. Wochenschr.* **73**, 446–452.

Wilsnack, R. E., and Parker, R. L. (1966). *Amer. J. Vet. Res.* **27**, 39–43.

Winkler, C., and Patzwaldt, H. G. (1966). *Zentralbl. Bakteriol., Parasitenk. Infektionskr. Hyg.* **200**, 179–190.

Zimmermann, T. (1968). *Deut. Tieraerztl. Wochenschr.* **75**, 91–95.

CHAPTER 21

The Serum Neutralization, Indirect Fluorescent Antibody, and Rapid Fluorescent Focus Inhibition Tests

J. B. Thomas

I. Introduction

The body's immunologic protective mechanisms serve to eliminate parasitic microorganisms and produce an immune response, thus enabling the host to recognize a parasite as a foreign body, and activating the defense mechanism to protect the individual from repeated infections as long as immunity is maintained. The immune

417

response is dependent on three types of cells: (1) reticuloendothelial cells; (2) macrophages and dendritic cells; and (3) immune-competent cells. The first cells, which provide an environment for the two remaining types, are the fibroblasts, endothelial cells, and reticulin-producing cells. Macrophages are found in the medulla of the lymph nodes and in the red pulp and marginal zone of the spleen and function to trap and concentrate antigen. The dendritic cells are found in the lymph nodes and white pulp of the spleen and serve to concentrate the antigen on their external membrane. The cells capable of synthesizing immunoglobulins are the immunoblasts which in turn give rise to plasma cells and lymphocytes. These cells are found in the bone marrow, spleen, lung, and lymph nodes.

II. Rabies Antibody

Rabies antibody appears to be most closely associated with the IgM and IgG classes of immunoglobulins (Fujisaki *et al.*, 1968; Matsumoto, 1970; Rubin *et al.*, 1971; Gough and Dierks, 1971; Cho *et al.*, 1972). During a primary response the IgM antibody can apparently be detected as early as 3 or 4 days (Fujisaki *et al.*, 1968), whereas the IgG apparently cannot be detected until approximately the tenth day (Rubin *et al.*, 1971). The IgM usually starts declining within 41 days (Rubin *et al.*, 1971), whereas the IgG appears to start declining before 225 days, but may remain detectable up to 20 years (Fox, 1958; Greenberg and Childress, 1960). The persistence of these antibodies has made possible the use of various serologic tests for determining the immune status of the host.

Serologic tests for detection of rabies antibody provide valuable tools for epidemiologic studies, including the determination of the immune status of man and animals, and the diagnosis of rabies infection by the presence of antibody in specimens from live or dead animals. The mouse neutralization and indirect fluorescent antibody tests have been those most frequently used for determining antibody levels in persons immunized against rabies. Other methods reported include (1) inhibition of cytopathic effect in cell cultures (Atanasiu and Lépine, 1959; Fernandes *et al.*, 1963; Kissling and Reese, 1963; Abelseth, 1964; Wiktor *et al.*, 1964); (2) inhibition of fluorescent foci in cell cultures (King *et al.*, 1965; Lennette and Emmons, 1971; Debbie *et al.*, 1972; Smith *et al.*, 1973); (3) inhibition of plaque formation in cell cultures (Sedwick and Wiktor, 1967); (4) lytic rabies antibody tests (Wiktor *et al.*, 1968); (5) hemagglutination-inhibition test (Halonen *et al.*, 1968); (6) gel-diffusion precipitation test (Grasset and Atanasiu, 1961; Lépine, 1973); (7) complement-fixation tests (Sever, 1962); (8) passive hemagglutination test (see Chapter 6, this volume).

III. Relation of Neutralizing Antibody to Protection

Neutralization tests have been used to correlate measurable antibody with resistance to challenge of dogs, cats, cattle, foxes, and other animals (Koprowski and Black, 1952; Fenje, 1960; Otto and Heyke, 1962; Dean *et al.*, 1964; Cabasso *et al.*, 1965). It has been reported (Schneider *et al.*, 1973; Wiktor *et al.*, 1973) that neutralizing antibodies in mice, guinea pigs, and rabbits were produced by the envelope glycoprotein of rabies virus, and that this antibody appears to protect against subsequent challenge with rabies virus. These antibodies did not appear to be produced when purified nucleocapsid was inoculated into rabbits, although indirect fluorescent antibody and complement-fixation antibodies were produced. These authors suggest that only the envelope glycoprotein is capable of eliciting a protective response to challenge.

IV. Experiments Employing Serum Neutralization Tests

Numerous studies have shown the therapeutic value of antirabies serum as discussed in Chapter 20, Volume II, this treatise. The neutralizing antibody is developed during an immune response resulting from single or multiple injections of rabies antigen (Hattwick *et al.*, 1972). Various tests have been used to determine the presence of the neutralizing antibody (Atanasiu and Lépine, 1959; Fernandes *et al.*, 1963; Kissling and Reese, 1963; Abelseth, 1964; Wiktor *et al.*, 1964; King *et al.*, 1965; Lennette and Emmons, 1971; Debbie *et al.*, 1972; Smith *et al.*, 1973).

A virus protection test in mice was first developed by Webster and Dawson (1935) to study the immunizing value of commercial antirabies vaccines. The following year Webster (1936) reported the use of this test to measure the amount of neutralizing antibody in humans given routine vaccination and in experimentally vaccinated mice. In these latter studies a varying amount of virus was used along with a constant quantity of serum; this method can also be used for virus identification (Johnson, 1973). By keeping the virus dose constant and varying the serum dilutions (Atanasiu, 1973), the neutralization test can be used for antibody titer determination, thus making it of value in studying the efficacy of human and animal vaccines.

The immune response to the varying doses, routes, and types of human vaccines (HEP Flury, Harris, or Semple) has been determined by the neutralization test (Fox *et al.*, 1957; Atanasiu *et al.*, 1957). This test was used by Tierkel and Sikes (1967), Greenberg and Childress (1960), and Farrar *et al.* (1964) to compare the human antibody response to vaccination with duck embryo or HEP Flury vaccines. Other studies have been conducted to determine the presence of neutralizing antibodies in individuals administered antisera soon after their exposure to rabies (Koprowski and Cox, 1951; Baltazard and Bahmanyar, 1955) or to determine the rapidity of the immune response following a booster (Cohen *et al.*, 1964).

The neutralization test has also been used to determine the antibody response in animal vaccine studies. In one study dogs were vaccinated with various rabies vaccines and the neutralization test was used to determine antibody in the prevaccination sera and sera taken 43 and 60 days after vaccination and 1 day before challenge (Tierkel *et al.*, 1949). Koprowski and Black (1952) reported the decline in antibody titer and resistance to challenge 2 years after the administration of chick embryo-adapted rabies virus to dogs. In 1954, Koprowski and Black reported on the antibody response of guinea pigs vaccinated with Flury strain LEP. Dean *et al.* (1964) reported a correlation between antibody response, vaccine dosage, and resistance to challenge in dogs, mice, guinea pigs, and hamsters. In this study of 162 dogs, 39.5% had antibody and resisted challenge, 1.9% had antibody but did not resist challenge, and 64.3% without antibody died when challenged. This test has also been used to determine neutralizing antibody in foxes, skunks, raccoons, bats, and opossums (Sikes, 1962; Constantine, 1966; McLean, 1971).

V. Performance of the Mouse Serum Neutralization Test

The laboratory mouse is used for a variety of viral and serologic tests because of its susceptibility and availability, and is recommended as the test animal for determining rabies neutralizing antibody. For the rabies neutralization test a standard rabies challenge virus (CVS, challenge virus standard) and the weanling mouse (3–4 weeks of age) are used. It should be noted, however, that mice of this age are resistant to certain strains of rabies virus, such as HEP Flury and Kelev vaccines, to which suckling (1- to 7-day-old) mice are susceptible. The CVS is a passage from the original Pasteur fixed virus; ampules of the virus can be obtained from the U. S. National Institutes of Health* or the World Health Organization†. The freeze-dried stock virus is reconstituted with a suitable diluent and inoculated intracerebrally (usually a 1:100 or 1:1000 dilution) into a sufficient number of 3-week-old mice to prepare a sufficient pool of stock virus. When the mice show signs of rabies (humping, paralysis, prostration), the brains are harvested aseptically, pooled, and a 20% tissue suspension is prepared using a suitable diluent (Sikes, 1962). The virus suspension is aliquoted and quickly frozen at $-70°C$. This is the first passage material, and in those laboratories where large numbers of serum neutralization (SN) tests are run, the virus is again passed in a similar manner to prepare a larger challenge virus stock. The second passage material is used in the neutralization test and should contain a minimum titer of 10^6 $LD_{50}/0.03$ ml for intracerebral mouse inoculation; when it is depleted more is prepared from the first stock virus passage.

A. Preparation of Serum to be Tested

The blood is allowed to clot and the serum (decanted or pipetted off within 24 hours to avoid hemolysis) is tested soon after collection. Prolonged storage at 4°C may result in degradation of the antibody and multiplication of contaminating organisms; therefore, if storage is required, the sample should be kept frozen until tested. Repeated freezing and thawing may also cause a decrease in the amount of detectable antibody.

B. Diluent

Rabies virus is relatively labile and requires protein stabilization such as 2–10% egg yolk, 0.4% bovine albumin, 1–10% rabbit serum, 1–10% horse serum, or other protein material which does not inhibit rabies virus. The protein is added to a balanced salt solution along with penicillin (1000 units/ml) and streptomycin (2 mg/ml). This type diluent will keep the virus titer from falling during laboratory testing procedures.

* Address: National Institutes of Health, Bureau of Biologics, Food and Drug Administration, NIH Building 29A, Bethesda, Maryland 20852.
† Address: World Health Organization, 1211 Geneva 27, Switzerland.

C. TEST PROCEDURES

The serum neutralization test is performed by adding the virus to the serum, incubating the mixture, and then inoculating it into mice which are then observed for later signs of rabies. Antibody, which neutralizes the virus, is detected by its ability to prevent mouse deaths. The test should be performed by an individual experienced in virus procedures.

The test serum prepared as described above may be tested undiluted or diluted as follows:

The serum specimen is inactivated at 56°C for 30 min in order to reduce the inhibitors and is then diluted in the following manner (see Fig. 1):

1. Serum (0.4 ml) is added to 0.6 ml of diluent to obtain a 1:2.5 dilution (this, when later diluted with an equal volume of virus, will result in a final dilution of 1:5).
2. Two-tenths ml of the 1:2.5 dilution is added to 0.8 ml diluent to obtain a 1:12.5 dilution.
3. Two-tenths ml of the 1:12.5 dilution is added to 0.8 ml diluent to obtain a 1:62.5 dilution.
4. Dilutions are continued beyond the probable endpoint (that point where no antibody can be detected, and the virus, not neutralized by antibody, is once again mouse lethal).

The standard virus dilution which is to be mixed with the varying serum dilutions is now prepared; specifically, a virus dilution is prepared in which 0.03 ml contains approximately 1.5 logarithms (64 LD_{50}) of virus. If the virus stock has an average titer of $10^{6.5}$ the virus will be diluted $10^{-5.0}$. The virus dilution may be prepared as follows:

1. Three-tenths ml of the 20% CVS working stock is diluted with 0.3 ml of diluent to make a 10^{-1} dilution.
2. Three-tenths ml of virus is diluted with 2.7 ml of diluent to make a 10^{-2} dilution, and 10-fold dilutions are then continued to at least 1.0 $\log_{50}$ past the virus endpoint (e.g., if the virus is expected to titer $10^{6.5}$, a $10^{-7.5}$ dilution is made).

The serum is now mixed with the virus; 0.2 ml of virus (containing approximately 64 $LD_{50}/0.03$ ml) is added to 0.2 ml of each of the desired test serum dilutions. A known positive serum (positive control) is tested in a similar fashion as the test serum to show that the test is specific (known antibody neutralizing the standard virus dose). A known negative serum (negative control) is also used to testify to the fact that virus neutralization does not result without antibody.

The serum–virus dilution is then agitated and incubated at 37°C for 90 min; after this incubation the dilutions are placed in an ice bath and then inoculated intracerebrally into mice using at least five mice per dilution.

The mice are observed daily for 14 days for signs of rabies. Those mice that die during the first 4 days are recorded as nonspecific deaths, whereas mice that die during the next 10 days are recorded as dying of rabies. Serum from persons administered a preexposure regimen or others in which time is not a critical factor may be "screened" at a 1:2 dilution; if the sample is shown to contain antibody, a titration is

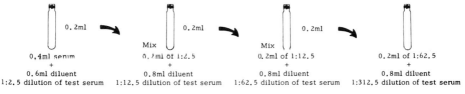

0,4ml serum
+
0.6ml diluent
1:2.5 dilution of test serum

0.2ml of 1:2.5
+
0.8ml diluent
1:12.5 dilution of test serum

0.2ml of 1:12.5
+
0.8ml diluent
1:62.5 dilution of test serum

0.2ml of 1:62.5
+
0.8ml diluent
1:312.5 dilution of test serum

Serial 10-fold dilutions of pre-titered CVS test rabies virus to give one dilution with 64 $LD_{50}/0.03ml$ and two to three additional dilutions beyond endpoint.

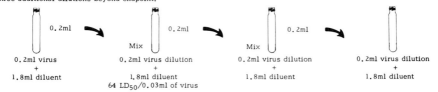

0.2ml virus
+
1.8ml diluent

0.2ml virus dilution
+
1.8ml diluent
64 $LD_{50}/0.03ml$ of virus

0.2ml virus dilution
+
1.8ml diluent

0.2ml virus dilution
+
1.8ml diluent

Combine 0.2ml of CVS virus (64 $LD_{50}/0.03ml$ of virus) to each dilution of serum to be tested. This gives a final 2-fold dilution of the virus and a 2-fold dilution of each dilution of test serum.

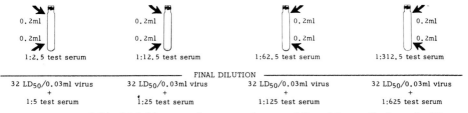

0.2ml
0.2ml
1:2.5 test serum

0.2ml
0.2ml
1:12.5 test serum

0.2ml
0.2ml
1:62.5 test serum

0.2ml
0.2ml
1:312.5 test serum

———————————————— FINAL DILUTION ————————————————

32 $LD_{50}/0.03ml$ virus
+
1:5 test serum

32 $LD_{50}/0.03ml$ virus
+
1:25 test serum

32 $LD_{50}/0.03ml$ virus
+
1:125 test serum

32 $LD_{50}/0.03ml$ virus
+
1:625 test serum

Fig. 1. Serial five-fold dilutions of serum to be tested for rabies antibody and addition of 64 $LD_{50}/0.03$ ml of CVS virus for serum neutralization test.

done to determine the level present. The antibody titer is then calculated [the Reed Muench method may be used (Reed and Muench, 1938)] after determining the 50% mortality endpoint. If desired a neutralizing index can be determined (e.g., a serum with a titer of $1:25/0.03$ ml against 32 LD_{50} of virus would indicate that each 0.03 ml of test serum could neutralize 800 LD_{50} of rabies virus).

VI. Indirect Fluorescent Rabies Antibody Test

The indirect fluorescent antibody technique (Thomas *et al.*, 1963) is another serologic test that has been reported as a rapid, sensitive, and reproducible method for measuring rabies antibody. Goldwasser and Kissling (1958) first reported the specificity of the indirect method for detecting rabies antibody; since then it has been primarily used for detecting the antibody response in vaccinated individuals. This rapid technique may be used to demonstrate antibody in individuals who have become allergic to rabies vaccine during past treatment, those persons at a definite risk of severe vaccine reaction. It is also used to determine whether antibodies are being ac-

Table I

Summary of Serum Neutralization (SN) and Indirect Fluorescent Rabies Antibody (IFRA) Tests[a]

Test group	IFRA positive, SN positive	IFRA positive, SN negative	IFRA negative SN negative	IFRA negative, SN positive	Total
1961	120	76	49	1	246
1962	160	149	29	4	342
TOTAL	280	225	78	5	588

[a] After Thomas *et al.*, 1963. By permission of *Journal of Immunology*.

tively produced in individuals administered nonhuman hyperimmune globulin (usually equine globulin) prior to vaccination. This test was also used in Colombia (D. I. Clemmer, personal communication, 1967), where antibody levels in dogs from various areas of the country were correlated with their vaccination history to determine the possible occurrence of nonfatal rabies infection.

Because it had been shown that the indirect fluorescent rabies antibody technique (IFRA) was specific (Goldwasser and Kissling, 1958), Thomas and associates (1963) developed it for routine examination of sera. These latter authors tested 588 human sera by this test and the mouse neutralization test (SN; Table I), and showed that there was only one false positive (1:2 titer by SN) in 166 sera from individuals having no history of rabies immunization. Of the 422 postvaccinal sera, 60 showed no demonstrable antibody by either test and 280 were positive by both tests, indicating a total correlation of 80%. There were 76 (13.7%) sera positive by IFRA and negative by the SN test and 4 (0.9%) sera negative by IFRA and positive by the SN test. These last four sera, however, were positive by IFRA upon reexamination, suggesting a technical error rather than a fallacy of the test. There was thus an overall agreement of 505 of 588 sera (86%) between the two tests. The IFRA test has since been employed in various other studies (Gispen and Saathof, 1964; Larsh, 1965; Leffingwell and Irons, 1965; Emmons, 1973).

The neutralizing and indirect fluorescent antibody response of individuals vaccinated with suckling rabbit brain vaccine was reported by Gispen and Saathof (1964) (Table II). These individuals were tested by both techniques and had neutralizing and fluorescent antibody responses at some period after vaccination. In serum samples taken 14 days after the initial vaccination, 11 out of 11 demonstrated fluorescent antibody titers, whereas only 9 of 11 showed

Table II

Neutralizing and Fluorescent Antibody Response of Patients 14 Days after Antirabies Treatment with Suckling Rabbit Brain Vaccine[a]

Patient number	Titer of neutralizing antibodies, serum dilution endpoint	Titer of immunofluorescence, serum dilution
3	1:8	1:64
4	1:48	1:1024
5	Neg	1:16
6	Neg	1:16
7	1:43	1:256
8	1:45	1:64
9	1:165	1:128
10	1:51	1:32
11	1:307	1:256
12	1:55	1:64
13	1:90	1:64

[a] After Gispen and Saathof, 1964. By permission of *Arch. Gesamte Virusforsch.*

SN antibody titers. At that time the mean indirect fluorescent antibody titer was 1:180, whereas the mean SN titer was 1:74.6. These authors reported that the indirect fluorescent antibody test appeared to be a convenient and rapid method for titrating rabies antibodies, and that it also appeared to be more sensitive than the neutralization tests.

In another study, Larsh (1965) reported using both SN and IFRA tests to measure the antibody response of 38 individuals receiving preexposure vaccination with duck embryo vaccine (Table III). The

Table III

Comparison of Old and New Standard Duck Embryo Vaccine by Serum Neutralization and Indirect Fluorescent Rabies Antibody (IFRA) Tests[a]

Type of vaccine (number of cases)	Results[b]			
	Prebooster serum neutralization	IFRA	Prebooster serum neutralization	IFRA
Old (19) Standard	14/19 (74)	14/19 (74) 1 Doubtful	15/18 (84)	18/19 (95)
New (19) Standard	13/19 (69)	15/19 (79) 2 Doubtful	16/19 (84)	19/19 (100)
TOTAL (38)	27/38 (78)	29/38 (76)	31/37 (84)	37/38 (97.4)

[a] After Larsh, 1965. By permission of *Ann. Intern. Med.*
[b] Number of positive tests in numerator; total number of cases in denominator; percent positive in parentheses.

IFRA test appeared to be more sensitive than the SN in both the prebooster and postbooster sera; 76 versus 71% positive in the prebooster bleeding, and 97.4 versus 84% at the postbooster bleeding. Eight of 50 sera (18%) were positive by the IFRA and negative by the SN test, whereas only 3 of 50 (6%) were positive by SN and negative by the IFRA test, further substantiating the value of the IFRA test.

Leffingwell and Irons' study (1965) of 85 sera from individuals immunized with either DEV or HEP vaccine further supports the specificity of the IFRA test: 29 sera were negative by both tests, 5 were positive by IFRA and negative by SN, 1 was negative by IFRA and positive by SN, and 49 were positive by both tests. There was complete agreement between the two tests on 78 (93%) of the sera with no false positives, again supporting the usefulness of the indirect method.

In conclusion, these studies support previous data on the value of the IFRA test for detection of rabies antibody. It is a test that can be completed in 1 day and is thus more economical than the mouse neutralization test, making it valuable for both diagnosis and rabies research. It also appears to be more sensitive than the SN test in detecting an early antibody response, as well as an overall higher resultant antibody titer.

VII. Performance of the Indirect Fluorescent Rabies Antibody Test

In the IFRA test the dye absorbs light at one wavelength and emits it almost immediately at another (see Chapter 20). A dye is chosen that absorbs the wavelength of the light produced by the lamp; fluorescein has most frequently been used in the fluorescent antibody technique. Fluorescein emits a yellow-green color light at a wavelength of 520 nm, and is usually preferred since the human retina appears to be more sensitive to the yellow-green color than to others. Another reason for this choice is that the autofluorescence of tissue is generally blue, gray, or white (occasionally red), in striking contrast to the yellow-green specific fluorescence.

In the direct fluorescent rabies antibody test an antispecies antibody is labeled with fluorescein isothiocyanate molecules that serve as the indicator and fluoresce a yellow-green color. For examining human sera, for instance, a tagged antihuman globulin is used to stain human rabies antibodies. This is a two-step technique

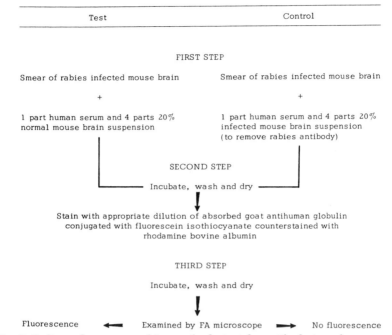

Test	Control

FIRST STEP

Smear of rabies infected mouse brain   Smear of rabies infected mouse brain

\+   +

1 part human serum and 4 parts 20% normal mouse brain suspension   1 part human serum and 4 parts 20% infected mouse brain suspension (to remove rabies antibody)

SECOND STEP

Incubate, wash and dry

Stain with appropriate dilution of absorbed goat antihuman globulin conjugated with fluorescein isothiocyanate counterstained with rhodamine bovine albumin

THIRD STEP

Incubate, wash and dry

Fluorescence   ⟵   Examined by FA microscope   ⟶   No fluorescence

Fig. 2. Indirect fluorescent rabies antibody test for antibody in unknown serum.

in which the human rabies antibody first reacts with the rabies antigen and the tagged antihuman globulin then reacts with the antigen–antibody combination (Fig. 2).

Test slides with rabies antigen are prepared from prostrate mice previously inoculated with either street or fixed rabies virus (two impression areas per slide), then fixed in acetone and either used immediately or stored at −20°C for future use.

Test (and control) sera are inactivated at 56°C for 30 min before testing. Aliquots of each serum to be tested are diluted 1:5 in either suspensions of normal brain (20%) or infective mouse brain (20%) and the suspensions are incubated to permit the antigen–antibody reaction to take place. The impressions on the test slides (which have been warmed to room temperature) are ringed with a marking pencil* to contain the liquid, and then are overlaid with the appropriate dilution of serum (serum and normal brain on one side, serum and infective brain on the other), then incubated, washed, and dried (Fig. 2).

* Mark-Tex pen (Mark-Tex Corp., Englewood, New Jersey).

If the sera contains rabies antibody, a reaction takes place between the antigen and antibody (Fig. 2, first step). This bond in turn behaves as an antigen toward the antispecies fluorescein labeled immune globulin (Fig. 2, second step); this latter is added to the impression, incubated, washed and dried. The tagged antibodies react with the antigen band of the test sera and are not washed off (Fig. 2, third step). The impression is examined using a fluorescent microscope, just as in the direct technique, as described in Chapter 20.

The test (and control) sera and labeled antispecies globulin are each diluted in 20% normal mouse brain suspension to minimize nonspecific reactions in the tissue impressions. A rhodamine or Evans Blue counter stain can be used as an additional step to give a red background fluorescence.

In a positive reaction, the labeled antispecies globulin reacts with the previously formed antigen–antibody complex, and yellow-green color is observed. If no rabies antibody is present in the test serum the tagged globulin cannot react and washes off, resulting in a negative test. The high degree of fluorescence makes this a sensitive test and a positive diagnosis can be made with a minimal amount of antibody.

VIII. Rabies Antibody Determination by Tissue Culture

Research in cell culture systems for rabies virus propagation (see Chapter 9) has led to the development of *in vitro* neutralization tests. Yoshino *et al.* (1966) and Sedwick and Wiktor (1967) reported the use of chick embryo fibroblast cultures and baby hamster kidney cell lines (BHK-21-13S), respectively, in a plaquing method for detecting rabies antibody. Hyperimmune sera and normal sera were diluted 1:20 with phosphate buffered saline and each mixed with equal volumes of serial dilutions of virus (Yoshino and Morishima, 1971). An interference test using chick embryo fibroblast has also been used to test sera. The presence of neutralizing antibodies prevented rabies virus from infecting the test cells, thus allowing infection by the subsequent challenge with cytopathic western equine encephalitis virus (Kaplan *et al.*, 1960).

The fluorescent antibody (FA) technique (see Chapter 20) has also been used for neutralization testing in cell cultures. King *et al.* (1965) reported the use of FA staining in chick embryo fibroblast infected with fixed (CVS) virus for the determination of rabies antibodies. This test could be completed within 72 hours after inoculation. Debbie *et al.* (1972) developed a similar test using BHK-21 (13S) cells grown in Lab-Tek TC chamber slides with ERA virus. A confluent monolayer of cells (formed within 24 hours) was inoculated with the serum–virus mixture. After 5 days of incubation, the slides were harvested, stained by FA, and examined. In this study 29 of 30 sera gave titers within a single fivefold dilution of the mouse neutralization test.

IX. Fluorescent Focus Inhibition Test

The California State Department of Health has reported the use of fluorescent focus inhibition test (FFIT) using BHK cell monolayers, low egg passage (LEP) Flury rabies virus, and FA staining in determining rabies antibody (Lennette and Emmons, 1971). A confluent monolayer was formed on glass slides within 48 hours, these were then inoculated with the virus–serum mixture, further incubated for 4 days, and harvested, stained by FA, and examined. When this test was compared to the mouse neutralization test, 111 of 126 sera tested were positive by the first versus 109 by the mouse neutralization test.

X. Rapid Fluorescent Focus Inhibition Test

Working along similar lines to those of the California State Department of Health, the Center for Disease Control (CDC) has developed a rapid fluorescent focus inhibition test (RFFIT; Smith *et al.*, 1973). The need for a monolayer is eliminated by adding a suspension of BHK-21 13S cells to the already incubated serum–virus mixture in the Lab-Tek TC Chamber slides. The infected monolayers in the TC chamber slides are stained and examined within 24 hours, thus reducing the total incubation time from 4 days to 24 hours. The RFFIT appears to measure the neutralizing antibody since it measures the ability of the serum antibody to block the infection of BHK-21 cells with a tissue culture BHK-21 adapted CVS rabies virus.

There was a 95% correlation between the RFFIT and Mouse neutralization test in 512 human sera tested (Table IV). Of the 512 sera tested, 487 were either positive by both tests or negative by both tests, but 25 were positive by RFFIT and negative by the mouse neutralization test. Neither test found any positive sera in 100 preim-

Table IV

Correlation of Results of Antibody Determination of 512 Human Sera by Rapid
Fluorescent Focus Inhibition Technique and Mouse Serum Neutralization Test[a]

	Results			
RFFIT	+	−	+	−
SN	+	−	−	+
No. of sera	366	121	25	0

[a] After Smith *et al.*, 1973. By permission of the *Bulletin of the W.H.O.*

munization samples. The RFFIT using human sera appears to be at least as sensitive as the mouse neutralization test (Table IV). Human cerebrospinal fluid and animal sera have also been tested by the RFFIT and mouse neutralization test (Smith *et al.*, 1973), and there seems to be no significant difference between the antibody titers by either method.

XI. Performance of the RFFIT

A. Serum

The sera for the RFFIT are processed and stored as are the sera used for the mouse neutralization test. The same serum dilutions used for the mouse neutralization tests can also be used for the RFFIT.

B. Virus

The CVS-11 strain of rabies virus (Kissling, 1958) was used to prepare a pool of virus in BHK-21 13S cells. A dilution of the eighth passage of this virus containing 16,000 PFU/0.1 ml was determined to be a good challenge dose and gave good cell infectivity at 24 hours as indicated by FA staining.

C. Tissue Culture

BHK-21 clone 13 cultures are grown using Eagle's MEM growth media modified by MacPherson and Stoker (1962) and supplemented with 10% inactivated fetal calf serum and 10% tryptose phosphate broth. One- to 4-day-old BHK monolayers are used in the RFFIT. Suspensions containing 1×10^5 cells/0.2 ml are added to each of the eight chambers of the Lab-Tek TC chamber slides.

D. DEAE-Dextran Treatment

A stock 1% solution of DEAE-Dextran is prepared in distilled water and kept under refrigeration. Cells are treated with a concentration of 10 μg/ml for 10 min at room temperature immediately before use in the RFFIT.

E. Performance of the RFFIT Test

An equal volume of challenge virus is added to all serum dilutions, incubated for 90 min at 35°C in a Lab-Tek TC chamber slide and held in a controlled humidity carbon dioxide chamber. A suspension of 1×10^5 cells in 0.2 ml growth medium is then added to each of the eight slide chambers, and the slide returned to the CO_2 chamber.

The slides are ready for FA staining after 24 hours of incubation. The growth medium is removed, the slides are rinsed once in phosphate-buffered saline, once in acetone at room temperature, and fixed in acetone at −20°C for 5 min. The FA staining (Goldwasser and Kissling, 1958) is performed as described by Dean and Abelseth (1973). Twenty low power (160×) microscopic fields are observed for each of the eight dilution chambers, and the number of fields containing fluorescing cells are tabulated. The control slides should contain fluorescing cells in at least 90% of the fields observed. A reduction of 50% or more in the number of fields with fluorescing cells is considered indicative of neutralizing antibody in the serum tested.

XII. Summary

Rabies antibody appears to be most closely associated with the IgM and IgG immunoglobulins. The IgM antibody is the first to appear during an immune response and is gradually replaced by the IgG antibodies. The neutralizing antibody found in both IgG and IgM appears to protect against subsequent challenge with rabies virus. The envelope glycoprotein of the virus induces neutralizing antibody and elicits a protective response to challenge. Neutralizing antibodies do not appear to be produced when purified nucleocapsid is inoculated into rabbits, although indirect fluorescent antibody and complement-fixation antibody are produced.

Serologic tests have been valuable in determining the antibody status of man and animals. Immune response to a vaccine in individuals can be determined by the serum–virus neutralization test, the indirect fluorescent antibody test, or the rapid fluorescent focus inhibition test. These tests can measure the immunologic response qualitatively and quantitatively, thus determining the efficacy of a vaccine and route of administration. Such studies have given a better understanding of the behavior of rabies virus and the factors related to infectivity and immunity.

References

Abelseth, M. K. (1964). *Can. Vet. J.* **5**, 84–87.

Atanasiu, P. (1973). *In WHO, Monogr. Ser.* **23**, 314–318.

Atanasiu, P., and Lépine, P. (1959). *Ann. Inst. Pasteur, Paris* **96**, 72–78.

Atanasiu, P., Bahmanyar, M., Baltazard, M., Fox, J. P., Habel, K., Kaplan, M. M., Kissling, R. E., Kamarov, A., Koprowski, H., Lépine, P., Gallardo, F. P., and Schaeffer, M. (1957). *Bull. WHO* **17**, 911–932.

Baltazard, M., and Bahmanyar, M. (1955). *Bull. WHO* **13**, 747–772.

Cabasso, V. J., Stebbins, M. R., Douglas, B. A., and Sharpless, G. R. (1965). *Amer. J. Vet. Res.* **26**, 24–32.

Cho, H., Fenje, P., and Sparkes, J. (1972). *Infec. Immunity* **6**, 483–486.

Cohen, D., Tierkel, E. S., and Sikes, R. K. (1964). *Bull. WHO* **31**, 426–429.

Constantine, D. G. (1966). *Amer. J. Vet. Res.* **27**, 20–23.

Dean, D. J. Abelseth, M. K. (1973). *WHO, Monogr. Ser.* **23**, 73–84.

Dean, D. J., Evans, W. M., and Thompson, W. R. (1964). *Amer. J. Vet. Res.* **25**, 756–763.

Debbie, J. G., Andrulonis, J. A., and Abelseth, M. K. (1972). *Infec. Immunity* **5**, 902–904.

Emmons, R. W., Leonard, L. L., DeGenaro, F., Protas, E. S., Bazeley, P. L., Giammona, S. T. and Sturckow, K. (1973). *Intervirology*, **1**, 60–72.

Farrar, W. E., Warner, A. R., Vivona, S. (1964), *Military Medicine*, **129**, 960–965.

Fenje, P. (1960). *Can. J. Microbiol.* **6**, 605–610.

Fernandes, M. V., Wiktor, T. J., and Koprowski, H. (1963). *Virology* **21**, 128–131.

Fox, J. P. (1958). *Ann. N. Y. Acad. Sci.* **70**, 480–494.

Fox, J. P., Koprowski, H., Conwell, D. P., Black, J., and Gelfand, H. M. (1957). *Bull. W.H.O.* **17**, 869–904.

Fujisaki, Y., Sekiguchi, K., and Hirasama, K. (1968). *Nat. Inst. Anim. Health Quart.* **8**, 132–139.

Gispen, R., and Saathof, B. (1964). *Arch. Gesamte Virusforsch.* **15**, 377–386.

Goldwasser, R. A., and Kissling, R. (1958). *Proc. Soc. Exp. Biol. Med.* **98**, 219–223.

Gough, P. M., and Dierks, K. E. (1971). *Bull. WHO* **45**, 741–745.

Grasset, N., and Atanasiu, P. (1961). *Ann. Inst. Pasteur* **101**, 639.

Greenberg, M., and Childress, J. (1960). *J. Amer. Med. Ass.* **173**, 333–337.

Halonen, P. E., Murphy, F. A., Fields, B. N., and Reese, D. R. (1968). *Proc. Soc. Exp. Biol. Med.* **127**, 1037–1042.

Hattwick, M. A., Weis, T. T., Stechschulte, C. J., Baer, G. M., and Gregg, M. B. (1972). *Ann. Intern. Med.* **76**, 931–942.

Johnson, H. N. (1973). *WHO., Monogr. Ser.* **23**, 94–97.

Kaplan, M. M., Wecker, E., Forsek, Z., and Koprowski, H. (1960). *Nature (London)* **186**, 821–822.

King, D. A., Croghan, D. L., and Shaw, E. L. (1965). *Can. Vet. J.* **6**, 187–193.

Kissling, R. E. (1958). *Proc. Soc. Exp. Biol. Med.* **98**, 223–228.

Kissling, R. E., and Reese, D. (1963). *J. Immunol.* **91**, 362–368.

Koprowski, H., and Black, J. (1952). *Proc. Soc. Exp. Biol. Med.* **80**, 410–415.

Koprowski, H., and Black, J. (1954). *J. Immunol.* **72**, 85–93.

Koprowski, H., and Cox, H. R. (1951). *Amer. J. Pub. Health* **41**, 1483–1489.

Larsh, S. (1965). *Ann. Intern. Med.* **63**, 955–964.

Leffingwell, L., and Irons, J. V. (1965). *Pub. Health Rep.* **80**, 999–1004.

Lennette, E. H., and Emmons, R. W. (1971). *In* "Rabies" (Y. Nagano and F. Davenport, eds.), p. 77–90. Univ. Park Press, Baltimore, Maryland.

Lépine, P. (1973). *WHO., Monogr. Ser.* **23**, 151–157.

McLean, R. G. *J. Infec. Dis.* **123**, 680–681.

MacPherson, I., and Stoker, M. (1962). *Virology* **16**, 147–151.

Matsumoto, S. (1970). *Advan. Virus Res.* **16**, 257–301.

Otto, G. L., and Heyke, B. (1962). *Vet. Med.* **57**, 613–616.

Reed, L. J., and Muench, H. A. (1938). *Amer. J. Hyg.* **27**, 493–497.

Rubin, R., Dierks, R. E., Gough, P., Gregg, M., Gerlach, H., and Sikes, R. (1971). *Lancet* **2**, 625–628.

Schneider, L. G., Dietzschold, B., Dierks, R. E., Matthaeus, W., Enzmann, P. J., and Strohmaier, K. (1973). *J. Virol.* **11**, 748–755.

Sedwick, W. D., and Wiktor, T. J. (1967). *J. Virol.* **1**, 1224–1226.

Sever, J. L. (1962). *J. Immunol.* **88**, 320–329.

Sikes, R. K. (1962). *Amer. J. Vet. Res.* **23**, 1041–1047.

Smith, J., Yager, P., and Baer, G. M. (1973). *Bull. W.H.O.* **48**, 535–541.

Thomas, J. B., Sikes, R., and Ricker, A. (1963). *J. Immunol.* **91**, 721–723.

Tierkel, E., Koprowski, H., Black, J., and Gorrie, R. (1949). *J. Vet. Res.* **10**, 361–367.

Tierkel, E. S. and Sikes, R. K. (1967), *J.A.M.A.*, **201**, 911–914.

Webster, L. (1936). *Amer. J. Pub. Health* **26**, 1207–1210.

Webster, L., and Dawson, J. (1935). *Proc. Soc. Exp. Biol. Med.* **32**, 570–573.

Wiktor, R., Fernandes, M. V., and Koprowski, H. (1964). *J. Immunol.* **93**, 362–368.

Wiktor, T., Kuwert, E., and Koprowski, H. (1968). *J. Immunol.* **101**, 1271–1282.

Wiktor, T., György, E., Schlumberger, H., Sokol, F., and Koprowski, H. (1973). *J. Immunol.* **110**, 269–276.

Yoshino, K., and Morishima, T. (1971). *Arch. Gesamte Virusforsch.* **34**, 40–50.

Yoshino, K., Taniguchi, S., and Arai, K. (1966). *Arch. Gesamte Virusforsch.* **3**, 370–373.

AUTHOR INDEX

Numbers in italics refer to the pages on which the complete references are listed.

M

SUBJECT INDEX

A 5
B 6
C 7
D 8
E 9
F 0
G 1
H 2
I 3
J 4